ANXIETY AND RELATED DISORDERS

Edited by **Ágnes Szirmai**

Anxiety and Related Disorders
Edited by Ágnes Szirmai

Published by InTech
Janeza Trdine 9, 51000 Rijeka, Croatia

Technical Editor Sonja Mujacic

Cover Designer InTech Design Team

Additional hard copies can be obtained from orders@intechopen.com

Anxiety and Related Disorders,
Edited by Ágnes Szirmai
p. cm.
ISBN 978-953-307-254-8

For EU product safety concerns:
IN TECH d.o.o., Prolaz Marije Krucifikse Kozulić 3, 51000 Rijeka, Croatia,
info@intechopen.com or visit our website at intechopen.com.

Meet the editor

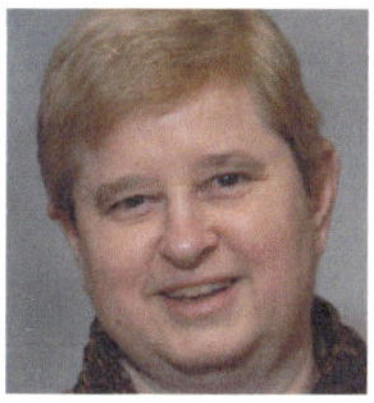

Dr. Ágnes Szirmai is an associate professor at the Department of Otorhinolaryngology and Head and Neck Surgery of Semmelweis University in Budapest. Her specialties are otorhinolaryngology, neurology, audiology, and neurootology. She has been the chief of the neurootological outpatient department of the University since 1989. She has been teaching medical students in Hungarian language since 1983 and in English since 1989. Dr. Szirmai holds postgradual courses for otorhinolaryngologist, neurologists, audiologists, and family doctors. She has wide range of publications about vertigo and vestibular system disorders (53 articles, 62 abstracts, 2 books, 18 book-chapters). Dr. Szirmai is a member of several Hungarian and International Scientific Societies (Hungarian Society of Otorhinolaryngologists, Hungarian Stroke Society, Hungarian Headache Society, Neurootological and Equilibriometric Society, which has its seat in Bad Kissingen, Germany and Barany Society (Uppsala, Sweden). She has been the president of the Otoneurological Section of Hungarian Society of Otorhinolaryngologists since 2008.

Contents

Preface

What do we know about anxiety?

Anxiety is one of the most frequent nosologic entities encountered not only in psychiatric but in general practice as well. It was defined by Janet as "fear without object". Anxiety, fright, fear, worry, dread, anguish, terror - this is a long list of approximate synonyms!

The very fine differences separating these notions may often generate confusion: it is normal to feel worried or scared, but is it all right to be anxious? If it is, then there is normal anxiety. What about anguish? On the other hand, could we live without anxiety?

Anxiety disorders are one of the most common psychiatric disorders world wide. Before the 1980s, Generalized Anxiety Disorder (GAD) was labelled as 'anxiety neuroses'. Anxiety disorders cover several different forms of abnormal and pathological fear and anxiety. Current psychiatric diagnostic criteria recognize a wide variety of anxiety disorders. Psychological conditions are highly prevalent among adults in general, and among adults with chronic diseases, in particular.

Many aspects of anxiety can be observed; epidemiological and genetics, biological bases, cognitive neuroscience, co-morbid mental and physical disorders, treatment resistance, biochemical and animal studies, experimental and behavioral aspects. Advancement has been made in the development of medication and psychosocial treatment strategies, but many patients still remain symptomatic.

General Anxiety Disorder falling into the category of anxiety disorders with symptoms of anxiety, worry and apparent alertness, displays a fairly constant prevalence (5-6.5%) in the general population.

Anxious patients often consult primary care physicians for their treatment, but in most cases they do not accept the diagnosis of anxiety disorder. The anxiety disorder diagnosis could result in a longer period of hospitalization, more frequent use of diagnostic tests and medication, and therefore, a heavy financial burden. This decreases the quality of life, and provokes serious family problems and prolonged absence from work.

Anxiety is a symptom that can be seen in many organic disorders and can accompany almost any psychiatric disorder. Anxiety disorders are frequent and are associated with significant distress and dysfunction. The dominant symptoms are variable but include complaints of persistent nervousness, trembling, muscular tensions, sweating, light-headedness, palpitations, dizziness, and epigastrial discomfort. Anxiety disorders represent a disabling condition and a social disability as severe as chronic somatic disorders such as arthritis, hypertension, asthma, or diabetes. Mostly, patients complain of somatic and sleeping problems. Accompanying symptoms include muscle tension, headache, muscle aches, restlessness, irritability, gastrointestinal symptoms, and difficulty in concentrating, fatigue, and insomnia. Fears that the patient or a relative will shortly become ill or have an accident are often expressed.

Stigmatization is an important factor in insufficient diagnosis and this can account for why a significant number of patients does not express the emotional problems to their physicians.

The relationship between anxiety and cardiovascular system is known since the 19th century. We often say, when we have anxiety, that it is a heartaache, and we often use the term "broken heart" after a severe sorrow, or anxious period.

In everyday medical practice co-morbidity and consecutive anxiety disorder could be often seen in patients with moderate to severe osteoarthritis, which is a painful disabling joint disease.

In our everyday life the eating is a very important thing, not only for supporting our body, but we might enjoy every meal. The eating disorders could also be dangerous. Nowadays, obesity is recognized to be one of the greatest public health problems worldwide. A connection between anxiety disorders and obesity is observed. Obesity is considered to be a modern disease. It seems that it is rapidly spreading worldwide, as is the anxiety. The disorders of eating, like anorexia and bulimia, could be connected not only to the fashion models, but the psychiatric disorders, like anxiety.

Research in the past 20 years has shown that the patients with epilepsy commonly have coexisting psychiatric conditions including mood disorders, anxiety disorders, and psychotic disorders.

The balance system is often affected. Anxious patients often say: "I've lost my balance". A frequent question in neurootological expertise is whether the vertigo of psychiatric patients suffering from anxiety disorders is caused by vestibular dysfunction or the vertigo is originated from psychiatric disease. A high degree of psychiatric disorders has repeatedly been described among patients with organic vertigo syndromes and attributed to vestibular dysfunction. The differential diagnosis can only be attained by a careful interdisciplinary way of thinking and activity, given the fact that the vestibular, neurological and psychiatric disorders - considered as pathogenic factors - are being present simultaneously in triggering the symptoms, and there can be overlaps between certain pathological processes.

So, we can see that the problems of anxiety cover all fields of our life in medical and everyday senses, too. This book intends to describe the epidemiological aspects and the main co-morbidities and consecutive diseases of the anxiety disorders.

Ágnes Szirmai
Associate Professor, PhD
Semmelweis University, Faculty of Medicine
Department of Otorhinolaryngology and Head and Neck surgery, Budapest, Hungary

Part 1

Nosology and Epidemiology

1

Anxiety Disorders

Delia Marina Podea and Florina Ratoi
"Vasile Goldis" Western University of Arad
Romania

1. Introduction

Modern man spends a lot of time, money and energy on alleviating his anxiety. In the Unites States the number of people who see clinicians because of anxiety complaints exceeds by far that the patients who see help for their colds. Tranquilizers prescribed either by psychiatrists or by general physicians, are among the top sellers both in Europe and in US. There hardly seems to be anyone who has not used tranquilizers at least once in his life in order to relieve stress.

What do we know about anxiety? Anxiety, fright, fear, worry, dread, anguish, terror-this is a long list of approximate synonyms! The very fine differences separating this notions may often generate confusion: it is normal to feel worried or scared, but is it all right to be anxious? If it is , then there is normal anxiety. What about anguish? On the other hand, could we live without anxiety? Quite a number of philosophers, psychologists and psychiatrists think that the answer is negative. Anxiety, like love, joy, hope, anger, disgust or hatred, is an integral part of life. It may act as a creative impulse or a muse, friend or foe, destroyer or advisor. Just think how many hasty decisions, how many mistakes we have all made because we felt anxious. The reverse is also true: there have been quite a few times in our lives when we passed a difficult exam, wrote a good paper or created a work of art because of anxiety.

Anxiety is one of the most frequent nosologic entities encountered not only in psychiatric but in general practice too. It was defined by Janet as "fear without object".

Anxiety is characterized by a diffuse, unpleasant, vague sensation of fear or anguish accompanied by autonomic symptoms such as head ache, sweating, palpitations, tachycardia, gastric discomfort, etc. Therefore it includes both a physiological and a psychological component, anxious individuals being usually aware of both. Anxiety may affect thinking, perception and learning, it can generate distortion of perception, impairment in concentration, recall and associations. Another important aspect is the effect it may have on selective attention, anxious individuals select certain things or events around them and exaggerate the importance of others, in an attempt to justify their anxiety as reaction to a fearful situation.

(Feraru R, Podea D, 1998, *Panic Disorder*, MAIKO, ISBN 973-95649-6-8, Bucharest)

The perception of an event as stressful depends both on the nature of the event and on the subject's resources. Individuals with an adequate ego are in a state of adaptive balance between the outer world and their inner world. The upsetting of this balance generates anxiety. The anxiety plays the role of an alarm signal that warns the person about impending danger and helps him to prepare to face it. Fear, another signal alerting the body, appear as a response to a familiar, external, well-defined threat or nonconflictual at origin, while anxiety is a response to an unfamiliar, internal, vague threat or may be conflictual at origin. The two notions came to be differentiated absolutely by chance, as the first translators of Freud into English chose to translate German concept "angst" by "anxiety" rather than "fear". Anxiety and fear have in common lots subjective and physiological aspects, that's why the difference between the two terms is still debated. (Marinescu M, Udristoiu T, Podea D., Ciucu A,2008, *Tulburarea depresiva si anxioasa-actualitati*, AIUS, ISBN 978-973-1780-97-9, Craiova)

2. Comparative nosology DSM-IV to ICD-10

DSM (Diagnostical and Statistical Manual of Mental Disorders) is the official classification system of mental disorders used in the United States, while ICD (International Classification of Diseases and Related Health Problems) in the counterpart of that system in Europe. Each of them sets clear and accurate diagnostic criteria; the system are correlated in order to provide a common language to mental health professional all over the world.

The first edition of DSM was published in 1952 and the second in 1968. The third one came out in 1980 and brought along five important innovations. First there was a heavy emphasis on operational criteria for each disorder, with rules for inclusion and exclusion.

The second important feature was a multiaxial system including five axes:

- clinical syndromes and other conditions that require follow-up and treatment
- developmental and personality disorders
- physical disorders
- severity of psychosocial stressors
- degree of adaptive functioning during the last year

The third innovation was a review of the terminology and regrouping of some syndromes (thus, for instance, the notions of neurosis and hysteria were abandoned, while all affective disorders were grouped together)

The fourth change was a restricted use of psychodynamic concepts in the substantiation of classifications, while the fifth was the inclusion among the diagnostic criteria of the duration of the disorder in some categories.

DSM-III-R released in 1987 was a intermediary scheme, before a comprehensive review was operated in DSM-IV in 1994. It coded pervasive development disorders on axis I, while axis II was limited only to personality disorders and mental retardation. DSM-IV includes an appendix that reflects the cultural and ethnic influences that may be relevant in evaluation and diagnosis.

In the same interval, the World Health Organization collaborated with psychiatric organizations of several countries in order to construct the 10th edition of Chapter V of the international classification (ICD-10) published in 1992.

ICD-10 reproduces many of the conceptual and taxonomic achievements of DSM-III.

ICD-10 is in many ways similar to DSM-II-R and DSM-IV, but contains clinical descriptions and diagnostic orientations that are less detailed and less restrictive. They are some important differences, such as those regarding terminology, the grouping of disorders and the definitions of some basic concepts. (see Table 1) (Feraru R, Podea D, 1998, *Panic Disorder,*MAIKO, ISBN 973-95649-6-8, Bucharest; Marinescu M, Udristoiu T, Podea D., Ciucu A,2008, *Tulburarea depresiva si anxioasa- actualitati*, AIUS, ISBN 978-973-1780-97-9, Craiova)

DSM-IV	ICD-10 CHAPTERV
Panic disorder -without agoraphobia -with agoraphobia	Panic disorder (episodic paroxysmal anxiety) Agoraphobia with panic disorder
Agoraphobia without history of panic disorder	Agoraphobia (without panic disorder)
Specific phobia	Specific (isolated) phobia
Social phobia	Social phobia
Generalized anxiety disorder	Generalized anxiety disorder
Anxiety disorder NOS	1. Mixed anxiety and depressive disorder 2. Other mixed anxiety disorders 3. Other specified anxiety disorders 4. Anxiety disorder, unspecified

Table 1. Comparative nosology between DSM-IV-TR and ICD-10 (American Psychiatric Association, 1994, *Diagnostic and Statistical Manual of Mental Disorders*, fourth edition , American Psychiatric Association, ISBN 0-89042-064-5, Washington, DC; WHO, 1998, ICD-10 Clasificarea tulburarilor mentale si de comportament, ALL, ISBN 973-9392-73-3, Romania)

3. Epidemiology

Epidemiological data about anxiety disorders in general are varied and controversial due to differences on the screening method and instruments used.

The overall lifetime prevalence of anxiety disorders was 14,6% and annually was 12,6 % in the Epidemilogical Catchement Area compared with national Comorbidity Survey where the prevalence of anxiety disorders was 25% (19% at men and 31% at women)

The prevalence is ranged around 3.8% for panic disorders and 5.6% for panic attacks. For agoraphobia the prevalence ranges between 0.6-6 %; the higher prevalence rate in the last decade does not seem to reflect a true increase: it is more indicative of a higher level of education and the uniformity of diagnostic criteria. At any rate , one of the most fascinating mysteries of agoraphobia remains its distribution by sexes: approximately 75% of agoraphobics are women.

The prevalence of OCD is around 2% in general population.

Social anxiety is the most frequent of the anxiety disorders with lifetime prevalence of approximately 13%.

When examining prevalence of PTSD, two conditional probabilities are important: the probability of PTSD in the general population and the probability of PTSD within specific trauma populations. General population prevalence estimates range from 1% to 9 %. Among individuals who have traumatic events higher rates of PTSD where found (24%). (Marinescu M, Udristoiu T, Podea D., Ciucu A,2008, *Tulburarea depresiva si anxioasa- actualitati*, AIUS, ISBN 978-973-1780-97-9, Craiova)

4. Etiopathogeny

Three theoretical schools, three different trends intersect, contradict and complete one another in an attempt to explain the etiology of anxiety disorders: psychoanalytic, cognitive behavioral and biological theories.

4.1 Psychoanalytic theories

One of Freud's major contributions to psychoanalytic thinking was the conceptualization of anxiety, a concern that stayed with him throughout his career. A careful analysis of Freud's neurophysiological model of anxiety, one of the first models created by him towards the end of the 19th century, reveals that anxiety neurosis described at the time is easily comparable to panic disorder as it is described today in DSM-IV. In the early period, Freud grouped neuroses into two major classes: actual neuroses and psychoneuroses.

4.1.1 Actual neuroses

Actual neuroses include neurasthenia, anxiety neurosis and hypochondriasis. They were considered somatic in origin, anxiety being attributed to a sexual disorder; in other words, direct transformation of sexual energy into anxiety was thought to be responsible for actual neurosis. The premise upon which this theory was based was that an increase in sexual tension which is a psysiological phenomenon, leads to a correspondent increase of the libido, namely of its mental representation. The normal release of sexual tension and implicitly of the libido is the sexual intercourse. In Freud's view, abnormal practices, sexual dissatisfaction or frustration resulting from abstinence, or "coitus interruptus" prevent this release of tension thus triggering actual neurosis.

4.1.2 Psychoneuroses

Psychoneuroses were represented by hysteria, fobias and obsession neurosis. Unlike actual neurosis which were somatically determined, psychoneurosis were psychological in nature, tension being generated by an unacceptable sexual impulse, there for by an intrapsychic conflict. According to Freud this anxiety was less intense then that occurring in actual neurosis.

Subsequently Freud abandoned the concept in favor of a psychological one. With the replacement of the topographic model by the tripartite structural model of the mind, which divides the psychic apparatus into the id, the ego and the super ego, a second theory of anxiety was born: "signal anxiety". The hypothesis was subsequently expanded by classifying this signals into:

- internal or neurotic, coming from the id or the ego, and
- external or real threats. Finally, Freud generalized this concept by identifying two types of anxiety traumatic and signal anxiety.

a. traumatic anxiety appears in response to actual traumatic situations. More frequently encountered in childhood, when the ego is insufficiently developed, it may also appear in adults in panic or in psychotic states when the ego has suffered massive disorganization.

b. Signal anxiety, which is more common, appears in anticipation of danger, not as a result thereof. Produced as a subconscious or an unconscious level, it plays a protective role warning the ego about impending internal or external dangers. It appears in adults whos defense mechanisms are mature. It may be useful to repeat here that defense mechanisms are psychological mechanisms design to mediate between individual wishes, impulses, needs and emotions, on one hand, and internalized interdictions and external reality, on the other.

Departing from Freud's early theory, where anxiety neurosis was seen as somatically conditioned subsequent psychoanalytic theories have conceptualized panic disorder as a result of failed defense, a partial failure of the ego to face the stimuli endangering it. Although in the later part of it's career Freud devoted more attention to anticipatory

anxiety, he always maintained the distinction between the two forms of anxiety, one mediated mainly biologically and the other psychologically.
Recent biological research has also confirmed the existence of two forms of anxiety one predominantly psychological in nature, appearing as anticipatory anxiety or signal anxiety, and the other predominantly neurophysiological, assuming the form of panic disorder.

4.2 Cognitive-behavioral theories

Like psychoanalysts, the supporters of cognitive-behavioral theories considered that biological hypotheses are insufficient to explain all the clinical manifestations of panic disorder. Starting from the premise that anxiety is a learned response, with learning occurring either as a result of classical conditioning or by following parental behavioral models (social learning theory), they have proposed a variety of etiologic explanations for panic disorder. In a similar way to Freud's theories, cognitive-behavioral theories have undergone numerous modifications and improvements over time. Some of these are:

4.2.1 Classical conditioning

Systematic exposure to anxiogenic situations has been observed to reduce avoidance behavior in agoraphobic patients and to alleviate panic attacks. In their attempts to explain the phenomenon, researchers have invoked classical conditioning as the etiology of panic disorder.
Let us remember that the first stage of conditioning is the association of a noxious stimulus, such as an electric shock (unconditioned stimulus) to an event perceived as neutral, such as entering a crowded shop or crossing a bridge (conditioned stimulus). Concomitant and repeated association of the two event induces fear (conditioned response). Which subsequently appears even in the absence of the unconditioned stimulus.
The second stage involves the subject's attempts to avoid the fear produced by dangerous and unpleasant situations by escape or by avoidance.
Although interesting, the theory of classical conditioning has numerous limitations, the most significant being that the most panic disorder patients external noxious elements (unconditioned stimuli) cannot be identified.

4.2.2 The "fear of fear" principle and interoceptive conditioning

As unconditioned external stimuli were hard to detect, subsequent cognitive-behavioral theories focused on more indepth research on internal stimuli, starting from the observation that the symptoms of panic disorder patients were in fact produced by internal and not external stimuli.
In panic disorder patients the interoceptive stimuli represented by harmless somatic sensations, such as dizziness or palpitations, become conditioned stimuli following association with panic attacks, generating fear or future attacks. After the first panic attack, patients frightened by the experience they experience, become hypervigilant concerning their own body. They may thus observe sensations they would have ignored or would have failed to notice otherwise; once this was observed they increase their anxiety. This closes the vicious cycle and may trigger new attacks.
The theory has its limitations too, the most serious objection being the overlap between conditioned stimuli and conditioned responses.

4.2.3 Catastrophic misinterpretation

The interpretation of harmless sensations as evidence for imminent catastrophe lies at the foundation of cognitive theories. According to these theories, panic attacks are caused by the individual's tendency to interpret somatic sensations in a catastrophic manner; palpitations for example are perceived as a symptom if imminent myocardial infarction, dizziness as a symptom of imminent fainting. The perception of imminent disaster triggers panic attacks.The theory, although interesting it fails to offer a full satisfactory explanation for panic attacks.

4.2.4 Anxiety sensitivity

This theory claims that panic disorder patients develop or maintain a mistaken interpretation of their harmless somatic sensations because of high anxiety sensitivity. Anxiety sensitivity reflects a pathological belief connected to anxiety symptoms; it appears before the onset of the disease and is a predisposing factor of panic disorder.

4.3 Neurobiological factors

The biology of anxiety and panic represents one of the biggest and most interesting fields of current research. Biological theories are based on experimental studies performed on animals and on comparative clinical research. The unprecedented accumulation of knowledge in neurochemistry, pharmacology, genetics and neuroendocrinology has helped researchers clarify many aspects of anxiety.

The stimulation of the Autonomic Nervous System (ANS) produces cardiovascular, respiratory, muscular and gastrointestinal symptoms such as dizziness, tremor, diarrhea, hypertension, palpitations, tachycardia, mydriasis and gastric discomfort. These are in fact the peripheral manifestations of anxiety.

It is generally accepted that central nervous system anxiety precedes its peripheral manifestation.

Some panic disorder patients exhibit increased sympathetic tone, adapt slowly and with difficulty to repeated stimuli, and respond excessively to moderate stimuli.

Epinephrine and norepinephrine were among the first panic-inducing agents known. Both are secreted in response to stress. Epinephrine stimulates beta-adrenergic receptors, while norepinephrine is a alpha-adrenergic agonist producing peripheral vasoconstriction, increased blood pressure and decreased heart rate. Epinephrine and norepinephrine do not cross the blood-brain barrier.

Isoproterenol, an agonist of beta-adrenergic receptors, has a more specific action than epinephrine. It induces attacks in panic disorder patients but not in normal subjects. It does not cross the blood-brain barrier.

The major neurotransmitters involved in anxiety are nor-epinephrine, serotonin and gamma-aminobutyric acid (GABA).

The noradrenergic hypothesis stresses the role of hyperactivity of the central noradrenergic system in the occurrence of panic disorder. The noradrenergic hyperactivity in the locus ceruleus produces both psychic and somatic symptoms of anxiety. The theory stipulates that patients with panic disorder have a dysfunction of the noradrenergic system manifested by occasional hyperactivity of the system. It is known that most noradrenergic neurons are located in locus ceruleus of the pons. They establish multiple connections with the cerebral cortex, the limbic system, the thalamus, the hypothalamus, the brainstem and the spinal cord. The locus ceruleus receives information on potential dangers and activates the cerebral areas.

The serotonergic hypothesis focuses on the role of this system in the etiology of panic disorder. Most of serotonergic neurons are found in the raphe nucleus, in the caudal locus ceruleus, in the area postrema and in the interpeduncular area. The raphe nucleus is situated in the brainstem; it sends impulses to the cerebral cortex , the limbic system, the thalamus, the hypothalamus, the locus ceruleus, the cerebellum and the spinal cord. Initially, serotonergic drugs may aggravate anxiety, as the anxiolytic effect appears only three ti six weeks later; their therapeutic action is supposed to be biphasic.

The GABA-ergic hypothesis of panic disorder is based on the observation that benzodiazepines increases the activity of GABA-A receptors. Benzodiazepines have proven their efficacy in the treatment of anxiety, and high-potency benzodiazepines are used successfully in panic disorder.

In the etiology of anxiety disorders are involved also other neurotransmitters (histamine, acetylcholine, adenosine, cholecystokinin) psycho-neuroendocrinological aspects, genetic ones. The neuroanatomical basis of anxiety disorders is still a topic of considerable interest.

The locus ceruleus, the raphe nucleus, the limbic system and cerebral cortex (the frontal cortex) are all involved in the etiology of anxiety disorders.

Anatomical images of the human brain can be produced by the use of X-ray computed tomography (CT) or of magnetic resonance imaging (MRI). For exploring neuroanatomical aspects can be utilized positron emission tomography(PET), single photon emission computed tomography (SPECT), functional MRI, magnetic resonance spectroscopy (MRS).

Studies have shown that persons with an asymmetric increase of regional cerebral flow (more on the right side) in the parahippocampal area of the temporal lobe and in the inferior prefrontal areas are more susceptible to sodium lactate-induced panic attacks. MRIs performed in panic disorders patient indicate abnormalities of the right temporal lobe, especially cortical atrophy.

(Marinescu M, Udristoiu T, Podea D., Ciucu A,2008, *Tulburarea depresiva si anxioasa-actualitati*, AIUS, ISBN 978-973-1780-97-9, Craiova)

5. Symptoms

The anxiety can take different aspects. It can be perceived as an inexplicable feeling of eminent death, as an unfounded and exaggerated worry from daily life (health of children, professional or financial problems, etc.) or un unjustified fear of certain situations (traveling by bus) of an activity (driving the car) or of un object (fear of sharp objects, of animals). Usually patients describe the following physical or psychical signs:

- excessive and unrealistic worries
- fear without a cause
- unreal fear about an unknown danger
- flash-backs of some past trauma
- compulsive behavior (rituals) as a way of minimize the anxiety
- shaking, muscular pain, sweating, nausea, tension, fatigue, palpitations, dry mouth, digestive discomfort, feeling of chocking, heart pounding
- losing the ability to relax
- insomnia

Into the anxiety disorders are specified disorders that have anxiety as a principal symptom (panic disorder and generalized anxiety disorder) and disorders in which anxiety is secondary to cognitive routes and inadequate conduits (obsessive-compulsive disorder and phobic disorder). Also in anxiety disorders are described anxiety feelings as an abnormal response to different stress factors (adaptive disorders), psychological reactions to traumatic events (acute stress disorder and posttraumatic stress disorder).

In classic psychiatry, after the symptomatology was recognized, before a diagnose was established, the grouping of the symptoms in syndromes was mandatory. In this way, was defined the anxious syndrome that is encountered not only in different forms of anxiety disorders but also in others psychic and somatic illnesses.
Nowadays is considered that exists a clear separation of anxious syndromes in different anxious disorders. This can be exactly diagnosed but there are vary comorbidities between them and each one can complicate with depression and abuse or substance dependence.
In general medicine, in classic acception, the anxious syndrome can be encountered an a compound of clinic image of an organic illness, function of organic and toxicological causes. In actual acception according to DSM-IV-TR, secondary anxious symptoms to an organic illness corresponds to anxious disorder due to a general medical condition and anxious disorder substance induced (see table 2). The correspondent in ICD-10 for this disorders if Organic anxious disorder (F06.4). (Marinescu M, Udristoiu T, Podea D., Ciucu A,2008, *Tulburarea depresiva si anxioasa- actualitati*, AIUS, ISBN 978-973-1780-97-9, Craiova)

Endocrinologic and metabolic disorders	dysfunction of the pituitary gland, thyroid, adrenals and parathyroid glands, changes in serum calcium, serum sodium and potassium, premenstrual syndrome, hypoglycemia
Cardiac diseases	Angina pectoris, arrhythmias, heart failure, arterial hypertension, hypovolemia, myocardial infarction, valvular heart disease
Respiratory diseases	asthma, respiratory failure, chronic obstructive pulmonary disease, pneumonia, pneumothorax, pulmonary edema, acute pulmonary embolism
Neurological disorders	brain neoplasms, brain injury, postcontuzionale syndromes, cerebrovascular disease, intracranial hemorrhage, migraine, encephalitis, cerebral syphilis, multiple sclerosis, epilepsy temporal, Wilson disease, Hungtington disease
Inflammatory and immune system diseases	systemic erythematosus lupus, rheumatoid arthritis, polyarthritis nodosa, temporal arteritis, anaphylactic shock
Carential states	pellagra, iron deficiency anemia, vitamin B12 deficiency
Secreting tumors	carcinoid syndrome, pheochromocytoma, insulinom
Intoxications	amphetamines and other sympathomimetics, anticholinergics, caffeine, theophylline, Yohimbine, cocaine, cannabis, hallucinogens
different substance withdrawal syndromes	alcohol withdrawal, hypertensive, caffeine, opioids, sedative / hypnotics

Table 2. Organic and toxic etiologies of anxiety syndrome

To recognize pathologic anxiety is necessary to establish if there is an organic, toxicological cause or is a psychic disorder. The differentiation is sometimes hard to be done, because the organism can react to anxiety through a somatic participation. (see table 3), the anxiety can be primary in psychic disorder or secondary (organic, drug induced or toxic)

RESPIRATORY sensation of breathlessness or suffocation chest tightness tachypnea chocking	CARDIOVASCULAR tachycardia palpitations precordial pain "sine materia" syncopate	MUSCULAR tremor muscle contractures muscle weakness startles muscle back pain
VEGETATIVE dry mouth pale face redness on skin "in cleavage" sweating Hot flashes	NEUROLOGICAL headache vertigo paresthesia visual illusions blurred vision hyperesthesia	GASTROINTESTINAL acceleration of intestinal transit cramps nausea vomiting abdominal pains

Table 3. Somatic symptoms of anxiety

6. Diagnostic criteria according to DSM-IV-TR

6.1 Panic attacks

is a discrete period of intense fear, anxiety, discomfort or apprehension during which at least four of the following 13 symptoms develop abruptly are exacerbated and reach a peak within 10 minutes of onset:

- Palpitations or tachychardia
- Sweating
- Tremor
- Sensation of dyspnea or smothering
- Feeling of choking
- Thoracic pain, constriction or discomfort
- Nausea or abdominal distress
- Sensation of dizziness, instability or fainting
- Derealization (feeling of unreality), or depersonalization (self-detachment)
- Fear of losing control or going crazy
- Fear of dying
- Paresthesias (numbness or tingling)
- Hot or cold flushes

6.2 Panic disorder without agoraphobia

a. Both (1) and (2) have to be met:
   1. Unexpected recurrent panic attacks
   2. At least one of the attacks should be followed for a month (or several) by:
   a) persistent concern for the recurrence of the panic attacks
   b) worry about the implications or consequences of the panic attack (such as fear of losing control, of being seized by a heart attack or of going crazy)
   c) significant modification in behavior related to panic attack
b. Absence of agoraphobia

c. Panic attacks are not a result of the direct physiological effects of a substance (as in the case of dug abuse, medication) or of a general medical condition (such as hyperthyroidism)
d. Panic attacks are not caused by another mental disorder, such as social phobia (for instance occurring on exposure to social circumstances the patient is afraid of), specific phobia (caused by exposure to a specific phobic situation), obsessive-compulsive disorder (occurring for instance on exposure to dirt of an individual with an obsession about contamination), post-traumatic stress disorder (occurring in a response to a stimuli associated with a severe stressor) or separation anxiety disorder (in response to being separated from home or close relatives)

6.3 Panic disorder with agoraphobia

a. Both (1) and (2) have to be met:
   1. Unexpected recurrent panic attacks
   2. At least one of the attacks should be followed for a month (or several) by:
   a) persistent concern for the recurrence of the panic attacks
   b) worry about the implications or consequence of the panic attack (such as fear of losing control, of being seized by a heart attack or of going crazy)
   c) significant modification in behavior related to panic attack
b. presence of agoraphobia
c. Panic attacks are not a result of the direct physiological effects of a substance (as in the case of dug abuse, medication) or of a general medical condition (such as hyperthyroidism)
d. Panic attacks are not caused by another mental disorder, such as social phobia (for instance occurring on exposure to social circumstances the patient is afraid of), specific phobia (caused by exposure to a specific phobic situation), obsessive-compulsive disorder (occurring for instance on exposure to dirt of an individual with an obsession about contamination), post-traumatic stress disorder (occurring in a response to a stimuli associated with a severe stressor) or separation anxiety disorder (in response to being separated from home or close relatives)

6.4 Agoraphobia

NOTE: Agoraphobia is not coded separately. The code is specific to disorders in which it occurs.

a. The anxiety about being in places from which the escape might be difficult (or embarrassing) or where help would be inaccessible in the case of having an unexpected or situationally predisposed panic attack or panic-like symptoms. Agoraphobics are afraid of a set of characteristic situations such as being outside the home alone, being in a crowed or standing in a line, on a bridge, traveling in a bus, train or automobile.

NOTE: If the avoidance is limited to only one or a few specific situations the diagnoses considered will be specific phobia, while if the avoidance is limited to social situations, the diagnosis will be social phobia.

b. The situation are avoided or endured with severe distress or with anxiety about recurrent panic attacks or panic-like symptoms, or else the presence of a companion is required.
c. Anxiety or avoidance behavior are not caused by another mental disorder such as: social phobia, specific phobia, obsessive-compulsive disorders or separation anxiety disorder.

6.5 Agoraphobia without history of panic disorder

a. The presence of agoraphobia related to fear of developing panic-like symptoms (e.g., dizziness or diarrhea).
b. Criteria have never been met for Panic Disorder.
c. The disturbance is not due to the direct physiological effects of a substance (e.g., a drug of abuse. a medication) or a genera l medical condition.
d. If an associated general medical condition is present. The fear described in Criterion A is clearly in excess of that usually associated with the condition.

6.6 Specific phobia

a. Marked and persistent fear that is excessive or unreasonable, cued by the presence or anticipation of a specific object or situation (e.g., flying, heights, animals, receiving an injection, seeing blood).
b. Exposure to the phobic stimulus almost invariably provokes an immediate anxiety response, which may take the form of a situationally bound or situationally predisposed Panic Attack. Note: In children, the anxiety may be expressed by crying, tantrums, freezing, or clinging.
c. The person recognizes that the fear is excessive or unreasonable. Note: In children, this feature may be absent.
d. The phobic situation(s) is avoided or else is endured with intense anxiety or distress.
e. E. The avoidance, anxious anticipation, or distress in the feared situation(s) interferes significantly with the person's normal routine, occupational (or academic) functioning, or social activities or relationships, or there is marked distress about having the phobia.
f. In individuals under age 18 years, the duration is at least 6 months .
g. The anxiety, Panic Attacks, or phobic avoidance associated with the specific object or situation are not better accounted for by another mental disorder, such as Obsessive Compulsive Disorder (e.g., fear of dirt in someone with an obsession about contamination), Posttraumatic Stress Disorder (e.g., avoidance of stimuli associated with a severe stressor), Separation Anxiety Disorder (e.g., avoidance of school), Social Phobia (e.g., avoidance of social situations because of fear of embarrassment), Panic Disorder With Agoraphobia, or Agoraphobia Without History of Panic Disorder.

Specify type:
Animal Type
Natural Environment Type (e.g., heights, storms, water)
Blood-Injection-Injury Type
Situational Type (e.g., airplanes, elevators, enclosed places)
Other Type (e.g., fear of choking, vomiting, or contracting an illness; in children, fear of loud sounds or costumed characters

6.7 Social phobia

a. A marked and persistent fear of one or more social or performance situations in which the person is exposed to unfamiliar people or to possible scrutiny by others.

The individual fears that he or she will act in a way (or show anxiety symptoms) that will be humiliating or embarrassing.

Note: In children, there must be evidence of the capacity for age-appropriate social relationships with familiar people and the anxiety must occur in peer settings, not just in interactions with adults.

b. Exposure to the feared social situation almost invariably provokes anxiety, which may take the form of a situationally bound or situation ally predisposed Panic Attack.

Note: In children, the anxiety may be expressed by crying, tantrums, freezing, or shrinking from social situations with unfamiliar people.

c. The person recognizes that the fear is excessive or unreasonable.

Note: In children, this feature may be absent.

d. The feared social or performance situations are avoided or else are endured with intense anxiety or distress.
e. The avoidance, anxious anticipation, or distress in t he feared social or performance situation(s) interferes significantly with the person's normal routine, occupational (academic) functioning, or social activities or relationships, or there is marked distress about having the phobia.
f. In individuals under age 18 years, the duration is at least 6 months.
g. The fear or avoidance is not due to the direct physiological effects of a substance (e.g., a drug of abuse. a medication) or a general medical condition and is not better accounted for by another mental disorder (e.g ., Panic Disorder With or Without Agoraphobia. Separation Anxiety Disorder, Body Dysmorphic Disorder, a Pervasive Developmental Disorder, or Schizoid Personality Disorder).
h. If a general medical condition or another mental disorder is present, the fear in Criterion A is unrelated to it, e .g., the fear is not of Stuttering, trembling in Parkinson's disease, or exhibiting abnormal eating behavior in Anorexia Nervosa or Bulimia Nervosa.

Specify if:

Generalized: if the fears include most social situations (also consider the additional diagnosis of Avoidant Personality Disorder)

6.8 Obsessive compulsive disorder

a. Either obsessions or compulsions:

Obsessions as defined by (1), (2), (3), and (4):

1. recurrent and persistent thoughts, impulses, or images that are experienced, at some time during the disturbance, as intrusive and inappropriate and that cause marked anxiety or distress
2. the thoughts, impulses, or images are not simply excessive worries about real life problems
3. the person attempts to ignore or suppress such thoughts, impulses, or images, or to neutralize them with some other thought or action
4. the person recognizes that the obsessional thoughts, impulses, or images are a product of his or her own mind (not imposed from without as in thought insertion)

Compulsions as defined by (1) and (2):

1. repetitive behaviors (e.g., hand washing, ordering, checking) or mental acts (e.g., praying, counting, repeating words silently) that the person feels driven to perform in response to an obsession, or according to rules that must be applied rigidly
2. the behaviors or mental acts are aimed at preventing or reducing distress or preventing some dreaded event or situation; however, these behaviors or mental acts either are not connected in a realistic way with what they are designed to neutralize or prevent or are clearly excessive

At some point during the course of the disorder, the person has recognized that the obsessions or compulsions are excessive or unreasonable. Note: This does not apply to children.

b. The obsessions or compulsions cause marked distress, are time consuming (take more than 1 hour a day), or significantly interfere with the person's normal routine, occupational (or academic) functioning, or usual social activities or relationships.

c. If another Axis I disorder is present, the content of the obsessions or compulsions is not restricted to it (e.g . preoccupation with food in the presence of an Eating Disorder; hair pulling in the presence of Trichotillomania; concern with appearance in the presence of Body Dysmorphic Disorder; preoccupation with drugs in the presence of a Substance Use Disorder; preoccupation with having a serious illness in the presence of Hypochondriasis; preoccupation with sexual urges or fantasies in the presence of a Paraphilia; or guilty ruminations in the presence of Major Depressive Disorder).

d. The disturbance is not due to the direct physiological effects of a substance (e.g . a drug abuse or medication abuse) or a general medical condition.

Specify if:

With Poor Insight: if, for most of the time during the current episode, the person does not recognize that the obsessions and compulsions are excessive or unreasonable

6.9 Posttraumatic stress disorder

a. The person has been exposed to a traumatic event in which both of the following were present:

 1. the person experienced, witnessed, or was confronted with an event or events that involved actual or threatened death or serious injury, or a threat to the physical integrity of self or others

 2. the person's response involved intense fear, helplessness, or horror.

Note: In children, this may be expressed instead by disorganized or agitated behavior

b. The traumatic event is persistently reexperienced in one (or more) of the following ways:

 1. recurrent and intrusive distressing recollections of the event, including images, thoughts, or perceptions. Note: In young children, repetitive play may occur in which themes or aspects of the trauma are expressed.

 2. recurrent distressing dreams of the event.

Note: In children, there may be frightening dreams without recognizable content.

 3. acting or feeling as if the traumatic event were recurring (includes a sense of reliving the experience, illusions, hallucinations, and dissociative flashback episodes, including those that occur on awakening or when intoxicated).

Note: In young children, trauma-specific reenactment may occur.

 4. intense psychological distress at exposure to internal or external cues that symbolize or resemble an aspect of the traumatic event

 5. physiological reactivity on exposure to internal or external cues that symbolize or resemble an aspect of the traumatic event

c. Persistent avoidance of stimuli associated with the trauma and numbing of general responsiveness (not present before the trauma), as indicated by three (or more) of the following:

 1. efforts to avoid thoughts, fee lings, or conversations associated with the trauma

 2. efforts to avoid activities, places, or people that a rouse recollections of the trauma

3. inability to recall an important aspect of the trauma
4. markedly diminished interest or participation in significant activities
5. feeling of detachment from others
6. restricted range of affect (e.g., unable to have loving feelings)
7. sense of a foreshortened future (e.g., does not expect to have a career, marriage, children, or a normal life)

d. Persistent symptoms of increased arousal (not present before the trauma), as indicated by two (or more) of the following:
1. difficulty falling or staying asleep
2. irritability or outbursts of anger
3. difficulty concentrating
4. hypervigilance
5. exaggerated startle response

e. Duration of the disturbance (symptoms in Criteria B, C, and 0) is more than 1 month.

f. The disturbance causes clinically significant distress or impairment in social, occupational, or other important areas of functioning.

Specify if:
Acute: if duration of symptoms is less than 3 months
Chronic: if duration of symptoms is 3 months or more
Specify if:
With Delayed Onset: if onset of symptoms is at least 6 months after the stressor

6.10 Acute stress disorder

a. The person has been exposed to a traumatic event in which both of the following were present:
(1) the person experienced, witnessed, or was confronted with an event or events that involved actual or threatened death or serious injury, or a threat to the physical integrity of self or others
(2) the person's response involved intense fear, helplessness, or horror

b. B. Either while experiencing or after experiencing the distressing event, the individual has three (or more) of the following dissociative symptoms:
1. a subjective sense of numbing, detachment, or absence of emotional responsiveness
2. a reduction in awareness of his or her surroundings (e.g., "being in a daze ")
3. derealization
4. depersonalization
5. dissociative amnesia (i .e., inability to recall an important aspect of the trauma
The traumatic event is persistently reexperienced in at least one of the following ways: recurrent images, thoughts, dreams, illusions, flashback episodes, or a sense of reliving the experience; or distress on exposure to reminders of the traumatic event.

c. Marked avoidance of stimuli that arouse recollections of the trauma (e.g ., thoughts, feelings, conversations, activities, places, people).

d. Marked symptoms of anxiety or increased arousal (e.g., difficulty sleeping, irritability, poor concentration, hypervigilance, exaggerated startle response, motor restlessness).

e. The disturbance causes clinically significant distress or impairment in social, occupational or other important areas of functioning or impairs the individual's ability to pursue some necessary task, such as obtaining necessary assistance or mobilizing personal resources by telling family members about the traumatic experience.

f. The disturbance lasts for a minimum of 2 days and a maximum of 4 weeks and occurs within 4 weeks of the traumatic event.
g. The disturbance is not due to the direct physiological effects of a substance (e.g., a drug of abuse, a medication) or a general medical condition, is not better accounted for by Brief Psychotic Disorder, and is not merely an exacerbation of a preexisting Axis I or Axis II disorder.

6.11 Generalized anxiety disorder

a. Excessive anxiety and worry (apprehensive expectation), occurring more days than not for at least 6 months, about a number of events or activities (such as work or school performance).
b. The person finds it difficult to control the worry.
c. The anxiety and worry are associated with three (or more) of the following six symptoms (with at least some symptoms present for more days than not for the past 6 months), Note: Only one item is required in children.
   1. restlessness or feeling keyed up or on edge
   2. being easily fatigued
   3. difficulty concentrating or mind going blank
   4. irritability
   5. muscle tension
   6. sleep disturbance (difficulty fall ing or staying asleep, or restless unsatisfying sleep)
d. The focus of the anxiety and worry is not confined to features of an Axis I disorder, e.g., the anxiety or worry is not about having a Panic Attack (as in Panic Disorder), being embarrassed in public (as in Social Phobia), being contaminated (as in Obsessive Compulsive Disorder), being away from home or close relatives (as in Separation Anxiety Disorder), gaining weight (as in Anorexia Nervosa), having multiple physical complaints (as in Somatization Disorder), or having a serious illness (as in Hypochondriasis), and the anxiety and worry do not occur exclusively during Posttraumatic Stress Disorder.
e. The anxiety, worry, or physical symptoms cause clinically significant distress or impairment in social, occupational, or other important areas of functioning.
f. The disturbance is not due to the direct physiological effects of a substance (e.g., a drug of abuse, a medication) or a general medical condition (e.g., hyperthyroidism) and does not occur exclusively during a Mood Disorder, a Psychotic Disorder, or a Pervasive Developmental Disorder.

6.12 Anxiety disorder due to

[Indicate the General Medical Condition]

a. Prominent anxiety, Panic Attacks, or obsessions or compulsions predominate in the clinical picture.
b. There is evidence from the history, physical examination, or laboratory findings that the disturbance is the direct physiological consequence of a general medical condition.
c. The disturbance is not better accounted for by another mental disorder (e.g., Adjustment Disorder With Anxiety in which the stressor is a serious general medical condition).
d. The disturbance does not occur exclusively during the course of a delirium.

e. The disturbance causes clinically significant distress or impairment in social, occupational, or other important areas of functioning.

Specify if:

With Generalized Anxiety: if excessive anxiety or worry about a number of events or activities predominates in the clinical presentation

With Panic Attacks: if Panic Attacks predominate in the clinical presentation

With Obsessive-Compulsive Symptoms: if obsessions or compulsions predominate in the clinical presentation

Coding note: Include the name of the general medical condition on Axis I

Anxiety Disorder Due to Pheochromocytoma, With Generalized Anxiety

Diagnostic criteria for Substance-Induced Anxiety Disorder

a. Prominent anxiety, Panic Attacks, or obsessions or compulsions predominate in the clinical picture.
b. There is evidence from the history, physical examination, or laboratory findings of either (1) or (2):
   1 the symptoms in Criterion A developed during, or within 1 month of, Substance Intoxication or Withdrawal
   2 medication use is etiologically related to the disturbance
c. The disturbance is not better accounted for by an Anxiety Disorder that is not substance induced. Evidence that the symptoms are better accounted for by an Anxiety Disorder that is not substance induced might include the following: the symptoms precede the onset of the substance use (or medication use); the symptoms persist for a substantial period of time (e.g., about a month) after the cessation of acute withdrawal or severe intoxication or are substantially in excess of what would be expected given the type or amount of the substance used or the duration of use; or there is other evidence suggesting the existence of an independent non-substance-induced Anxiety Disorder (e.g., a history of recurrent non-substance-related episodes).
d. The disturbance does not occur exclusively during the course of a delirium.
e. The disturbance causes clinically significant distress or impairment in social, occupational, or other important areas of functioning.

Note: This diagnosis should be made instead of a diagnosis of Substance Intoxication or Substance Withdrawal only when the anxiety symptoms are in excess of those usually associated with the intoxication or withdrawal syndrome and when the anxiety symptoms are sufficiently severe to warrant independent clinical attention.

Specify if:

With Generalized Anxiety: if excessive anxiety or worry about a number of events or activities predominates in the clinical presentation

With Panic Attacks: if Panic Attacks predominate in the clinical presentation With Obsessive-Compulsive Symptoms: if obsessions or compulsions predominate in the clinical presentation

With Phobic Symptoms: if phobic symptoms predominate in the clinical presentation

Specify if :

With Onset During Intoxication: if the criteria are met for Intoxication with
the substance and the symptoms develop during the intoxication syndrome

With Onset During Withdrawal: if criteria are met for Withdrawal from the substance and the symptoms develop during, or shortly after. a withdrawal syndrome

(American Psychiatric Association: Diagnostic and Statistical Manual of Mental Disorders, Fourth Edition, Text Revision , American Psychiatric Association,2000, ISBN 0-890-12-025-4, Washington, DC)

7. Evaluation

A special sub-chapter is dedicated to the psychological assessment of anxiety disorders (structured or semi-structured interviews, psychometric tests).
The diagnosis of anxiety disorders is established mainly through clinical interviews. We will therefore review some aspects related to interviews, without however going into the specifics of technique, methods, time influencing factors circumstances or setting.
The interview usually is structured or semi-structured. The interview may be free or standardized. Some of the best standardized interviews are: SCID, SADS, DIS, PSE.
Generally, in evaluation of anxiety disorders is used psychometric assessment having a diagnostic role, helping the clinician to establish a positive or differential diagnosis and it evaluates progress during therapy.
The tests used in anxiety may be objective and projective. Objective tests are: MMPI, MCMI, ADIS-R, HAM-A, STAI, SADS-LA, API, Cognitive Questionnaire for Agoraphobia, Daily Activity Form, Zung, Beck and Sheehan anxiety scales and so on.
Projective tests evaluate the individual's personality in its complexity assessing so the level of current anxiety. Some of this tests are the Rorschach, TAT, SCT, Draw-a-Person.

8. Treatment

Treatment of anxiety disorder is carried out in several stages:

- Acute phase. The goal of treatment in this phase is a rapidly reduce symptoms and allow better control, if not a complete remission of panic attacks. It has a duration of 4 to 6 weeks with benzodiazepines, but usually takes 2 to 3 months of treatment with tricyclic antidepressants, SSRIs or monoamine oxidase inhibitors (MAOIs), time in which the appropriate dose is reached. If improvement does not occur within 8 to 10 weeks after starting pharmacotherapy, requires a reassessment of drug therapy.
- Stabilization phase. Its purpose is to maintain and expand the response obtained in the acute phase; and extend is focused specifically on improving the avoidant behavior. Stabilization phase is between the second and sixth months of treatment, dosage of medication is adjusted to obtain maximum clinical response with minimal side effects.
- Maintenance phase. Includes 6-24 months of treatment, the main purpose being to maintain and improve the socio-professional rehabilitation. In this phase, the patient returns to a normal life, both professionally and socially. Drug doses can be reduced, taking care not won away in the early symptomatic phase.
- The discontinuation phase. In general, most authors agree that 12 to 24 months after drug therapy can be stopped. Stopping will be a gradual decline, particularly slow, which will stretch over two to four months. So gradual reduction aims at preventing the occurrence of benzodiazepine withdrawal symptoms, and also enables temporary readjustment of dosage for panic recurrence of complaints.

A great number of therapeutic agents have proved their efficacy in anxiety disorders. For didactic purposes, we shall attempt a systematic presentation in what follows:
Antidepressants:

- tricyclics
- serotonin specific reuptake inhibitors (SSRI)
- monoamine oxidase inhibitors (MAOI)
- recently introduced agents -venlafaxine
- nefazodone
- High-potency benzodiazepines:
  - alprazolam
  - Clonazepam

Other agents

None of this drug groups has been proven to be more efficient than the others in the treatment of anxiety disorders, each having both advantages and disadvantages. Tricyclics, for instance, can be described in a single dose to be taken in the evening before going to bed, but improvements can only appear 6 to 12 weeks later, and in the most cases side effects are difficult to tolerate. MAOIs also have several potential side effects and are accompanied by severe dietary restrictions. SSRIs develop fewer side effects and are safer than tricyclics, owing to their lower toxicity giving rise to a reduced mortality rate in overdose; as is the case for tricyclics, however, clinical improvement only becomes apparent after 6 to 12 weeks of treatment. Benzodiazepines act faster (one to two weeks), they have a significant effect on anticipatory anxiety, they are more easily tolerated by patients, but due to their short duration of acting the administration of several daily doses is required, and they produce dependence and withdrawal syndromes(see Table 4).

Advantages	Disadvantages
• rapid effect • safety in overdosing • improvment in sleep quality	• sedative effect • balance disorders • memory disorders • potentiating of alcohol effects • depresogen effect • addictive potential • Paradoxical reactions

Table 4. Advantajes and disadvantajes of benzodiazepine use in anxiety therapy

Nowadays, the most widely used drugs are SSRIs. In the tables below we present the efficacy of SSRIs in different types of anxiety disorders, their side effects, the dosage and the advantages and disadvantages of SSRI versus Venlafaxine (see table 5, 6, 7).

8.1 Panic disorder

Pharmacological and psychotherapeutic treatment in most cases leads to a dramatic improvement of agoraphobic and panic disorder symptoms. Goals of treatment are:

- reducing the number and intensity of panic attacks
- reduction of anticipatory anxiety
- treatment of comorbid disorders
- identification and treatment of agoraphobia

ISRS		Anxiety disorders				
Generic name	Trade name	PD	OCD	SAD	GAD	PTSD
Paroxetină	ALS-Paroxetin, Arketis, Paroxat, Paroxetin Stada, Paroxetin Teva, Paxetin, Rexetin, Seroxat	X	X	X	X	X
Fluvoxamină	Fevarin, Fluvoxamin Stada, Fluvoxamine Teva	X	X	X		
Fluoxetină	Fluohexal, Fluoxetine, Fluoxin, Fluran, Magrilan, Prozac	X	X			
Sertralină	Asentra, Serlift, Sertralin, Sertralin Sandoz, Sertralina Dr. Reddy's, Stimuloton, Zoloft	X	X	X		X
Citalopram	Citalec, Citalomerk, Citalopram Stada, Citaloran, Dalsan, Linisan	X	X	X	X	
Escitalopram	Cipralex	X	X	X	X	

Table 5. ISRS efficacy in anxiety disorders.

Advantages	Disadvantages
• effectiveness in all anxiety disorders • antidepressant effect • safety in overdose • reduced weight gain	delayed onset of therapeutic effect • early treatment may increase anxiety • Gastrointestinal side effects especially at the beginning of treatment • Sexual dysfunction is maintained throughout treatment

Table 6. Advantages and disadvantages of Venlafaxine and ISRS use in anxiety disorders.

Citalopram	Fluoxetine	Fluvoxamine	Paroxetine	Sertraline
Headache	Nausea	Nausea	Nausea	Nausea
Nausea	Headache	Insomnia	Sedation	Headache
Dry mouth	Nervousness	Headache	Headache	Diarrhea
Insomnia	Insomnia	Dry mouth	Dry mouth	Sexual dysfunction
somnolence	Anxiety	somnolence	fatigue	insomnia

Table 7. The most common side effects of SSRIs

8.1.1 Pharmacological treatment

Tricyclic antidepressants

The first study demonstrated the efficacy of imipramine in TP therapy was developed by Klein and was published in 1964. This finding was confirmed by a further 15 controlled studies. Given the equivalence of tricyclic antidepressants is very likely, although there are few controlled studies, that other than tricyclic imipramine have similar effectiveness. In most trials, tricyclic antidepressant average dose was approximately 150 mg / day and maximum dose of 300 mg per day. Selective serotonin reuptake inhibitors (SSRIs). The main goals of therapy with an SSRI is to reduce the intensity and frequency of panic attacks, reduce anticipatory anxiety and to treat depression associated. Also, appropriate therapy leads to reduction of phobic avoidance. For all SSRIs are currently available randomized controlled trials demonstrating efficacy of this class compared with placebo. TP patients who are prescribed an SSRI, may appear during the first two weeks of treatment an increase in anxiety, which is why it is recommended that therapy with low doses: 5-10 mg for fluoxetine, 25 mg for sertraline, 10 mg 50 mg paroxetine and fluvoxamine. It is generally accepted that the effect of therapy with an SSRI does not occur until after about four weeks, 8-12 weeks is needed to install full effect.

Benzodiazepines

Alprazolam was the first treatment approved by the FDA for the treatment of PD and although effective in relieving symptoms quickly, it is difficult to cut the majority of patients. Alprazolam dose for PD therapy is 5-6 mg / day. Studies have been published suggesting that other benzodiazepines (especially diazepam, clonazepam and lorazepam), administered in doses equivalent, may be as effective as alprazolam in the treatment of TP(Table*). Due to the risk of dependence and tolerance that it involves therapy with benzodiazepines, benzodiazepines are currently recommended only as short-term therapy. (see table 8, 9)

Generic name	Trade name	Equivalent dose	Daily usual dose for adults and regimen
clonazepam	Rivotril	0,5	1-6mg/day, 2 times/day
diazepam	Diazepam	5	4 - 40 mg/day 2-4 times/day
alprazolam	Xanax, Alprazolam LPH, Frontin, Prazolex, Neurol SR (preparat retard)	0,25	0,5 - 10 mg/day 2-4 times/day
lorazepam	Anxiar	1	1 - 6 mg/day 3 times/day
oxazepam		15	30 - 120 mg/day 3 - 4 times/day
clordiazepoxid		10	10 - 150 mg/day 3-4 times/day
clorazepat	Tranxene	7,5	15 - 60 mg/day 2- 4 times/day
prazepam		10	20 - 60 mg/day 3- 4 times/day
halazepam		20	60 - 160 mg/day 3- 4 times/day

Table 8. Benzodiazepine used in anxiety treatment (Ballenger J,2005, Benzodiazepine receptor agonist and antagonist, Kaplan and Sadock's Comprehensive Textbook of Psychiatry, Eight edition, Lippincott Williams & Wilkins,ISBN 0-7817-3434-7, Philadelphia,Baltimore, New-York, London, Buenosaires, Hong-Kong, Sydney, Tokyo).

anxiety iritability insomnia fatigue headache spasms or muscular pain vertigo tremors sweating concentrating difficulty nausea sau loss of appetite * depression * depersonalization, derealisation * high senzorial perception (smell, light, taste, feel) * abnormal perception sensation of movement *
• symptoms that represent more likely a withdrawal syndrom rather than exacerbation or reaparance of initial anxiety symptoms

Table 9. Symptoms frequently observed during benzodiazepine withdrawal.

Also proved useful venlafaxine (mean dose 150 mg / day), nefazodone (300-500 mg / day), mirtazapine, gabapentin and pregabalin. In cases resistant to SSRIs or augmentation therapy have proven useful and MAOIs.

8.1.2 Psychotherapy

Should be encouraged in all patients participating in cognitive-behavioral psychotherapy sessions, which is recognized as the most effective psychotherapeutic techniques for patients with PD with or without agoraphobia. Can be used in combination with pharmacotherapy.

8.2 Generalized anxiety disorder

Currently we have a wide choice of treatment of GAD, both psychopharmacology and psychotherapy. However, although patients with GAD are frequent users of medical services, only about 25% of people who actually suffer from this disorder are treated.

8.2.1 Pharmacological treatment

Benzodiazepines

A long period of time, GAD has been treated with benzodiazepines. Several double-blind placebo controlled clinical trials have demonstrated the efficacy of certain benzodiazepines (diazepam, clorazepat, alprazolam, lorazepam) in the acute treatment (3-6 months) of GAD, but long-term efficacy (6 months - 1 year) is less robust. Primary anxiolytic effect of benzodiazepines is mainly aimed at somatic symptoms of GAD, leaving cognitive symptoms, such as concern, partly unresolved. Moreover, benzodiazepines do not reduce depressive symptoms, while often present in these individuals.

Main advantages of benzodiazepines in the treatment of GAD are fast effect, safety in overdose and rapid improvement of the quality of sleep.

In general, different benzodiazepines have equivalent efficacy in the treatment of GAD. Approximately 35% of patients obtain a marked benefit, and 40% achieved a moderate improvement. The response is rapid, usually within the first week. Equivalent to 15-25 mg daily doses of diazepam produced an adequate therapeutic effect (see Table 10).

Benzodiazepine	Recommended daily dose (mg)
Alprazolam	0,75 – 10
Clordiazepoxid	5 – 100
Clorazepat	15 – 60
Diazepam	4 – 40
Halazepam	60 – 160
Lorazepam	1 – 10
Oxazepam	30 – 120
Prazepam	20 - 60

Table 10. Recommended daily dose

Patients treated with benzodiazepines have a recurrence rate of symptoms two times higher than patients treated with medication nonbenzodiazepinic. Although benzodiazepines have a faster onset of action 3-6 weeks of treatment efficacy is similar to that of antidepressants or buspirone.
Due to the risk of physical dependence, rebound anxiety upon discontinuation of treatment and adverse effects, benzodiazepines are now considered as second choice treatment or as adjuvant agents in short-term treatment with other compounds.

Buspirone

Initial studies on the efficacy of buspirone in the treatment of GAD have suggested that buspirone would be an alternative to benzodiazepines in treating anxiety, with some specificity for psychiatric symptoms of the disorder. However, more recent studies questioning its effectiveness in the treatment of GAD. Some authors believe that patients often discontinue treatment with buspirone than patients treated with benzodiazepines. Not sure if this is due to decreased efficacy of this compound over time.
Buspirone effect occurs in about 2-3 weeks. Doses useful are between 30 mg and 60 mg, although sometimes they even used a dose of 90 mg. At doses below 30 mg, buspirone is not superior to placebo. The effect is weaker on patients previously treated with benzodiazepines.

Selective serotonin reuptake inhibitors (SSRIs)

Currently, data from the literature on the effectiveness of SSRIs is increasing. Most studies have focused on paroxetine (20-50 mg / day), which is currently approved by the FDA for the treatment of GAD. Positive results have been published and fluvoxamine, sertraline (50-150 mg/day) and escitalopram (10-20 mg/day). So far, three randomized placebo controlled

studies have demonstrated the efficacy of escitalopram in the treatment of GAD, which is why escitalopram is approved by the FDA for the treatment of GAD.
It was suggested that the effectiveness of SSRIs in the treatment of GAD was due, as in depression or other anxiety disorders, normalizing dysfunctional activity in certain neuroanatomic circuits involved in the pathophysiology of GAD.

Venlafaxine

Several studies have demonstrated venlafaxine (extended-release form) efficacy compared with placebo, in reducing somatic and psychological symptoms specific to TAG, both in acute treatment and long term, venlafaxine was approved by the FDA for the treatment of GAD. Doses up to 150 mg/day are needed for symptom control.
Antidepressants in the treatment of GAD have shown improvement in joint symptoms in about 2-4 weeks and, unlike benzodiazepines, mainly improves psychiatric symptoms of anxiety. Because anxious patients are particularly sensitive to the activating effects of some antidepressants, it is generally recommended that treatment be started with half the dose recommended for treatment of depression, with dose titration in 1-2 weeks. The optimal dose of antidepressant for the treatment of GAD is similar to that used in the treatment of depression.
Beta blockers can be used with high efficacy in anxious patients with cardio vascular symptoms; atenolol is preferred because it has less bronchoconstrictor effect. It is used for short periods of time associated with benzodiazepines.
Limited efficacy has riluzole also, a antiglutamatergic compound and pregabalin and tiagabina. In patients refractory to treatment with SSRIs, can be augmented with olanzapine, ziprasidone or risperidone.

Psychopharmacological treatment guide

- Antidepressants (SSRIs and venlafaxine), are now considered first-line therapy in the GAD treatment because of their proven efficacy, the possibility of concomitant comorbid depression often, lack of dependence, potential and favorable profile of adverse effects.
- buspirone is currently indicated for patients with a history of substance abuse that have not responded or have not tolerated treatment with antidepressants.
- The use of benzodiazepines should be limited to short-term administration due to the potential development of dependency.
- In case of lack of response to treatment given in appropriate dose and for a sufficient length of time, a rational approach would be a therapy change from another class. When this event does not get an adequate response could be given a combination of two drugs from different classes.
- Currently there is insufficient data on treatment duration for GAD after getting a favorable response. Relapse rates are significant if medication is discontinued in the early months after obtaining a response and it is not known at what point the risk of relapse is low enough to try stopping the medication. Since GAD tends to be chronic and often complicated by depression, the psychiatrist must be careful discontinuing of treatment. Some authors have suggested that patients should be treated with the lowest effective dose and for stopping medication reviewed every six months. At present, it is

considered that treatment should be continued for another 6 months to a year after remission of symptoms.

8.2.2 Psychotherapy

The most intensively studied modality of psychotherapy for GAD is cognitive-behavioral psychotherapy addressed to intolerance of uncertainty and danger, associated with concerns perceived by this patients as uncontrollable. Cognitive-behavioral psychotherapy has demonstrated efficacy in controlling symptoms, in both short and long term, associated with a low rate of relapse.

8.3 Specific phobias

Phobia, as the central symptom of phobic disorder, is defined as a persistent and irrational fear to specific stimuli. Exposure to these stimuli triggers an intense anxiety response (suggesting the panic attack) and the development of avoidance behavior. Phobias are classified as:

- Specific phobias
- agoraphobia
- social phobia.

We present only the specific phobias; agoraphobia and social phobia beeing presented separately.

While behavioral therapy is the main method of treatment for specific phobias that affect quality of life and interferes with daily functioning, studies have shown the efficacy of SSRIs in the treatment of phobias. Recent studies have demonstrated the efficacy of combining pharmacological treatment (especially the D-cycloserine dose of 50 mg/day) with psychotherapy.

8.4 Obsessive compulsive disorder (OCD)

Obsessive Compulsive Disorder (OCD) is an anxiety disorder characterized by the appearance of obsessive ideas and compulsive behaviors, and significantly affects quality of life. It is a chronic disorder with a typical evolution, with periods of improvement which alternate with periods of rebound symptoms.

OCD is likely psychological disorder for which the last 20 years of psychopharmacological and psychotherapeutic treatment have been most progressive. OCD anxiety disorder is probably the most difficult to treat, while having the highest rate of resistance to treatment.

Modern treatment of OCD consists of pharmacotherapy combined with cognitive-behavioral therapy.

The goal of treatment is to reduce symptoms and improve patients functioning in society, so that the patient have a normal life. A modest proportion of patients will achieve a complete release of symptoms.

Before prescribing drug therapy must take into account the following steps:

- assess the awareness that obsessions and compulsions are excessive and unjustified
- Assessment of comorbid conditions: affective disorders, other anxiety disorders, substance abuse, personality disorder
- identifying and exploring the patient's symptoms
- measurement of severity at baseline using the Yale-Brown scale

- patient and family education on OCD and its treatment

8.4.1 Pharmacological treatment

Of all the classes of drugs used in psychiatry, serotonin reuptake inhibitors are by far the most effective in treating OCD, as first line therapy in the treatment of this disorder. Of this group of drugs are clomipramine - tricyclic antidepressant (TCA) - and selective serotonin reuptake inhibitors (SSRIs) - fluoxetine, sertraline, paroxetine, fluvoxamine, citalopram and escitalopram. Although the response to treatment does not necessarily imply remission of symptoms, one can obtain a substantial improvement in quality of life. Among patients treated with SSRIs, 40 - 60% will have a good response and very good.

The therapeutic effect of SSRIs are of particular interest because, from a therapeutic perspective, OCD appears to be a single disorder. From numerous studies on the treatment of OCD is clear that only antidepressants with a specific action on the serotonin system have demonstrated efficacy. The efficacy of SSRIs in treating OCD does confirm that serotonin may be a specific condition. Unlike other mental disorders, the placebo response rate is typically low.

Clomipramine was the first effective treatment for OCD treatment. Its beneficial effect was seen in 60 years, but its effectiveness has been clearly demonstrated in studies compared with placebo in 80 years. Was also shown to have a beneficial effect in both adults and children. The consistency with which its effect was confirmed in studies anti-obsessive even small scale is a measure of the robustness of the effect. Positive results are in contrast to clomipramine with results for other tricyclic antidepressants have been tested for a possible positive effect, but without success. The dose used is: clomipramine 200-250 mg/day, which provides a clear antiobsessional effect in 4-6 weeks. Starting dose (25 mg/day given vesperal) will be increased gradually by 25 mg every four days or 50 mg weekly until reach maximum dose. If patients can not tolerate adverse effects (dry mouth, sedation, tremor, nausea and abnormal ejaculation), the administered dose will be 150-200 mg/day (Clomipramine Collaborative Study Group, 1991). For nonresponsive or multiple adverse effects cases can be used clomipramine i.v., a equivalent dose, with antiobsessional effect obtained in 4-5 days.

Given that there are currently no studies that compare the effectiveness of SSRIs in treating OCD, the choice of a particular SSRI should take into account the adverse effect profile, potential interactions with other drugs, pharmacokinetic properties and personal experience of each physician. In most cases the use of higher doses than those needed to treat depression were more likely to produce better therapeutic effect. If one starts with a lower dose patients should be reassessed and the dose should be increased if the response is not satisfactory. With higher doses, we can expect more side effects. The problem of adverse effects is extremely important because the negative influence on adherence to treatment, and efficacy also. Clomipramine usefulness is limited by side effects typical of tricyclic antidepressants.

Long-term studies conclusion is that SSRI efficacy is maintained. If treatment is interrupted, a considerable number of patients will relapse. For this reason, treatment should be followed for long periods of time. It was very clear that the antiobsessive efficacy of clomipramine and SSRIs is independent of their antidepressant activity. In this regard, OCD resembles other non-affective disorders such as panic disorder, bulimia, enuresis, migraine, chronic neuropathic pain, the tricyclic antidepressants are effective in the absence of depression.

A significant proportion of patients with OCD and depressive symptoms have been marked. From a therapeutic standpoint it is important to note that depressive symptoms associated with OCD have the same therapeutic specificity and OCD symptoms. Depressive symptoms do not respond to antidepressants that have a strong activity on the serotonin system. Symptoms improve in the same time with OCD symptoms only with anti-obsessive treatment. It is considered that depressive symptoms in people in which it appears, is a part of the TOC and not a secondary disorder.

The most important predictor of a possible negative response is early onset. The presence of a borderline type of personality disorder, schizotypal or avoided also have a negative predictive role. Also it was found that the severity, duration of disorder, gender, age and type of symptoms have no predictive value in this respect.

Recent studies (Denys et al., 2004, Grossman and Hollander, 1996) recommends the use of venlafaxine (a selective inhibitor of serotonin and norepinephrine reuptake) at a dose of 37.5 to 225 mg/day, maximum dose is 375 mg/day (March et al., 1997).

Treatment guide

1. Treatment of choice is represented by an SSRI. Principles of treatment:

- effective doses to treat OCD are generally higher than those used to treat depression;
- Many patients notice a clear benefit after about six weeks of treatment, lack of efficacy during this period should not be viewed as a discouraging sign;
- it takes several months, half a year, even more to achieve maximum response;
- patients not responding to low doses of SSRIs may respond to higher doses;
- treatment with an SSRI should be followed at least 10-12 weeks, including at least 6 weeks at maximum tolerated dose, before being replaced with another SSRI if the ineffectiveness of the former;
- patients who have never received treatment with SSRIs have a greater likelihood of response to treatment than patients who have received treatment with SSRIs, without obtaining a significant improvement in symptoms;
- SSRIs are better tolerated than clomipramine, all SSRIs are well tolerated by most patients, side effects are usually mild
- Because we can not predict which of the SSRIs to be effective in a given patient often requires a number of attempts to find the right medicine;

  If a patient treated with an SSRI does not tolerate appropriate dose or does not achieve a clinical response to a dose at the upper limit of the recommended therapeutic dose, the change of treatment with another SSRI is recommended, since there is evidence that patients that do not respond to a particular SSRI, often respond to another SSRI. Also to be considered clomipramine administration after trying unsuccessfully of one or more SSRIs. As with SSRIs, to determine the efficacy, increased doses should be administered, if tolerated, for 10-12 weeks.

2. In case of obtaining only a partial response to the second SSRI or no response to a third SSRI, augmentation is useful to test the therapeutic effect by combining SSRIs with other drugs.
3. Even if other compounds were tried to be used for this purpose - buspirone (20-60 mg/day), lithium (300-600 mg/day), gabapentin (300-2400 mg/day), inositol (16-18 mg/day), L-tryptophan (4-6 g/day), fenfluramine (20-60 mg/day), topiramate (250

mg/day) - only small doses of risperidone (1-2 mg 2 times/day) and pindolol (2.5 mg three times daily) have proved effective in double-blind comparative studies (Jenike and Rauch, 1994; Rassmusen, Eisen and Pato, 1993; Piccinelli et al., 1995, Saxena et al., 1996).

4. Clonazepam that has serotonergic action too, has proved to be effective as monotherapy in a double blind study. However, there were presented cases in which clonazepam augmentation was beneficial in cases resistant to treatment. For this reason, clonazepam can be a useful option that can be taken into account in some cases requiring augmentation.
5. There is evidence that the beneficial effects of treatment with clomipramine and SSRIs are maintained throughout treatment. Patients should be encouraged to continue treatment with the same dose with clinical response was obtained for periods of at least one year after they get this response. Discontinuation should be achieved by very slow gradual decrease in dosage (e.g, lowering the dose by 20-30% every 6-8 weeks).

8.4.2 Psychotherapy

For a long time it was considered that psychoanalysis would be effective in treating OCD. However, there are insufficient data to support the usefulness of the techniques of psychotherapy. Cognitive behavioral psychotherapy is the most frequently used psychological treatment for OCD.

Research in recent years have shown that behavioral therapy technique of exposure and response prevention (exposure and response prevention, to - ERP) is an extremely effective therapy for OCD in adults and children.

8.5 Social anxiety disorder (social phobia)

The initial problem in the treatment of SAD is to identify the disorder. Many patients affected by the SAD does not realize that they have a condition that is treatable. They consider their symptoms as extreme shyness or as an unpleasant feature of their personality, so they have to be convinced that a long-term treatment may be useful.

8.5.1 Partial form treatment

Partial form presents an unsatisfactory response to drug therapy, most appropriate treatment beeing behavioral psychotherapy in vivo exposure. Specific social phobias such as fear of speaking in public, respond quite well to β blockers drug administration, although most data come from isolated cases. They must be administered several hours before the performance. It is used a dose of 20 mg propranolol, atenolol dose of 50 mg.

8.5.2 Generalized form treatment

Pharmacological treatment

Only in recent years psychopharmacological treatment has been accepted by clinicians as a therapeutic option for SAD. In the 80s, when they began studying for the medical treatment of SAD, many clinicians regarded SAD as a personality disorder, which is why it was not considered appropriate psychopharmacological treatment.

Selective serotonin reuptake inhibitors (SSRIs) are effective antidepressants, widely used, which have a positive effect on depression and anxiety in the different anxiety disorders.

The class of drugs that has been the most extensively studied for TAS. Paroxetine, fluvoxamine, sertraline and escitalopram were studied in double-blind placebo for generalized form of SBP, demonstrating their effectiveness in treating this disorder.

Among SSRIs, paroxetine is the most studied, the first SSRI approved for the treatment of social phobia by the FDA. Preferred dose of paroxetine seems to be 20-40 mg / day.Today and sertraline has received approval from the FDA for the same indication. Because efficacy and safety of SSRIs are considered first-line treatment for SBP. Since about 60-70% respond to treatment with an SSRI, it is clear the need to expand and diversify ways of treatment.

Oxidase inhibitors (MAOIs) were the first drugs with proven efficacy in the treatment of TAS. Dietary restrictions and the many troublesome side effects is a significant disadvantage compared to SSRIs, which are much better tolerated. However, MAOIs can be used in case of resistance to other safer ways of treatment. Moclobemide, a reversible inhibitor of monoamine oxidase A, has proven effective in the treatment of SBP in most studies.

Among benzodiazepines, clonazepam alone is demonstrated efficacy in a double-blind study. Clonazepam has the advantage of twice daily administration and a lower potential than other benzodiazepines to be misused. However, clonazepam as monotherapy because of adverse reactions is not considered first-line treatment. Therapeutic effects appear quite quickly, with greater efficacy in less severe cases. It may be useful as an adjunctive therapy in patients with a high level of anxiety, but its use should be limited to initial clonazepam period of treatment. Used as adjunctive therapy could be an alternative in refractory cases.

Venlafaxine, a selective inhibitor of serotonin and norepinephrine reuptake, is approved by the FDA for the treatment of TAS.

Have been tested, obtaining encouraging results: mirtazapine, pregabalin (600 mg / day), topiramate, buspirone (30 mg / day), bupropion, gabapentin, citalopram, olanzapine, valproate and D-cycloserina (antagonist of NMDA receptor glutamate, and has proven effective in combination with behavioral therapy graduated exposure).

Most studies on the efficacy of pharmacotherapy in the treatment of SBP were of short duration. However, TAS is a chronic condition. It was shown that patients who discontinue paroxetine or phenelzine have a significantly increased risk of relapse than those who continued treatment for longer periods.

Most patients who responded to treatment achieved a reduction of anxiety and avoidance behavior, leading to improved social and occupational functioning. However, most patients do not obtain a complete and permanent disappearance of symptoms.

Treatment guide

1. Treatment of first choice is an SSRI. Treatment should be started at doses used to treat depression - such as paroxetine 20 mg/day, sertraline 50 mg/day. For SAD, as in OCD, there is a period of latency in onset of response to treatment and are often required higher doses than those used to treat depression. Control disorder is usually found after 6 to 8 weeks. To determine the effectiveness of SSRI administration is required for a period of 10-12 weeks.
2. Currently there are insufficient data to guide treatment choice if not get a satisfactory response after treatment with SSRIs first. You can try another SSRI. When this event does not get a response, is another option and then use of clonazepam, the gabapentin

or venlafaxine. Only if the latter inefficiency and treatment can try a MAOI (e.g phenelzine).

3. Having achieved a significant improvement of symptoms is recommended to continue treatment for at least a year. Interruption of treatment is achieved by gradually lowering the dose very slowly during several months (eg, lowering the dose by 20-30% every 6-8 weeks). During this period, physicians should be alert to symptoms of possible relapse.

Psychotherapy

Psychotherapy is effective in the treatment of SAD, but most of them are safe and cognitive-behavioral therapy group. They are geared to strengthen and affirm the patient's self, and lead to different social skills, to produce a cognitive restructuring and exposure to find appropriate techniques in different social situations. In two recent meta-effectiveness of pharmacotherapy and psychotherapy should be similar, with a slight superiority in the short term pharmacotherapy

8.4 Post traumatic stress disorder (PTSD)

An important component of treatment is to ensure psychoeducation, which should help the patient understand the nature of the condition of suffering and what is the process of recovery.

In addition to the choice of therapeutic modalities, the physician should take into account other factors that may influence the disorder: the stigma, ambivalence regarding treatment, shame, social support, attitudes and behaviors of family antitherapeutics possibility of legal action or the victim.

The psychopharmacological treatment, especially with SSRIs and psychotherapy have proven effective in relieving symptoms of PTSD, there are even studies showing superior efficacy of combining two therapeutic modalities, compared with each treatment method in part.

8.4.1 Pharmacological treatment

Psychopharmacological treatment of PTSD goals are: improvement of key symptoms, minimize disability and to comorbidities, quality of life and prevent recurrence.

Although the diagnosis of PTSD in DSM was introduced in 1980, the number of studies pharmacological treatment of this condition is surprisingly low. Have not yet developed pharmacological compounds that affect biological changes characteristic of PTSD, so that psychopharmacological treatment of this disease was limited to the administration of different compounds with proven efficacy in other anxiety disorders or depression.

SSRIs are the most studied antidepressants for the treatment of PTSD and are considered as first line therapy (Stein, 2006). The effectiveness of these compounds has been demonstrated in double blind studies for sertraline, paroxetine and fluoxetine in open studies for escitalopram (10-20 mg/day), citalopram (20-60 mg/day), fluvoxamine (100-300 mg/day) , nefazodone (200-600 mg/day), venlafaxine (150-225 mg/day) and mirtazapine (15-45 mg/day) .

SSRIs have proven efficacy clear cases of PTSD experienced by civilians, although there are conflicting data could be effective in cases arising after military conflicts. SSRIs results in an improvement in all PTSD symptoms, with the exception of sleep disorders. Improvement of symptoms seen in 2-4 weeks, but may improve irritability and dysphoria as the first week.

Paroxetine and sertraline are approved by the FDA for the treatment of PTSD. The doses used are higher than those commonly used, being 100-200 mg/day for sertraline and 30-50 mg/day for paroxetine (Ninan and Dunlop, 2006). Also, amitriptyline and imipramine (initial dose of 50-75 mg/day increased to 300 mg/ day) have proven their efficacy in the treatment of this disorder.

It has been suggested that patients with comorbid mental illness and another might show a better response to antidepressant treatment than patients who do not have other comorbid mental disorder, since the differences between active drug and placebo would be higher if a comorbidities. This might explain the higher rate of response to placebo if no other comorbid condition.

Of the anticonvulsants, lamotrigine has demonstrated efficacy for the treatment of PTSD in a double blind, mainly improving the symptoms of reliving the traumatic event and avoidant behavior. Have been published and smaller studies have demonstrated that other anticonvulsants (sodium valproate and carbamazepine) could play a role in PTSD therapy.

In the treatment of PTSD and have proven effectiveness and:

- MAOI - phenelzine at a dose of 45-75 mg/day in improving symptoms of intrusive (Davidson, 1994);
- α1 adrenergic blockers - prazosin vesperal administered at a dose of 1-4 mg in relieving nightmares, and intrusive symptoms
- benzodiazepines in improving sleep disorders

Treatment guide

- SSRIs are currently recommended as first choice therapy in the treatment of PTSD due to efficacy, safety and tolerability of this class of compounds.
- If a patient does not tolerate or respond to an SSRI, you can try another compound in this class. Nefazodone, amitriptyline, imipramine, lamotrigine are other options for these patients.
- Augmentation of drug treatment is necessary in cases where only get a partial answer to the second treatment tried (in this case you can try and replace it with another drug), or if no response is achieved or attempted in the third treatment. Thus, depending on each patient's specific symptoms, you can try taking lithium or an anticonvulsant in patients with fits of anger and an atypical neuroleptic (especially Olanzapine) in agitated patients. Quetiapine (100 mg/day) is recommended in the treatment of refractory severe insomnia (Robert et al., 2005; Ninan and Dunlop, 2006).
- Where the PTSD is a chronic evolution is continued treatment for at least a year after obtaining the response to treatment. Discontinuation of treatment, as with other anxiety disorders, it is recommended to achieve the slow decrease in dosage (eg 20-30% of the dose a few months). Currently there are no sufficient data on the maintenance of therapeutic effect compared with placebo or the long term development disorder after discontinuation of drug therapy.

8.4.2 Psychotherapy

Among the psychotherapeutic methods tested for PTSD treatment, the most effective is cognitive behavioral psychotherapy, which is indicated as first line therapy in the treatment of mild or moderate PTSD. Among the most effective techniques are used exposure therapy and cognitive restructuring.

8.5 Acute stress disorder

Acute stress disorder is a short transitional period - lasting less than a month - a significant severity characterized by intrusive memories that occurs shortly after a physically or emotionally stressful event exceptional. It is similar to post traumatic stress disorder, distinguishing evolutionarily. Occurs within 4 weeks after the traumatic event, lasting from 2 days to 4 weeks. Stresorul can be a traumatic experience involving a serious threat to the security or integrity of the subject or someone close (eg natural disasters, accidents, fights, criminal assault, rape, etc..), or an unusually sudden and threatening change social position and / or the subject's social network, for example: multiple losses of people close to the fire house, etc..

An important role in the occurrence and severity of side play individual vulnerability and capacity to cope with events.

Treatment of acute stress disorder include psychopharmacological and psychotherapeutic intervention, psychoeducation, and case management.

Currently there are few studies on the psychopharmacological intervention in acute stress disorder. However, it can be recommended selective serotonin reuptake inhibitors (SSRIs) and other antidepressants. Benzodiazepines are useful in cases where immediate cause persists (diazepam: 5-10 mg / day or i.m. dorazepam.: 1-2 mg / day). In patients who are contraindicated benzodiazepines can be used low doses of neuroleptic sedatives

8.6 Adjustment disorder with anxiety

(ICD-10 Clasificarea tulburarilor mentale si de comportament, ALL, ISBN 973-9392-73-3, Romania)

Adjustment disorder is defined as a maladaptive response, a response to an identifiable stressor, namely: a significant life change or a stressful life event (presence or possibility of a serious physical illness).

Treatment

Adjustment disorder requires a psycho-therapeutic approach centered on stress, on its significance and how the patient perceives and controls the stress. It is recommended bio feedback, relaxation techniques and hypnosis. Medications (anxiolytics) has an auxiliary role by reducing the severity of symptoms.

9. References

American Psychiatric Association, 1994, *Diagnostic and Statistical Manual of Mental Disorders*, fourth edition , American Psychiatric Association, ISBN 0-89042-064-5, Washington, DC; WHO, 1998,

American Psychiatric Association: Diagnostic and Statistical Manual of Mental Disorders, Fourth Edition, Text Revision , American Psychiatric Association,2000, ISBN 0-890-12-025-4, Washington, DC)

Ballenger J,2005, Benzodiazepine receptor agonist and antagonist, Kaplan and Sadock's Comprehensive Textbook of Psychiatry, Eight edition, Lippincott Williams & Wilkins, ISBN 0-7817-3434-7, Philadelphia, Baltimore, New-York, London, Buenosaires, Hong-Kong, Sydney, Tokyo).

Feraru R, Podea D, 1998, *Panic Disorder,*MAIKO, ISBN 973-95649-6-8, Bucharest

ICD-10 Clasificarea tulburarilor mentale si de comportament, ALL, ISBN 973-9392-73-3, Romania)

Marinescu M, Udristoiu T, Podea D., Ciucu A,2008, *Tulburarea depresiva si anxioasa-actualitati,* AIUS, ISBN 978-973-1780-97-9, Craiova

2

Epidemiological Patterns of Anxiety Disorders in Kenya

David M. Ndetei, Lincoln I. Khasakhala,
Anne W. Mbwayo and Victoria Mutiso
Africa Mental Health Foundation (AMHF)
Kenya

1. Introduction

The global burden of mental health problems including anxiety is enormous, neglected and under resourced, particularly in the developing nations [1-3]. People with untreated anxiety disorders are at dire risk of descending into other mental disorders since the anxiety symptoms interfere with social and occupational functioning and therefore lowers their self-esteem. While studies on the effects of untreated mental illness on national economic development have not been conducted in developing countries, research in developed countries provides an important framework and data for understanding these costs in developing countries [4]. Overally, lack of treatment for mental disorders results in much infallible expenses, as a result of the higher indirect costs associated with greater morbidity to untreated disorders [5]. Most of these costs are quantifiable and occur outside the health sector; loss of employment and income generation, increased absenteeism from work or school, poor performance within the workplace or school work and premature retirement [5]. People with mental disorders have higher unemployment rates, less access to treatment and face more discrimination [6-8].

Anxiety is, "one of the main motivating factors in most of human behaviour" and is a normal reaction to threatening or unthreatening situations in the environment. It produces a wide range of both physiological and psychological reactions that are often of sudden onset as the body prepares for 'fight or flight' response. These symptoms occur as a result of increased amount of adrenaline that is produced by the autonomic nervous system in response to a perceived threat from the environment. The increased level of adrenaline causes an increase in the heart respiration rate, elevation of the blood pressure and the contraction of blood vessels and intestines as blood is diverted to the heart, lungs and muscles. Although these reactions are appropriate when faced with incidents of threat or danger, the state of anxiety usually continue after the threat has been removed, or when there is no real threat existing. These physical and psychological symptoms occurring without a real stimulus in the person's environment can lead to the development of the different types of anxiety disorders. Anxiety disorders are therefore combinations of various physical and mental manifestations which are not attributable to real danger, but keep re-occurring in attacks or as a persisting hyper aroused state. Anxiety disorders include general anxiety (GAD), panic disorders, phobias, fears which keep repeating itself as acute, chronic or abnormal response states that become disabling on the individual's life.

2. Classification of anxiety disorders

A comprehensive review of available data worldwide has shown that 8-12% of children, youth and adults suffer from anxiety symptoms that are severe enough to interfere with daily life and functioning.[1] According to Diagnostic Statistical Manual for mental disorders fourth edition[2], anxiety disorders may be classified as follows:

1. separation anxiety disorder
2. Generalised Anxiety Disorder (GAD)
3. Panic Disorder
4. Phobic disorders - Agoraphobia, specific phobias and social phobia
5. Obsessive Compulsive disorder (OCD)
6. Post traumatic Stress Disorder (PTSD)
7. Secondary to General Medical Condition / substances

3. Anxiety disorders in childhood and adolescents

Recognizing anxiety symptoms in children is important because in most cases of anxiety disorders in youth and adults, the onset is usually during childhood [9]. In a school survey in Kenya among adolescent students utilizing different anxiety measuring instruments, several different types' of clinically significant anxiety syndromes were documented [10-12]. Multidimensional Anxiety Scale for Children (MASC) instrument revealed that definitive anxiety states was 12.9% where most of the students (>75%) had harm avoidance and social phobia[10,13]. Social anxiety for clinical pathology in this population of high students in a similar setting of 80% prevalence is not surprising since there are high levels of bullying in the same schools [12]. Utilising a questionnaire for screening a broad range of DSM-IV defined anxiety disorder symptoms in children and adolescents in the same setting, almost all students had separation anxiety, school phobia and obsessive or compulsive symptoms [12, 14-15]. The lowest anxiety symptoms (54.7%) were in specific phobia for animals [12]. However, some of these symptoms reported by the high school students can be reported as perfectly normal symptoms like; 'when frightened my heart beats fast'. Anxiety Disorders among children identified in Kenya include:

4. Panic disorder

- These are recurrent spontaneous episodes of panic associated with physiological and psychological symptoms. The physiological symptoms can be seen as emanating from circulatory, respiratory, gastro-intestinal, and urinary systems. Symptoms from respiratory system include: chest pains, shortness of breath, choking, dizziness/giddiness, fear of dying or going crazy and lapse into unconsciousness. The respiratory symptoms are related physiologically to changes in blood gaseous imbalance with a result of low levels of carbon dioxide. Symptoms from circulatory system include: palpitation, sweating, trembling, elevated blood pressure and muscle tension. Gastro-intestinal symptoms include nausea, butterfly feeling at the epigastria area and sometime diarrhoea and vomiting. While in the urinary system there is increased frequency of micturation, all these are in preparation for either fight or flight
- However, most instruments for measuring Anxiety Disorders in children do not screen for Panic Disorder

- In Kenyan setting, adolescents who have spontaneous panic attacks report greater severity of attacks, more depression and greater lifestyle changes as a result of the attacks

5. Selective mutism

- Lack of use of speech is specific to certain situations e.g. public places, with strangers or in presence of elements associated with traumatic event in the affected child (abuser)
- Common and usually characteristic with girls unlike boys
- Diagnosis most of the time missed out and child treated for a seizure disorder. In adolescent it is miss diagnosed as a conversion disorder
- Often children are shy, negative, controlling or oppositional. Been seen more common in family settings where mothers are overprotective; child develops fear of the environment and therefore cannot manipulate it.

6. Separation anxiety disorder

- The **essential features** of Separation Anxiety Disorder are excessive worry about separation from attachment figures. It is the commonest disorder in pre-pubertal children.
- Children with Separation Anxiety Disorder show different symptoms to those with other Anxiety Disorders. Fear of getting lost is common in separation Anxiety Disorder and fear of germs, illness and bee stings. Younger children report nightmares about separation.
- There may be a relationship between Separation Anxiety Disorder and later panic disorder or agoraphobia. Separation Anxiety Disorder seems to be a nonspecific precursor to a number of adult conditions including depression and anxiety disorders.

Children with separation anxiety disorder must have symptoms for at least half the time and this may cause interference in function (school work) or social communication. Separation anxiety was associated with symptoms of depression, such as sadness, withdrawal, apathy, or difficulty in concentrating. This explains some of the significant findings on the MASC scales and high score on the CDI in this Kenyan study; such as separation anxiety and depression at the age of 15-16 years for both boys and girls [12].Though the validity (convergent and divergent) of the MASC in the Kenyan text was not tested against any gold standard that can be acclaimed to be culturally appropriate in Kenya for either anxiety or depression, MASC has been acclaimed to concur with DSM-IV diagnosis of anxiety disorders and also Children Depression Inventory to DSM-IV diagnosis of dysthymia, as reviewed in the introduction [12, 15-16]

7. Generalized anxiety disorder (GAD)

- This was found to be characterized by excessive worry about the future and past events and behaviours, concern about competence and self-consciousness.
- Overanxious children reported more fears about social and performance concerns, being criticized, teased or making mistakes. Their worriers were unrealistic about the future.

- This was found in older age than Separation Anxiety Disorder, although there was equal sex ratio.
- 85% of those with Anxiety Disorders had features of GAD.
- The most common symptoms were:
  a. Unrealistic worry over future events.
  b. Preoccupation with appropriateness of individual behaviour in the past.
  c. Over-concern about competence in a variety of areas.
  d. Somatic complaints.
  e. Marked self-consciousness or susceptibility to embarrassment or humiliation.

8. Social phobia

- Persistent fear of social or performance situations when the person is exposed to unfamiliar people or scrutiny
- Social Phobia had all the features of panic disorder and was to be frequently co-morbid with other anxiety disorders

9. Simple phobia and fears [12]

- Simple phobias are specific, isolated, persistent fear of circumscribed stimuli e.g. school
- Associated avoidant behaviour interferes with the normal functioning of the child
- Mild fears are common in children. Girls fear more than boys do
- The commonest fears expressed by Kenyan children in Nairobi (urban setting) are:
  - Being confronted by bad news
  - Not being able to breathe
  - Being mugged
  - Getting burned by fire
  - Falling from a high place
  - Burglar breaking into the house
  - Death
  - Getting poor grades
  - being battered or watching a relative being battered (domestic violence)

10. Post traumatic stress disorder (PTSD)

- Children over the age of 3-4 years did not become amnestic for traumatic events and did not show psychic numbing, nor did they have intrusive flashbacks. However they commonly engaged in posttraumatic play or reenactment behaviour and had nightmares
- They also showed more distortion in their sense of time and a striking foreshortened view of the future.
- Children exposed to a single violent event - proximity to the event correlates directly with the severity of symptoms.
- Those with severe PTSD had more intrusiveness, emotional constriction and avoidance of reminders of the trauma. The difference between severe and mild PTSD has been associated with disturbances in sleep and concentration.

- In children with ongoing trauma (e.g. sexual abuse or domestic violence) there were complications to the diagnosis of PTSD because of complicating factors (poverty, neglect, alcoholism or drug abuse in the parents.) However many develop PTSD symptoms

In the school survey in Kenya, traumatic experience among the students was assessed to determine the levels of post traumatic stress disorder (PTSD [17]. Students indicated that being confronted with bad news was the commonest traumatic event they experienced (66.7%), followed by witnessing a violent crime and domestic violence at 23.2% and 16.5% respectively, where survivors of violence had serious bodily harm and sexual abuse. Accumulatively, PTSD symptoms were very common; avoidance and re-experiencing occurred in 75% of the students and hyper arousal reported in over 50% of the population [17]. The prevalence of PTSD was 50.5% with no gender difference; however students in boarding schools were more affected than day students ($p=0.005$) and there existed a difference in levels of PTSD between the different schools ($p<0.001$). Therefore school students in Kenya commonly experience traumatic events which are unnoticed and they therefore suffer PTSD and go without treatment [17]. Further, traumatic grief in which one looses a loved one through circumstances that are objectively traumatic and in which the trauma symptoms interfere with the normal grieving process causes the person to develop other mental disorders. In Kenya many human atrocities have occurred that have left many people with traumatic grief which affect both children and adults [18-20]. Results from these studies where a traumatised person also lost a loved one indicate the universality of emotions associated with trauma and grief and confirm an association between PTSD and grief.

The diagnosis of PTSD depended upon the child or adolescent first experiencing a traumatic event either by themselves or being witness to a traumatic event against another and there after exhibiting an intense fear, hopelessness or horror reaction in children, disorganized or agitated behaviour as specified in the Diagnostic and Statistical Manual of Mental Disorders [15]. PTSD among children is unique from the adult disorder in that children tend to re-experience the event through play or drawing and exhibit nightmares involving monsters rather than the traumatic event. Adolescent reactions include intense emotional distress and physiological reactions; more similar to adult reactions such as re-experiencing the event through intrusive thoughts, memories and flashbacks. The other symptoms of PTSD in children and youth included feeling disconnected from others or loss of interest in activities, and hyper-arousal (e.g. sleep disturbances and easy to startle) [20]. Assessment in children is particularly challenging because those less than 11 years old may not be able to conceptualize or verbalize their symptoms. Primary caregivers and teachers are often used as informants for the assessment of their child's feeling of hopelessness and loss of interest in previously enjoyed activities. Criteria for diagnosing PTSD among youth in Kenya included the presence of at least one symptom related to re-experiencing, three or more emotional numbing / avoidance symptoms, and two symptoms of hyper-arousal [20]. These symptoms must be present for more than 1 month and cause clinically significant distress or impairment in functioning. The symptoms of PTSD usually arise within three months from the experience of the traumatic event, yet clinical diagnosis of PTSD is made usually only if symptoms persist for six months after the event.

Posttraumatic stress and grief were examined in middle school children 8 to 14 months after experiencing loss in the Embassy bombing, adding to the growing body of literature that documents posttraumatic stress and grief in children who experience traumatic loss within and outside the immediate family [18-19]. With the exception of pre-bomb loss, the hypothesized predictors (physical exposure, acute response, type of bomb-related loss, post-bomb loss, and PTSS-Other) were significantly associated with bomb-related posttraumatic stress. The positive association of bomb-related PTSS with physical exposure and with acute response supports the stressor criterion of the diagnosis of PTSD. The finding that posttraumatic stress related to other negative life events was associated with higher bomb-related posttraumatic stress. Posttraumatic stress associated with prior negative experiences may increase the vulnerability of children exposed to later traumatic events. The results suggested that having additional negative life events and losses subsequent to the bombing may also have increased the children's vulnerability to posttraumatic stress [18-19]. Neither the time elapsed between the bombings nor subsequent loss, or the child relationship to the deceased in losses unrelated to the bombing, were assessed and should be addressed in further research. Thus, both posttraumatic stress and grief should be examined in children following mass casualty terrorist events. Consistent with a view of traumatic grief as a convergence of conditions rather than a distinct entity, posttraumatic stress and grief should be measured instead of unique reactions associated with a specific construct of traumatic grief [18-20].

A high level of PTSD was expected among children and youth at risk in the Kibera slum in Nairobi following disputed presidential election results of 2007 [20]. It was well known that this slum was acutely affected by violence during the month following the broadcast of the 2007 Kenya Presidential election results. The violence experienced in Nairobi following the 2007 elections was unique in that it involved clashes between neighbours of differing tribal heritage, excessive violence against girls/women, forced circumcisions on boys/men, and the concentration of violent activities (including murder) in certain urban slums. In addition to personal physical violence, many safe havens such as churches and schools and common areas such as kiosks and stores were burned or destroyed. The impact of the violence in the affected areas will be long lasting. It is important to note that if the above symptoms are present within two days after the event and less than a month is over, they are referred to as Acute Stress Disorder (ASD) and not PTSD, especially if within this period; those affected also have feelings of detachment of being alienated from themselves or the environment. If symptoms of PTSD occur for the first time six months after the traumatic event, then it is referred to as late onset PTSD. Although the variety of events capable of producing PTSD varies somewhat between children and adults, characteristics of the stresses remain primarily determinants of psychological reactions within and across a variety of settings. For example:

a. Exposure is directly related to the risk for PTSD symptoms
b. PTSD can result from direct, witnessed or verbal exposure to trauma
c. Aspects of the symptom picture may vary with stress-specific factors e.g. chronic physical and sexual abuse in childhood often results in severe psychopathology that bears little resemblance to the classical PTSD picture
d. There are two clinically useful distinctions in types of trauma which represent different literatures and sometimes approaches:
    i. Type I trauma - sudden, unexpected, unpredictable, single-incident stressor that may be multiply repeated
    ii. Type II trauma - chronic, expected, repeated stressor, usually childhood physical or sexual abuse.

There is high prevalence rate of PTSD found among sexually abused children in Kenya, which shows that as many as 100% of children who witness a parental homicide or sexual assault develop PTSD [21]. In this study by Syengo the rates of PTSD were much higher in children and adolescents recruited from at risk groups with the rates varying from 3 to 100%. It further indicated that 90% of sexually abused children, and 77% of children exposed to school shooting develop PTSD [21]. This study indicates that among sexually abused children, the prevalence of psychiatric morbidity measured by the DSM- IV - TR is high 69% [15,21]. The results of this study confirm that sexually abused children develop PTSD therefore putting credence to the fact that there is a relationship between the effects of traumatic events and psychological health. In this study, there were more female respondents than male suggesting that the girl child is more vulnerable to child sexual abuse than boys. This could be postulated to be a masculine / feminine stereotypic view of sexual power relations where the male exercises his dominance through sexual violence and threats on the female. The inferior social status of the female gender could also be a contributing factor that makes them be easily violated. This could also be attributed to some myths in Kenya that believe that having sex with a child or a virgin cures HIV/AIDS. The author postulates that exposure to traumatic events has the same distressing effects to everyone regardless of their age and the development of PTSD will depend on the individuals' personal characteristics among other environmental risk factors. Therefore sexually abused children are at a high risk of developing post traumatic stress disorder with adolescent girls being more at risk than their male counterparts. In this study, even though all the cases were reported in a timely manner and recruited into an intervention plan through the Rescue Centre, lack of support immediately after the incident may have played a major role in contributing to the development of PTSD [21].

11. Obsessive compulsive disorder (OCD)

- Features similar to adult symptoms
- Children had compulsions without associated obsession, this may been due to cognitive immaturity
- There was a strong association with other anxiety disorders, depression, ADHD, Conduct Disorder and substance abuse

In the school survey, obsessive compulsive disorder was also assessed by using the Leyton's symptom check list for OCD in Children and Adolescent, 69.1% of the students had obsessive symptoms while 81.1% had compulsive features, with a total of 40.7% having Obsessive compulsive symptoms [22-23]. This apparently high prevalence of obsessive and compulsive disorders in this age group could be a reflection of the first peak of maximum incidence obsessive and compulsive symptoms at ages 12-14 as reported in western countries which have been shown to be carried on into adulthood and present life OCD [24]. Harm avoidance - perfection (trait of obsessive compulsive) was at 81.5% on the MASC and OCD at 99.3% on the SCARED-R [10-11]. In the case of the SCARED-R some of the symptoms that contributed to high scores on the OCD could be regarded as normal for children who are subjected to a patterned way of doing things in a school environment, more so a boarding school, where obedience to school rules is not only a must but strictly enforced [11].

This trend of high prevalence of obsession-compulsive symptoms and syndromes and OCD was repeated on using a scale only for obsessive compulsive disorder symptoms. There was a prevalence of 40.7% clinical pathology for obsession disorder and 81.1% for compulsive disorder and 69.1% for both obsessive compulsive disorders. Although some but not all of the symptoms could be explained as already discussed, the presence of obsessive-compulsive symptoms cannot be ignored in African children. This is despite the fact that they are rarely recognized in routine clinical practice. This apparently high prevalence's at this age group could be a reflection of the first peak of maximal incidence of OC symptoms at ages 12-14 reported in the Western settings [24]. This is an important finding especially on obsessive-compulsion symptoms and syndromes in clinical situation since these traits are likely to be carried to adulthood where they present as obsessive compulsive disorder (OCD).

12. Anxiety disorders in adults

In communities, cases of PTSD are common. Following any traumatic event, affected individuals on assessment are found to have hyper-arousal symptoms, had startled responses, lacked sleep; re-experiencing the event beyond 6 months trauma [25].In December 2007 following post election violence in Kenya, many female rape survivors in Kibera informal settlement were left with shame and guilt, manifestations of anxiety and depressive symptoms. This has been observed by primary health workers at a health centre (Woodley- City Council Clinic) where about 200 female survivors of rape following 2007 post election sought psychological support. Observation by health workers and a study finding at the clinic by Nyaga indicate that although medical treatment was given to the rape survivors, depressive symptoms, PTSD and other anxiety symptoms were not given adequate psychological support [26]. Nyaga showed high prevalence of PTSD among the female rape survivors to be as high as above 80%.

According to human rights group, at least 1000 women across Kenya were raped during chaos that followed the country's December, 2007 elections. The UNHCR reported that the highest incidents of rapes in Kenya were witnessed in 2007 post election violence in most parts of the country [27]. An estimated 1200 victims of sexual assault who included women, men as well as girls and boys were reported [27]. According to the police spokesman 200 rape cases were reported to police but only 15 cases made it to court with only 12 convictions. The number of rape cases reported in Nairobi women's gender recovery centre was 341 which was a quarter of the one thousand women rapes reported in the country [27].

Anxiety disorders seen in general health facilities are more frequently associated with chronic medical conditions [28]. Using the Leeds Scale for the Self-Assessment for Anxiety and Depression (LSAD) in this study, 20 to 30% of patients who had cancer, HIV, diabetes and cardiovascular disease had features of general anxiety disorder. The high levels of anxiety disorders in this population were related to the chronicity of medical conditions. Among adults admitted in psychiatric hospital in Kenya, the leading anxiety disorder was shown to be general anxiety disorder, followed by panic attack with agoraphobia, obsessive compulsive disorder then social phobia [28]. The level of PTSD among motor vehicle accident survivors attending the orthopaedic and trauma clinic at Kenyatta National Hospital has been shown to be 13.3%. This is familiar to the 7%-39% PTSD rate found in the developed world [29]. Ongecha in this study identified some risk factors associated with PTSD such as younger age (20 to 39 years), being female, previously married for women and currently married for men, of post-primary education, being a driver, being involved in first accident, and perceived threat of a life at a time of accident especially the thought of being maimed [29]. Being previously married (widowed/divorced) is a major life event that can lead to PTSD, predisposing one to develop PTSD with a subsequent trauma. Being a driver seems to predispose one to PTSD since they are mainly in full view and tend to witness the whole or better part of the accident. The result in this study showed that there was more (26.6%) distress from avoidant symptoms compared to the hyper-arousal (15.7%) or re-experiencing (14.7%) symptoms. Thus avoidance symptoms were more prominent in this study group and this subscale may be a better measure for distress in this population [29]. In this study, the co-morbidity rate was found to be 28.6%. PTSD was found to be associated with the following psychiatric disorders; general anxiety disorder (11.4%), major depressive disorder (8.6%), bipolar I disorder - single manic phase (2.9%), bipolar I disorder mixed type (2.9%) and schizophrenia (2.9%). Lifetime substance use was found to be 50.8%, with increased amounts of nicotine and sedatives among respondents. Hence with PTSD prevalence rate of 13.3% and co morbidity rate of 28.6% there is need to institute a multidisciplinary approach in the care of Motor Vehicle Accident survivors from the emergency health facility setting [29].

In a study among inpatients at Mathari psychiatric Hospital[1], 63.9% of patients had experienced a traumatic event with 48% presenting with avoidance symptoms while 33.5% with hyper arousal features [30]. In the same setting 12.2% of the inpatients met the criteria for obsessive compulsive disorder [31]. Among these patients at Mathari Hospital, a wide variety of anxiety disorders were reported. The leading disorder was Generalised anxiety disorder (prevalence of 20.8%); the fourth common disorder after schizophrenia, bipolar mood disorder and alcohol abuse. The other anxiety disorders found in this population included panic attack, panic attack with agoraphobia, obsessive compulsive disorder and social phobia [31]. The prevalence rate of obsessive compulsive symptoms among the patients at the hospital reflects the ages of the respondents at the time of the interview and not the duration of the age at onset [32]. However the age structure of the respondents in the study reflected having anxiety disorders generally among the youth in Kenya, which was apparent that the onset starts early in life. The prevalence rates of obsessive and compulsive symptoms peaked at the 21- to 30-year age band. The finding that more than half (59.5%) of the respondents were single again reflects the youthful study population. In addition, the education levels of the respondents were also a true reflection of the literacy rates amongst the youthful population in Kenya, given that over 87% were literate [32].

One third of the patients recruited in the study at the Hospital experienced traumatic events [30-31]. The most common of these were violent events of different types, directed to the person or to another. Those who had been exposed to traumatic events experienced post-traumatic stress disorder (PTSD) symptoms such as avoidance (48%) and hyper arousal (33.5%). In spite of the above, only 7.4% of the patients scored for DSM-IV diagnoses of PTSD in past admissions, while only 4% reported PTSD at the time of the interview. These findings among African sample support the universality of emotions associated with trauma and grief and confirm an association between posttraumatic stress and grief, even with losses outside the immediate family. Future studies should further explore the construct of traumatic grief , delineate more carefully the two processes of trauma and loss, and examine developmental issues associated with traumatic loss.

Regrettably, various anxiety and obsessive compulsive symptoms in the patients in the study at Mathari Hospital had not been recognized in this psychiatric clinical setting [30-32].

---

[1] Referral National Psychiatric Hospital in Kenya

This is explained by a clinical preoccupation with the disturbed behaviour that often necessitates admission into the Psychiatric Hospital, and reveals the fact that an investigation into anxiety and OCD would elicit their prevalence. Co-morbidity with schizophrenia, bipolar mood disorders, substance-induced disorders, psychosis, schizoaffective disorders and depression as reported in this study was high [30-31]. This co-morbidity was also found between all the DSM-IV core syndromes, more than half of which were significantly associated with OC symptoms [15].

The recognition of this co-morbidity of anxiety and other severe psychiatric disorders is important since it calls for the appropriate management of each of the co-morbid disorders [30-32]. The authors have no explanation for why anxiety and OCD DSM-IV diagnosis are missed out, although it is possible that patients in the Kenyan socio-cultural context may have difficulties in differentiating between symptoms with a locus inside or outside their minds. Further research to clarify this is needed. It should be noted that the interviewers asked questions strictly on the DSM-IV definitions of the symptoms. Of particular significance is the association between Obsessive and Compulsive symptoms and passivity symptoms of schizophrenia. Whereas DSM-IV distinguishes between the clinical symptoms of OCD and passivity symptoms of schizophrenia, in clinical practice, the latter may camouflage the former. The clinical implication is that there is a need to adopt routine clinical tools that systematically enquire for all symptoms, including Obsessive and Compulsive symptoms. Missing them and therefore not treating them affects the overall prognosis of the patient.

13. Conclusion

Addressing anxiety disorders matters whether in hospital or community setting. Because anxiety disorders contribute to severe and significant morbidity, productivity and quality of life. Moreover, anxiety disorders usually co-exist with other chronic mental and physical conditions and may adversely influence the outcomes of these chronic conditions. These findings should stimulate clinical and epidemiological research on anxiety and depression in Africa with a view to improve clinical practice and formulating policy in mental health. Studying psychometric properties of instruments that assess anxiety is urgently required in African settings. Besides there is need for more research in epidemiology on mental health with an aim of developing several policies so that: inputs on mental health for all medical and paramedical personnel is ensured; there is a proactive identification of anxiety disorders in docile population or anxiety disorders co-existing with severe mental and physical disorders is proactively identified; and in place there is appropriate policy framework for promotion, prevention and clinical interventions within the national health strategic plans. In particular a policy in schools which should be in place to identify and provide intervention for children with mental problems. This role can best played by school resident counselors. This is more so since anxiety patterns clearly indicate that these problems exist right at the earlier ages of secondary school entry and by retrospective projection in primary school before joining secondary schools. The high prevalence of anxiety disorders continue and change in pattern across the whole spectrum of secondary school education into adulthood and co-exist with physical and other mental disorders. Of particular interest for a proactive enquiry is depression, alcohol abuse and suicide related symptoms.

In view of the large numbers of population with anxiety disorders, there is need to have in place simple self administrated screening tests to facilitate the identification of persons who need further assessment. This can be an important screening entry point among patients attending general and psychiatric health facilities where there is high prevalence of psychiatric morbidity which largely go undiagnosed and therefore, unmanaged in Kenya. The more specialized medical facilities get in the various general and surgical disciplines, the less recognized mental disorders become. Chronic conditions physical and mental conditions have been shown to have highest co-morbidity with mental disorders, in particular anxiety and depressive disorders. These findings call for continuing education on mental health at all levels of psychiatry, general and surgical facilities, and also for routine screening for mental disorders.

14. Reference

[1] Murray CJL, Lopez AD (eds). 1996. The global burden of disease: a comprehensive assessment of mortality and disability from diseases, injuries and risk factors in 1990 and projected to 2020. Global Burden of Disease and Injury Series. Cambridge, MA: Harvard School of Public Health on behalf of the World Health Organization and the World Bank.

[2] Lopez, D. A., Mathers, D. C., Ezzati, M., Jamison, T. D., & Murray, J. L. C. (2006). *Global Burden of Disease and Risk Factors*. New York: Oxford University Press and The World Bank.

[3] WHO (2004). *Prevention of mental disorders: effective interventions and policy options.* Geneva: WHO.

[4] Lund, C., Breen, A., Flisher, A. J., Swartz, L., Joska, J., Corrigall, J. et al. (2007). Mental health and poverty: a systematic review of the research in low and middle income countries. *The Journal of Mental Health Policy and Economics, 10, Supplement 1*,S26-S27

[5] Ndetei DM, Pizzo M, Khasakhala LI, Maru HM, Mutiso VN, Ongecha FA, Omar A, Kokonya DA. Perceived economic and behavioural effects of the mentally ill on their relatives in Kenya: a case study of the Mathari Hospital. Volume 12, Issue 4, Afr J Psychiatry 2009;12:293-299

[6] Ndetei DM, Ongecha FA, Khasakhala L, Mutiso V, Kokonya DA. The Prevalence of Mental Disorders and the Attitude in General Medical Facilities in Kenya - A WHO Monograph; 2006.

[7] Ssebunnya J, Kigozi F, Lund C, Kizza D, Okello E. Stakeholder perceptions of mental health stigma and poverty in Uganda. *BMC International Health and Human Rights.* 2009;9:5. [PMC free article] [PubMed]

[8] Adewuya AO, Makanjuola RO. Social distance towards people with mental illness in southwestern Nigeria. *Australian & New Zealand Journal of Psychiatry.* 2008;42(5):389–395. [PubMed]

[9] Bernstein, G.A., Borchardt, C.M., & Perwien, A.R. (1996). Anxiety disorders in Children and adolescents. A review of the past 10 years. Journal of the American Academy of Child and Adolescent Psychiatry, 35, 1110-1119.

[10] Ndetei DM, Seedat S, Syanda J, Ongecha-Owuor FA, Kokonya DA, Khasakhala LI, Mutiso VN. Psychometric properties of the Multidimensional Anxiety Scale for Children (MASC) amongst Nairobi public secondary school children, Kenya. *Journal of Child & Adolescent Mental Health* 2008, 20 (2) : 101–109

[11] Ndetei DM, Ongecha FA, Khasakhala L, Syanda J, Mutiso V, Othieno CJ, Odhiambo G, Kokonya DA. Bullying in public secondary schools in Nairobi, Kenya. J Child Adol Mental Health 2007; 19 (1), 45-55.

[12] Ndetei DM, Khasakhala L, Nyabola L, Ongecha-Owuor F, Seedat S, Mutiso V, Kokonya D, Odhiambo G. The prevalence of anxiety and depression symptoms and syndromes in Kenyan adolescents. *Journal of Child and Adolescent Mental Health* 2008; 20 (1): 33-51

[13] The Multidimentional Scale for Children (MASC). Factor structure, reliability, and validity. Journal of the American Academy of Child and Adolescent Psychiatry, 36, 554-565.

[14] Muris, P., Dreessen, L., Bogels, S., Weckx, M., and Van Melick M. (2004). A questionnaire for screening a board range of DSM-IV defined anxiety disorder symptoms in clinically referred children and adolescents. Journal of Child Psychology and Psychiatry 45: 4 pp. 813-820.

[15] American Psychiatric Association (1994), Diagnostic and Statistical Manual of Mental Disorders, 4th edition (DSM-IV). Washington, DC: American Psychiatric Association. March, J.S., Parker, JDA., Sullivan, K., Stallings, P. & Cornors, CK. (1997).

[16] Kovacs M, Gatsonis C, Paulauskas S, Richards C (1989), Depressive disorders in childhood: A longitudinal study of comorbidity with and risk for anxiety disorders. Arch Gen Psychiatry 46:776–782[Abstract/Free Full Text]

[17] Ndetei DM, Ongecha FA, Khasakhala L, Mutiso V, Othieno CJ, Syanda J, Odhiambo G, Kokonya DA. Traumatic Experiences of Kenyan Secondary School Students. J Child Adol Mental Health 2007; 19 (12): 147-55.

[18] Ndetei DM, Omar A, Mutiso VN, Ongecha FA, Kokonya DA. Profiles of referrals to a psychiatric service: a descriptive study of survivors of the Nairobi US Embassy terrorist bomb blast. Volume 12, Issue 4, Afr J Psychiatry 2009;12:280-283

[19] Pfefferbaum B, North CS, Doughty DE, Pfefferbaum RL, Dumont CE, Pynoos RS, Gurwitch OH, Ndetei DM. Trauma, Grief And Depression In Nairobi Children After The 1998 Bombing Of The American Embassy. Death Studies 2006, 30: 561–77

[20] Harder VS., Mutiso V., Khasakhala L., Burker H., Ivanova MY., Ndetei DM. Behavioral and Emotional Problems among Kenyan Youth from an Urban Slum. *Journal of Child Psychology and Psychiatry*

[21] Syengo-Mutisya CM, Kathuku DM, Ndetei DM. Psychiatric morbidity among sexually abused children and adolescents. *East Africa Medical Journal* 2008, 85 (2): 85-91

[22] Bamber D., Tamplin A., Park R.J., Kyte Z., and Goodyer, I. M. (2002). Development of a Short Leyton Obsessional Inventory for Children and Adolescents. Journal of Amrican Child and Adolescent Psychiatry, 41,10, pp. 1246-1252

[23] Ongecha FA, Khasakhala LI, Maru H, Mutiso V, Kokonya DA. Obsessive-Compulsive (OC) Symptoms in Kenyan high school students. *African Journal of Psychiatry* 2008, 11: 182-186

[24] Flament MF, Cohen D (2000), Child and adolescent obsessive-compulsive disorder: a review. In:Obsessive-Compulsive Disorder, Maj M, Sartorius, Okasha A, Zohar J, eds. Chichester, England: Wiley, pp 145-183

[25] Rasmussen SA, Tsuang MT (1986). Clinical characteristics and family history in DSM-III obsessive-compulsive disorders. American Journal of psychiatry, 143:317-322.

[26] Nyaga, I [2009]. Prevalence of PTSD, Depression, and other General Anxiety Symptoms among Female Survivors of Rape Following Post Election Violence 2007 Nairobi- Kenya. Thesis in Partial Fulfilment of the Requirement for Award of Master of Clinical Psychology of University of Nairobi

[27] UNHCR Report 2008. December 2007 Post Election Violence in Kenya

[28] Ndetei DM, Khasakhala L, Kuria M, Mutiso V, Ongecha FA, Kokonya D, The Prevalence of Mental Disorders in Adults in Different Level General Medical Facilities in Kenya: A Cross-Sectional Study. *Annals of General Psychiatry* 2009, 8:1. Available online at http://www.annals-general-psychiatry.com/content/8/1/1

[29] Ongecha-Owuor FA, Kathuku DM, Othieno CJ, Ndetei DM. Post traumatic stress disorder among motor vehicle accident survivors attending the orthopaedic and trauma clinic at Kenyatta National Hospital, Nairobi. East Afr Med J 2004; 81 (7):362-6. PMID: 15490709 [PubMed - indexed for MEDLINE]

[30] Ndetei DM, Khasakhala LI, Ongecha FA, Mutiso V, Kokonya DA. Outcome of a working diagnosis of "psychosis" in relation to DSM-IV diagnostic criteria in a Kenyan in-patient cohort at Mathari hospital, Nairobi. African Health Sciences 2007; 7 (3): 197-201

[31] Ndetei DM, Khasakhala LI, Maru H, Pizzo M, Mutiso V, Ongecha-Owuor FA, Kokonya DA. Clinical Epidemiology in Patients Admitted at Mathari Psychiatric Hospital, Nairobi, Kenya. *Social Psychiatry & Psychiatric Epidemiology 2008;* 43(9):736-742

[32] Ndetei DM, Ongecha FA, Khasakhala LI, Maru H, Mutiso V, Kokonya DA. Obsessive-Compulsive (OC) Symptoms in Psychiatric In-patients at Mathari Hospital, Kenya. *African Journal of Psychiatry* 2008, 11: 182-186

[33] Ndetei DM, Khasakhala L, Nyabola L, Ongecha-Owuor F, Seedat S, Mutiso V, Kokonya D, Odhiambo G. The prevalence of anxiety and depression symptoms and syndromes in Kenyan adolescents. *Journal of Child and Adolescent Mental Health* 2008; 20 (1): 33-51

[34] Ndetei DM, Ongecha FA, Khasakhala LI, Maru H, Mutiso V, Kokonya DA. Obsessive-Compulsive (OC) Symptoms in Psychiatric In-patients at Mathari Hospital, Kenya. *African Journal of Psychiatry* 2008, 11: 182-186

[35] Pfefferbaum B, North CS, Doughty DE, Pfefferbaum RL, Dumont CE, Pynoos RS, Gurwitch OH, Ndetei DM. Trauma, Grief And Depression In Nairobi Children After The 1998 Bombing Of The American Embassy. Death Studies 2006, 30: 561–77

[36] Ndetei DM, Omar A, Gakinya BG, Ongecha FA, Kokonya DA, Mutiso V, Mwangi J. Psychological reactions to and biopsychosocial impacts of a fire disaster: A naturalistic study of the student survivors and the staff at a Kenyan rural school. Journal of Traumatic Stress

[37] Ndetei DM, Khasakhala L, Kuria M, Mutiso V, Ongecha FA, Kokonya D, The Prevalence of Mental Disorders in Adults in Different Level General Medical Facilities in Kenya: A Cross-Sectional Study. *Annals of General Psychiatry* 2009, 8:1. Available online at http://www.annals-general-psychiatry.com/content/8/1/1

[38] Ndetei DM, Seedat S, Syanda J, Ongecha-Owuor FA, Kokonya DA, Khasakhala LI, Mutiso VN. Psychometric properties of the Multidimensional Anxiety Scale for Children (MASC) amongst Nairobi public secondary school children, Kenya. *Journal of Child & Adolescent Mental Health* 2008, 20 (2) : 101–109

[39] Ndetei DM, Ongecha FA, Khasakhala L, Mutiso V, Othieno CJ, Syanda J, Odhiambo G, Kokonya DA. Traumatic Experiences of Kenyan Secondary School Students. J Child Adol Mental Health 2007; 19 (12): 147-55

3

Intergeneration Familial Risk and Psychosocial Correlates for Anxiety Syndromes in Children and Adolescents in a Developing Country

Jorge Javier Caraveo-Anduaga
Instituto Nacional de Psiquiatría "Ramón de la Fuente Muñiz"
México

1. Introduction

In the last decade of the 20th century a growing body of data on psychiatric disorders, from both clinical an epidemiological settings, signalled toward the childhood onset of adult psychiatric disorders (Rapoport, 2000). Epidemiological studies included in the International Consortium of Psychiatric Epidemiology (ICPE) showed that anxiety disorders tend to be chronic and relatively stable as compared to affective and substance-use disorders (Kessler et al., 2003). Furthermore, some anxiety disorders such as specific phobias and separation anxiety disorder have an early lifetime-onset. Also, studies on adult populations have shown that at least one third of all cases are comorbid and that psychiatric comorbidity is proportionally higher among persons with anxiety disorders (Caraveo et al., 1999). The study of comorbidity between different types of disorders: anxiety, affective and substance-use showed that the onset of the former usually precedes use, abuse and dependence on alcohol and other substances (Merikangas et al., 1998). Also, the comorbidity of depressive episodes with all anxiety disorders was striking, showing that all primary anxiety disorders that were not in remission were powerful predictors of the emergence of a depressive episode. A question raised by these results was whether anxiety disorders are a causal factor for depressive episodes or simply markers of other causes (Andrade et al., 2003).

From a developmental perspective the interest in studying general psychopathology as well as specific psychiatric disorders, the sequence in which they develop, the form they take in childhood and adolescence, and how they evolve into adulthood, has important public health and preventive implications (Weissman et al., 2000; Kessler et al., 2003).

As a group, anxiety disorders are frequent and persistent in childhood and adolescence. A fair estimate of current prevalence for any anxiety disorder accompanied by impairment is between 5 and 10% (Klein & Pine, 2002) Separation anxiety disorder (SA), specific phobias SP) and generalized anxiety disorder (GA) (previously defined as overanxious disorder in DSM-III) are the most common. Anxiety disorders are especially susceptible to impairment thresholds; however, the importance of impairment is uncertain in early diagnoses. Moreover, anxiety symptoms that are not impairing in early childhood may become so as development and life-experiences continues (Malcarne et al., 2010).

Findings from family studies, either using a "top-down" design where the children of parents with anxiety disorders are evaluated or a "bottom-up" design which ascertain the parents of children with anxiety disorders, have clearly establish the cross-generation transmission of anxiety from parents to children (Klein & Pine, 2002). Kendler et al. (1995) attempted to disentangle genetic and environmental factors underlying several psychiatric adult disorders including phobias, GAD, panic disorder (PD), and major depression (MDD). They concluded from their study that:

1. The risk conferred by genes and environment for each disorder is distinctive.
2. Genetic influence on the disorders is not particularly highly specific or highly nonspecific.
3. Anxiety disorders are heterogeneous.
4. Regarding specific relationships, they find evidence for shared genetic risk factors for MDD and GAD, and for separate shared genetic risk factors for panic disorder and phobias.

Besides genetic risk factors, behavioural inhibition (a consistent tendency of children to display fear and withdrawal in unfamiliar situations) also deserves attention (Kagan et al., 1984). Results from different studies suggest that an inhibited temperament in early childhood is associated with the later development of anxiety disorders (Biederman et al., 2001; Schwartz, Snidman, & Kagan, 1999) as well as depression (Caspi et al., 1996; Hayward et al., 1998).

Also, as findings also reveal the importance of individual-specific environmental experiences on the risk of internalizing disorders, various aspects of parents-child interactions such as modelling of avoidant behaviour through parental overprotectiveness, harsh rearing practices and failure to soothe children, have been suggested as contributing to child anxiety disorders although these effects, by definition, cannot explain familial clustering (Kovacs M. & Devlin B, 1998).

All common psychiatric disorders where a genetic basis is suspected, corresponds to the so called "complex disorders". These are the result of the interaction between genetic liability and environmental factors. By this means, epidemiologist and genetic interests convey and there is a need for a common methodology. Intergenerational studies, have become of special interest and several prospective studies are underway (see Journal of Abnormal Child Psychology vol. 31 (2), 2003) Interest in this kind of studies is that heritable risk and biological markers (e.g., temperamental variables, elevated cortisol levels) of emotional disorder that are identifiable in early childhood may be passed across consecutive generations (e.g., Ashman el al., 2002; Goldsmith, Buss, & Lemery, 1997). In a like manner, psychosocial characteristics that increase the risk of emotional disturbances may be passed from parent to child via processes such as modelling and direct communications (Pettit et al., 2008).

To the extent that these genetic, biological, and psychosocial characteristics— and their attendant risk—are transmitted from one generation to the next, an intergenerational mediation model (i.e., G1 G2 G3) may best characterize the development of psychopathology in general as well as for emotional disorders.

As most of the studies published are based on Caucasian populations and in developed countries, there is the need for data from studies in other countries with different ethnicity, cultural and socio-economic conditions.

For this chapter, we will present results from an epidemiological study carried out in Mexico City where familial risk for developing psychopathology across three generations (Caraveo, et al., 2005) was included as a complementary objective.

2. The familial risk for developing anxiety disorders across three generations in Mexico City: A general population study

2.1 Background

In 1988, as part of the first National Addictions Survey, the National Mental Health Survey was applied in a sub-sample of 2025 adults aged between 18 and 65. This study was the first of its kind to attempt to estimate the prevalence of specific psychiatric disorders in Mexico (Caraveo et al., 1996). In that same study, it was decided to investigate the prevalence of probable psychiatric disorders in childhood using an instrument employed by the WHO, the Report Questionnaire for Children (Giel et al., 1981). The results indicated that 15.6% of the child population between 3 and 12 years old had mental health problems, half of which (7%) could be considered severe cases (Caraveo et al., 1993). Researchers also studied the association between the presence of psychopathology in children and the presence of depression and alcohol consumption in parents, highlighting the need to study and deal jointly with these problems in the population (Caraveo et al., 1994; 1995).

In 1994, with the experience and knowledge acquired and bearing in mind the experience from the National Comorbidity Survey in the United States (Kessler et al., 1994), a broadly comprehensive epidemiological project was submitted and approved to study the prevalence of specific psychiatric disorders among the general adult population in Mexico City (Caraveo et al., 1998). A version of CIDI 1.1 modified by the University of California in Fresno (CIDI-Fresno) (Vega et al., 1998) was used as the basic epidemiological clinical instrument. The translation, carried out by the Mexican Institute of Psychiatry, preserved the original official translation of CIDI 1.1., as well as the contents of all the necessary items for carrying out a diagnosis according to the International Classification of Diseases ICD-10 (WHO, 1993).

The methodological rigor with which this research project was planned and developed enabled the data obtained to be incorporated into the first generation of studies of the International Consortium in Psychiatric Epidemiology (ICPE) (Aguilar-Gaxiola, et al., 2000) which facilitated international comparison and yielded interesting, important results for the development of the discipline.

In Mexico, there are no epidemiological familial studies on the most common psychiatric disorders. The survey started the collection of data seven months after a very severe financial crisis in the country, thus, impact of ongoing psychosocial adjustments in the population are of special interest. A distinctive and original characteristic of the present study is that most epidemiological research about psychiatric disorders and mental health problems have not investigated the presence of adult psychopathology and mental health problems in their parents as well as in their children (Caraveo et al., 2005). Moreover, to our knowledge, when we started the research project there was not a family study that had examined familial risk across three generations from a large epidemiological sample. However, in the last decade several intergenerational studies have been published (Brook et al. 2003; Thornberry et al. 2003; Hammen et al., 2004; Weissman et al., 2005;Pettit et al., 2008; Warner et al., 2008) but none have focused primarily on anxiety disorders as an outcome in the offspring.

2.2 Objective

Our goal was to investigate the familial risk for the development of psychopathology, including anxiety syndromes, across three generations.

2.3 Method

For the present study, the family-history method was used. The study was designed as a household survey on a representative sample of the adult population aged 18 - 65 years in Mexico City (Caraveo et al., 1999). Briefly, a standardized assessment for adults' lifetime prevalence of psychiatric disorders was obtained via an amended version of the Composite International Diagnostic Interview, CIDI. 1.1. The diagnostic categories included were:

Anxiety disorders: Agoraphobia, social phobia, specific phobias, generalized anxiety, panic and obsessive-compulsive disorder.

Affective disorders: Depressive episodes, dysthymia, hypomania and mania.

Disorders due to the use of psychotropic substances: distinguishing between abuse and alcohol dependence and other substances that include: sedatives, tranquilizers, stimulants, analgesics, inhalants, marijuana, cocaine, hallucinogens and heroin.

Response rate was 60.4%. The total sample size was 1932 adult subjects (probands, Generation 2). In addition to the CIDI, all respondents provided information on the psychiatric history of their parents (Generation 1) about anxiety, affective and substance-use disorders following the Family-history research criteria (Andreasen et al., 1977; 1986; Kendler et al., 1997). Also, 925 respondents with children aged 4 - 16 years living at the same household were interviewed about them (1686 children and adolescents, Generation 3) using a standardized screening questionnaire for assessing psychopathology, the CBTD.

The Brief Screening and Diagnostic Questionnaire (CBTD for its initials in Spanish) is a 27-item questionnaire answered by the parents of the child exploring symptoms frequently reported as motives for seeking attention at the outpatient mental health services. Presence of the symptom requires that each item has to be reported as "frequently" presented. The internal consistency of the questionnaire showed a Cronbach's alpha of 0.81, range: 0.76 to 0.85 (Caraveo, 2006). Diagnostic algorithms in order to define probable DSM-IV disorders in children were created based on data from this epidemiological study (Caraveo, 2007).

For comparisons, adult probands' lifetime diagnoses (ICD-10) as well as psychiatric history of their parents were grouped as follows: 1. Only anxiety disorders; 2. Only affective disorders; 3. Only substance-use disorders; 4. Comorbid anxiety-affective disorders; 5. Comorbid anxiety-affective-substance use disorders; 6. No lifetime psychiatric diagnoses.

For children, caseness was defined first, based on the questionnaire score for those at the 9th decil and beyond ($\geq$ 5 symptoms) and second, two screening anxiety syndromes were identified: generalized anxiety and anxiety with inhibition (Caraveo, 2006; 2007).

The generalized anxiety screening syndrome was defined as follows: Key symptom: a positive response to the question: Does the child gets scared or nervous for no good reason?, and at least two of the following: can´t seat still, irritable, sleep problems, and frequent nightmares.

The anxiety with inhibition screening syndrome was defined as follows: Key symptom: a positive response to the question: Is the child excessively dependent or attached to adults?; and at least two positive answers on the following: aloof, frequent headaches, afraid of school, physical complains without a medical problem, sleep problems, low weight, overweight, do not work at school, and backward compared to other children.

Concurrent validity with DSM-IV anxiety diagnoses using the E-MiniKid standardized interview (Sheehan et al., 2000) showed Kappa agreement to be 0.53 and 0.68 respectively, and using Yule´s Y coefficient results were 0.65 and 0.92 respectively. Receiver Operating Characteristic Curves (ROC) analyses showed Area under the Curve (AUC) to be 0.82 and 0.78 respectively (Caraveo et al., 2011 accepted).

To estimate the familial morbid risk for children and adolescents with anxiety syndromes, interaction of familial psychopathology across generations was defined as follows:
Psychiatric history only in grandparents (G1); psychiatric history only in proband (mother or father, G2); psychiatric history on both previous generations (G1 & G2). The research general schema for this chapter is as follows:

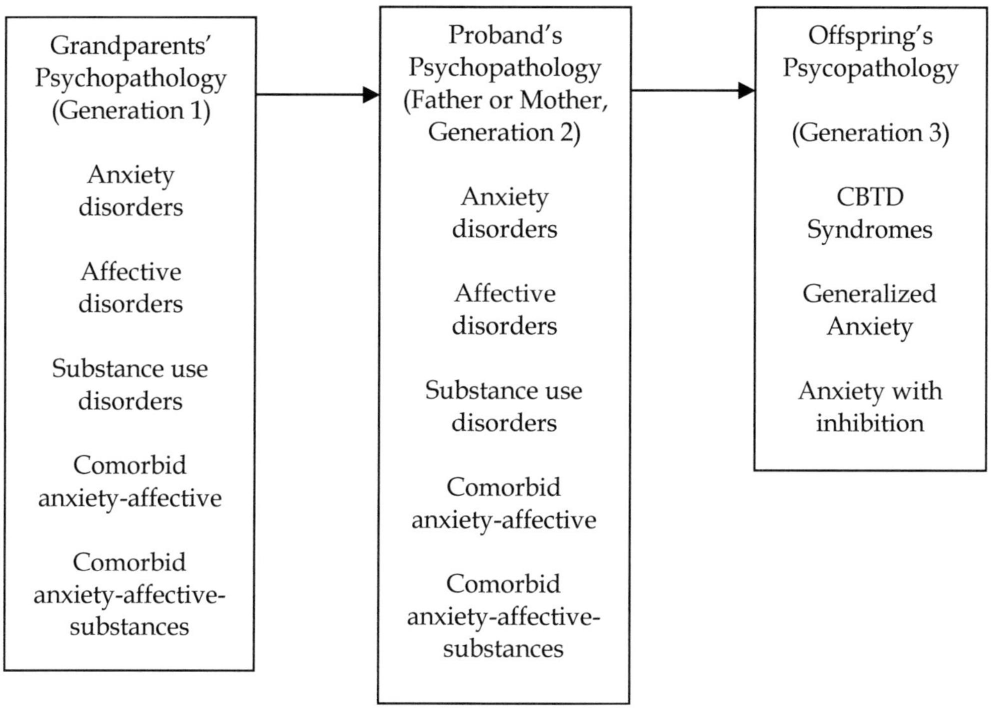

Analyses were done using the Stata 8.0 program. Variance and confidence interval estimation accounted for the complex stratified sampling of the survey, as well as for the clustering by family units that has been extensively described elsewhere (Caraveo et al., 1998, 2002; Vega et al., 2002).
Morbid risk in terms of the odds ratio was calculated using generalized estimating equations (GEE) population-averaged models with an exchangeable structure. GEE is an iterative procedure, using quasi-likelihood to estimate the regression coefficients; the relationships between the variables of the model at different time-points are analysed simultaneously. Because the repeated observations within one subject are not independent of each other, a correction must be made for these within-subject correlations choosing a correlation structure. In an exchangeable structure, as used in this study, the correlations between subsequent measurements are assumed to be the same, irrespective of the length of the time interval (Twisk, 2003).
Analyses were carried out controlling for the effect of different potential confounding variables. The first group included: grandparents' gender, proband's gender and age, children's gender and age, proband's labour status, and household income. The second group included the following proband's psycho-social variables: relationship with spouse, stress at work, couple's total work hours per week, worries between home and work, perception of family support (not living at the same household), perception of community

support, own health's perception, and social isolation. On these, the survey included specific sections with questions and scales that were used by Dr. Kessler at the NCS and described elsewhere (Caraveo et al., 1998). Scores were converted into dummy variables using quartiles.

As a multi-nominal sampling was used, and the odds ratios are always an over-estimation of the real population's relative risk, GEE population-averaged analysis with Poisson regression was performed based on the results of the most complete previous models (McNutt et al., 2003). Also, as the data are representative of the population and a wide comprehensive approach of psycho-social variables was included, the attributable risk in the population was also obtained from the complete models with GEE population-averaged logistic analysis.

2.4 Results

Characteristics of the sample are shown in Table 1. Proband's mean age was 34.8 years old, 55% had one offspring, 30.5% had two, 11.3% had three, 3.2%had up to six offspring. Children mean age was 9.7 years old; distribution by age groups was as follows: 4–5 years old 16.3%, 6-8 years old 25.5%, 9-12 years old 30.9%, and 13-16 years old 27.4%. The estimated household income was divided into 5 levels (Caraveo et. al, 1998): 26.04 % were at the bottom, 27.35%, 26.09%, 16.94% in subsequent levels, and only 3.6% at the top.

	Males	**Females**	**Total**	**Cases**	**Non cases**
Probands (Gen 2)	871	1061	1932	552	1380
Grandparents (Gen 1)	1339	1404	2743	647	2096
Probands (Gen 2) with offspring aged 4 to 16 years	381	544	925	292	633
Children & adolescents (Gen 3)	865	821	1686	269	1416

Table 1. Sample Characteristics

Prevalence of psychiatric disorders by groups in G1 and G2 are shown in Table 2

Psychiatric Antecedents	Grandparents % (95% CI)	Parents % (95% CI)
Anxiety only	1.0 (0.2, 1.9)	6.2 (4.1, 5.8)
Depression only	7.4 (4.9, 9.9)	5.4 (3.6, 7.2)
Substances only	6.4 (4.2, 8.7)	0.6 (0.0, 1.3)
Anxiety & depression	10.6 (8.4, 12.9)	3.8 (1.8, 5.8)
Anxiety, depression & substances	11.9 (9.2, 14.7)	3.5 (2.2, 4.9)

Table 2. Prevalence of psychiatric disorders on G1 and G2

Prevalence of the screening anxiety syndromes in children an adolescent is 4.1% (CI: 2.7, 5.6) and 4.0% (CI: 2.7, 5.3) for generalized anxiety and anxiety with inhibition, respectively. Both syndromes are more prevalent in boys, 5.4% and 5.0%, than in girls, 2.9% and 3.1%, respectively.

2.4.1 Does familial psychopathology, that is, any type of disorder in the two previous generations is associated with the report of screening anxiety syndromes in the offspring?
Results on Table 3 show that psychopathology on G1 is not significantly associated with the report of any of the two screening anxiety syndromes in G3. However, the probability for developing the generalized anxiety syndrome in the offspring is significantly associated, in terms of the odds ratio, 6-fold increase, when there is history of psychiatric disorders in the parent, Gen-2, and considerably increases to 24-fold increase when there are also psychiatric antecedents in grandparents (G2 & G3). The screening syndrome anxiety with inhibition in the offspring is marginally associated with familial psychopathology in G1 & G2.

Any Psychiatric Antecedents	Generalized anxiety OR (95% CI)	P	Anxiety with inhibition OR (95% CI)	P
G 1	2.5 (0.4, 15.0)	.325	1.1 (0.3, 3.8)	.926
G 2	6.0 (1.0, 36.1)	.049	---	
G 1 & G 2	24.3 (5.4, 109.8)	.000	3.2 (0.98,10.3)	.055

No. obs.: 739; No. gps.:419; Wald chi2=26.15;gl=3; p= 0.000; Wald chi2=5485;gl=3; p= 0.000

Table 3. Familial psychiatric antecedents and anxiety syndromes in the offspring, crude

2.4.2 Do gender, age, household income and work status explain, in whole or in part, the association between anxiety syndromes in the offspring and familial psychopathology?
Results on Table 4 show that for generalized anxiety the strength of the association increases notably when there is psychopathology interaction between G1 and G2. The contribution of G1 seems to arise from grandmother's psychopathology, as when controlling for sex, grandfather's psychopathology is inversely associated. The rest of the variables, not included on the Tables, did not show a statistical significant association.
For the anxiety with inhibition screening syndrome, interestingly, mother's psychopathology emerged showing a 7-fold increase, which is similar in magnitude to the G2 association with the generalized anxiety syndrome. Also, psychopathology interaction between G1 and G2 became significantly associated on the anxiety with inhibition syndrome, as well as low household income.

Any Psychiatric Antecedents	Generalized anxiety OR (95% CI)	P	Anxiety with inhibition OR (95% CI)	P
G 1	4.4 (0.6, 29.0)	.128	1.4 (0.3, 6.0)	.638
G 2	6.8 (1.1, 40.3)	.034	---	
G 1 & G 2	41.9 (8.4, 208.3)	.000	4.9 (1.3,18.2)	.016
Grandfather	0.1 (0.01, 0.84)	.033	NS	
Mother	NS		7.5 (1.7, 32.8)	.007
Household income			0.6 (0.4, 0.9)	.008

No. obs.: 728; No. gps.:413; Wald chi2=51.80; gl=10; p= 0.000; Wald chi2=5411; gl=10; p= 0.000

Table 4. Familial psychiatric antecedents and anxiety syndromes in the offspring, 1st. adjustment

2.4.3 The final model incorporated the group of proband's psychosocial variables. On Table 5, results show that for general anxiety the odds ratio for G 2 increases considerably, from almost a 7-fold increase in the previous model to a 20-fold increase, although it is important to note that the confidence interval is very wide. A little increase in the odds ratio is also observed for the association with psychopathology on both previous generations. Stress at work emerged as an important proband's psychosocial variable associated with the generalized anxiety syndrome in the offspring, while more total working hours per week is associated with the syndrome anxiety with inhibition. Having worries between home and work is inversely associated with the presence of both anxiety syndromes, while for anxiety with inhibition, relationship with spouse is also inversely associated.

	Generalized anxiety OR (95% CI)	P	Anxiety with inhibition OR (95% CI)	P
G 1	5.6 (0.5, 56.8)	.113	1.1 (0.2, 4.8)	.937
G 2	20.4 (1.5, 282.7)	.023	7.7 (1.04, 56.5)*	.046
G 1 & G 2	47.0 (5.5, 405.0)	.000	2.2 (0.6, 7.5)	.208
Stress at work	6.5 (1.9, 22.0)	.003	--	
Worries between home and work	0.24 (0.07, 0.8)	.020	0.21 (0.06, 0.76)	.017
Working-hours per week	--		1.8 (1.04, 3.0)	.034
Relationship with spouse	--		0.45 (0.26, 0.79)	.006

No. obs.: 698; No. gps.:396; Wald chi2=47.67; gl=17; p= 0.000; Wald chi2=4197; gl=17; p= 0.000
*only mother's psychiatric antecedents

Table 5. Familial psychiatric antecedents and anxiety syndromes in the offspring, 2nd. Adjustment

As the odds ratios are always an over-estimation of the real relative risk, GEE population-averaged analysis with Poisson regression was performed to obtain the prevalence risk ratios, PRR. Results on Table 6 show that PRR are smaller than previous adjusted odds ratios. Also, for anxiety with inhibition, besides the variable working more hours per week, being employed and living in a low income household, completed the risk picture. Considering all the variables studied in the population, familial psychopathology interaction between G1 & G2 explains most of the risk for the generalized anxiety syndrome in the offspring, along with higher stress at work on G2. In contrast, for the anxiety with inhibition syndrome, psychiatric familial atributable risk is low, but most important is that a better couple's relationship is a considerable protective factor.

2.4.4 What specific groups of psychiatric familial disorders are associated with the development of anxiety syndromes in the offspring?

In order to answer this question, groups of psychiatric disorders in G1 and G2 were entered in the analyses as independent covariates. Because of the extremely low prevalence of G 3 anxiety syndromes in the non-comorbid grandparents' antecedents groups, the analysis was restricted to the comorbid-anxiety groups. Results on Table 7 shows that comorbid anxiety either with depression or with it and substance abuse in grandparents are significantly associated with the generalized anxiety syndrome in G3, but not with the screening syndrome anxiety with inhibition. All groups of parent's psychiatric disorders are associated with generalized anxiety, and odds ratios are quite consistent for all groups, except for the depression-only group. For anxiety with inhibition, parent's comorbid anxiety-depression as well as anxiety-only, show significant association.

	Generalized Anxiety		Anxiety with Inhibition	
	PRR (95% CI)	Attributable risk %	PRR (95% CI)	Attributable risk %
G 1	5.5 (0.6, 52.4)	1.2	1.0 (0.2, 4.3)	0.5
G 2	17.8 (1.5, 213.7) 1	3.5	6.8 (1.1, 41.6)* 1	2.2*
G 1 & G 2	35.0 (4.7, 259.3) 2	10.6	2.0 (0.6, 6.0)	3
Stress at work	5.2 (1.8, 14.7) 3	1,2-31.9	--	
Household income	NS		0.5 (0.3, 0.99) 1	0.3-2.5
Employed			9.8 (1.01, 95.4) 1	1.2
Worries between home and work	0.26 (0.09, 0.8) 1	1-1.6	0.21 (0.06, 0.76) 1	0.6-2.4
Working-hours per week	NS		1.7 (1.07, 2.7) 1	0.1-0.9
Relationship with spouse	NS		0.47 (0.28, 0.79) 3	0.2-4.1

No. obs.: 698; No. gps.:396; Wald chi2=58.98; gl=17; p= 0.000; Wald chi2=4865; gl=17; p= 0.000
*only mother's psychiatric antecedents; 1 p<0.05; 2 p<0.001; 3 p< 0.005

Table 6. Familial antecedents and anxiety syndromes in the offspring, Adjusted Risk Ratios

Antecedents in grandparents	Generalized anxiety OR (95% CI)	P	Anxiety with inhibition OR (95% CI)	P
Anxiety & depression	7.1 (2.8, 17.9)	.000	1.8 (0.8, 4.2)	.162
Anxiety, depression & substances	8.2 (3.3, 20.7)	.000	1.7 (0.7, 4.3)	.262
Antecedents in parents				
Anxiety- only	5.7 (2.1, 15.9)	.001	3.3 (1.2, 8.8)	.019
Depression - only	3.5 (1.2, 10.1)	.022	1.6 (0.4, 7.1)	.532
Anxiety & depression	5.7 (2.3, 14.1)	.000	7.7 (2.8, 21.0)	.000
Anxiety, depression & substances	5.5 (1.1, 27.0)	.038	--	

No. obs.: 1100; No. gps.:608; Wald chi2=59.05; gl=6; p= 0.000; Wald chi2=22.62; gl=5; p= 0.000

Table 7. Specific familial antecedents and anxiety syndromes in offspring, crude.

2.4.5 Does the magnitude of the association remains or is it modified when adjustment for the first block of covariables is introduced to the model? Do gender, age, household income and labour status play a role for the development of anxiety syndromes in the offspring?

The odds ratios between grandparents' history of anxiety-comorbid disorders and the presence of both anxiety syndromes in their grandchildren as shown in Table 8 are practically the same as in the previous model. That is, history of anxiety-comorbid disorders on G1 is significantly associated with general anxiety screening syndrome on G3, but not with the screening syndrome anxiety with inhibition.

Although none of the first group of potential confounding variables was found significantly associated with anxiety syndromes on G 3, some effects on the magnitude of the association between groups of psychiatric disorders on G 2 and the screening anxiety syndromes on G 3 became evident. The strength of the association between anxiety-only, depression-only and comorbid anxiety-depression disorders with the generalized anxiety syndrome in the offspring increases, while an antecedent of comorbid anxiety-depression and substance abuse is no longer significant. For the anxiety with inhibition screening syndrome, only history of comorbid anxiety-depression remains significantly associated.

Antecedents in grandparents	Generalized anxiety OR (95% CI)	P	Anxiety with inhibition OR (95% CI)	P
Anxiety & depression	7.3 (2.9, 18.4)	.000	1.9 (0.8, 4.4)	.134
Anxiety, depression & substances	8.6 (3.4, 21.4)	.000	1.7 (0.7, 4.3)	.238
Antecedents in parents				
Anxiety- only	6.6 (2.2, 19.8)	.001	2.3 (0.9, 6.5)	.092
Depression - only	4.0 (1.3, 12.7)	.018	1.1 (0.2, 5.2)	.857
Anxiety & depression	7.1 (2.5, 20.6)	.000	5.3 (1.9, 15.2)	.002
Anxiety, depression & substances	4.4 (0.7, 26.7)	.105	--	

No. obs.:1083; No. gps.:599; Wald chi2=74.21;gl=12; p= 0.000; Wald chi2=30.63; gl=11; p= 0.001

Table 8. Specific familial antecedents and anxiety syndromes in offspring, first adjustment.

2.4.6 When adjustment for the proband's psychosocial variables is introduced in the analysis, results on Table 9 show that female children and adolescents develop less generalized anxiety syndrome than males. Also, as previous results have shown in Table 5, the relationship with spouse is inversely associated with the presence of anxiety with inhibition in the offspring. The strength of the association between comorbid anxiety on G 1 and both anxiety syndromes on G3 remain more or less the same. However, changes emerged between G2 and G3: Anxiety-only, became associated with the syndrome anxiety with inhibition; depression-only is marginally associated with generalized anxiety.

GEE population-averaged analysis with Poisson regression was performed to obtain the PRR. Results on Table 10 show that depression-only reaches statistical significance, as it was only marginally associated in the precedent analysis with generalized anxiety in the offspring. However, PRR is almost half compared to parent´s antecedents of anxiety-only disorders.

Attributable risk in the population relies on familial antecedents of anxiety, either alone or comorbid, mainly, with depression.

Anxiety with inhibition in the offspring show only marginal significant PRR with antecedents of anxiety-only in parents, and no other type of psychiatric history has a significative associated risk with this anxiety screening syndrome. However, its worth to note that attributable risk in the population follows the same path as for generalized anxiety, although roughly at half the risk.

Antecedents in grandparents	Generalized anxiety OR (95% CI)	P	Anxiety with inhibition OR (95% CI)	P
Anxiety & depression	8.1 (2.9, 22.4) 1	.000	2.2 (0.9, 5.1)	.070
Anxiety, depression & substances	7.1 (2.5, 19.9) 1	.000	1.4 (0.4, 5.2)	.630
Antecedents in parents				
Anxiety- only	7.4 (2.4, 22.9) 1	.001	2.7 (1.0, 7.1) 3	.050
Depression - only	3.3 (0.99, 10.9)	.051	1.3 (0.3, 6.4)	.705
Anxiety & depression	6.1 (1.8, 20.5) 1	.004	2.6 (0.8, 8.5)	.110
Anxiety, depression & substances	1.5 (0.1, 18.4)	.733	--	
Daughter	0.4 (0.2, 0.98) 3	.044	NS	
Relationship with spouse	NS		0.6 (0.4, 0.9) 4	.010

No. obs.:1025; No. gps.:567; Wald chi2=99.04; gl=20; p= 0.000; Wald chi2=42.49; gl=19; p= 0.001

Table 9. Specific familial antecedents and anxiety syndromes in offspring, second adjustment

Antecedents	Generalized Anxiety		Anxiety with Inhibition	
in grandparents	PRR (95% CI)	Attributable Risk %	PRR (95% CI)	Attributable Risk %
Anxiety & depression	7.0 (2.7, 18.1)	6,7	2.0 (0.9, 4.5)	3.5
Anxiety, depression & substances	6.2 (2.4, 15.8)	8.8	1.4 (0.4, 4.8)	1.5
Antecedents in parents				
Anxiety- only	5.8 (2.1, 15.8)	10.2	2.4 (0.98, 6.0) *	5.4
Depression - only	3.0 (1.04, 8.8)	3.3	1.3 (0.3, 5.8)	1.4
Anxiety & depression	4.7 (1.6, 13.6)	15.4	2.4 (0.8, 6.9)	7.7
Anxiety, depression & substances	1.5 (0.1, 18.4)	1.1	--	
Daughter	0.5 (0.2, 0.97)	1.6	NS	
Relationship with spouse	NS		0.6 (0.4, 0.9)	0.3 - 4.3

No. obs.:1025; No.gps.:567; Wald chi2=123.3; gl=20; p= 0.000; Wald chi2=50.01; gl=19; p= 0.000
1 $p \leq 0.001$; 2 $p<0.005$; 3 $p<0.05$; 4 $p=0.01$; * $p= 0.54$

Table 10. Specific familial antecedents and anxiety syndromes in offspring, adjusted risk ratios

2.4.7 Psychosocial variables are closer to actual and on-going circumstances. As in the method used for the analysis of the data the correlations between subsequent measurements have been assumed to be the same, and this does not hold for psychosocial variables, the final analysis included only information between probands (G 2) and their children (G 3).

Results presented on Table 11 show that parent's history of anxiety-only as well as comorbid anxiety-depression are significantly associated with both screening anxiety syndromes in their offspring. Also, as in the previous model, male children develop more generalized anxiety as compared to females, and the relationship with spouse is inversely associated with the presence of anxiety with inhibition in the descendant. Interestingly, two variables, one from each adjustment's group, became associated with anxiety syndromes in the offspring: household income and proband's own health perception. The first, only associated with the generalized anxiety syndrome, while the second with both.

For generalized anxiety in the offspring, it is worth noting that the strength of the association with parents' anxiety-only disorders diminishes more than a half as compared when grandparents antecedents were included in the previous analysis, while comorbid anxiety-depression antecedents shows a slight increase in the odds ratio, and depression-only diminishes one-fold.

Comparatively, for the anxiety with inhibition syndrome in the offspring the strength of the association with parents' comorbid anxiety-depression increases one-fold and becomes significantly associated, while anxiety-only and depression-only show a very slight increase.

Antecedents in parents	Generalized anxiety OR (95% CI)	P	Anxiety with inhibition OR (95% CI)	P
Anxiety- only	3.5 (1.6, 7.9)	.002	3.0 (1.3, 6.8)	.012
Depression- only	2.0 (0.6, 6.0)	.234	2.2 (0.8, 5.7)	.108
Anxiety & depression	6.7 (3.0, 14.7)	.000	3.7 (1.6, 9.0)	.003
Anxiety, depression & substances	2.1 (0.6, 7.6)	.251	--	
Daughter	0.5 (0.3, 0.9)	.015	NS	
Household income	1.3 (1.04, 1.7)	.022	NS	
Health perception	1.3 (1.04, 1.8)	.026	1.4 (1.1, 1.8)	.005
Relationship with spouse	NS		0.7 (0.5, 0.9)	.021

No. obs.:1550; No. gps.:849; Wald chi2=67.16; gl=18; p= 0.000; Wald chi2=62.93; gl=18; p= 0.000

Table 11. Parent´s disorders, psychosocial variables and anxiety syndromes in offspring

Adjusted PRR obtained with GEE population-averaged analysis with Poisson regression show only a noticeable adjustment for the risk between parent's comorbid anxiety-depression and generalized anxiety in the offspring (Table 12). However, for the anxiety with inhibition syndrome, parent's antecedents of anxiety-only and comorbid anxiety disorders show a significant risk. Noteworthy, is that risk between each screening anxiety syndrome in the offspring and parent's antecedents of depression-only, is not significant.

Antecedents in parents	Generalized Anxiety		Anxiety with Inhibition	
	PRR (95% CI)	Attributable risk %	PRR (95% CI)	Attributable risk %
Anxiety-only	3.2 (1.6, 6.5) 2	7	2.7 (1.3, 5.9) 4	5.8
Depression-only	1.9 (0.7, 5.3)	1.9	2.1 (0.9, 5.1)	3.4
Anxiety & depression	5.1 (2.6, 9.7) 2	16.6	3.3 (1.5, 7.1) 1	10.5
Anxiety, depression & substances	2.1 (0.6, 6.6)	1.6	2.9 (1.1, 7.8) 3	3.4
Daughter	0.51 (0.3, 0.9) 3	2	NS	
Household income	1.3 (1.03, 1.6) 3	1.4-4.9	NS	
Health perception	1.3 (1.02, 1.7) 3	1.1-4.6	1.4 (1.1, 1.7) 4	1.2-4.8
Relationship with spouse	NS		0.7 (0.6, 0.96) 3	0.4-4.1

1 $p \leq 0.005$; 2 $p<0.001$; 3 $p< 0.05$; 4 $p \leq 0.01$

Table 12. Parent´s disorders, and anxiety syndromes in offspring, adjusted risk ratios

3. Discussion

This epidemiological study in the general population of Mexico City has shown evidence, consistent with results from studies on Caucasian populations in developed countries (Klein & Pine, 2002), that familial risk for developing anxiety disorders is a fact, thus not limited by ethnicity or culture, but mediated by socio-economic conditions. Our contribution is that to our knowledge, there are no other studies that have analyzed familial risk for anxiety disorders in children and adolescents across three generations in the general population. However, some considerations and limitations of the study should be kept in mind before discussing the results.

Assessments of psychiatric history in grandparents, G1, and lifetime psychiatric diagnoses on probands, G 2, were made with accepted international criteria and epidemiological instruments (Kendler et al., 1997; Kessler et al., 2002). Screening for caseness in children and adolescents, G 3, was made with a new questionnaire: The Brief Screening and Diagnostic Questionnaire (CBTD for its initials in Spanish). It is important to highlight that the CBTD includes symptoms that are frequently reported as motives for consultation at outpatient mental health services. So, the instrument does not merely translate diagnostic criteria into questions but rather use the way that the population perceives and express concern about their children's behaviour, in order first, to define caseness and second, to identify probable disorders.

Screening syndromes for several children's psychiatric disorders were obtained from this general population study (Caraveo, 2006; 2007). The hypothesis was that data would be able to identify a generalized anxiety syndrome as well as a separation anxiety syndrome. The first was fully accomplished but not the second one. Instead of it, what has been presented as the anxiety with inhibition syndrome, emerged from the cluster analysis and do not resemble any accepted diagnostic category. Nonetheless, concurrent validity with DSM-IV anxiety diagnoses has been found to be good (Caraveo et al., 2011 accepted for publication). As the principal objective of the survey was focused on adult population, only one adult was selected at each household, and so familial risk across generations, is lacking on information about one parent. However, as the sample was representative of the adult population aged 18 to 64 years; morbid risk was calculated using GEE averaged-population models, in which the interest is the population and not the individual's risk (Twisk, 2003).

Other limitations are: This was a cross-sectional study. All information was obtained from only one person and retrospectively. Comorbidity between anxiety and other syndromes in children and adolescents were not considered for control during the analyses, and impairment associated with the screening anxiety syndromes was not assessed.

3.1 Do the results show sufficient evidence supporting the hypothesis of a familial risk between the screening anxiety syndromes in children and adolescents and familial antecedents of psychopathology in the two precedent generations?

From the more general standpoint, that is the association between the two screening anxiety syndromes in the offspring, G3, and any familial psychiatric history on G1, G2, and the interaction between G1 and G2, results suggest that for the generalized anxiety syndrome familial risk is more plausible than for the anxiety with inhibition syndrome.

Crude odds ratios showed that generalized anxiety is 6 times more frequent in G3 when there is history of any psychiatric disorders in the proband, G2, with a statistical significance of $P<.05$, and considerably increases up to 24 times more, $P<.001$, when there is also history of psychiatric disorders in grandparents, G1 and G2. Controlling the effects of potential confounding variables increased the odds ratios as well as confidence intervals indicating high variability, altough and very important, statistical significance of these morbid risks, $P<.05$ and $P<.001$ respectively, persisted throughout all the analyses.

Adjusting for the first block of confounders suggested that the interaction between G2 and G1 relies more on grandmothers' psychopathology. However, its statistical significance was lost when control for other variables was included. Nonetheless, its relevance should be kept in mind for further studies as the mother´s figure is very important in familial relationships. An intergenerational study (Hammen et al., 2004) have presented very interesting data on how major depressive disorder (MDD) in grandmothers have an effect on grandchildren by maternal, G2, chronic interpersonal stress. On this, there is the fact that grandmothers help their descendants in nurturing and raising grandchildren especially if both parents have to work, or when their offspring are single parents.

Most important, and certainly a distinctive contribution from this study, is the documentation of the enormous increase in the association between psychopathology in G 2 and generalized anxiety in G 3 when controlling for the proband's psychosocial variables. Odds ratio raised from a 7-fold increased risk to a 20-fold increased risk between any parent's psychiatric disorder and generalized anxiety in their offspring, along with the variable stress at work with a 6-fold increased risk, $P<.005$, thus indicating the impact of the financial crisis on the mental health status and well-being of the population. Moreover, the attributable risk of the variable stress at work showed a range, according to quartiles, from 1.2% to a high 31.9%. To have an idea of how important the financial crisis was, here are some data: Money exchange rate increased from 3.49 pesos x dollar to 9.42; devaluation represented 173.82%; inflation 225.32%, and acquisitive power diminished 34.79 %(Fernández-Torres, 2005).

Adjusted prevalence risk ratios clearly shows that morbid risk for the generalized anxiety syndrome in descendants is almost the double when there is interaction between history of psychiatric disorders on G1 and G2 as compared to only having psychiatric antecedents on G2. These first results follow the path reported on major depressive disorder, MDD, across three generations by Weissman et al. (2005) that found a 5.4-fold increased risk for any disorder in the offspring when interaction between grandparental MDD and parental MDD was present. Also, Pettit et al. (2008) using linear regression procedures reported that the interaction of G1 MDD x G2 MDD significantly predicted Anxious/Depressed scores on the Children Behavior Check List (CBCL).

Compared to the generalized anxiety syndrome, associations of the anxiety with inhibition sydrome as related to any familial psychiatric antecedents across generations and potential confounding variables, results suggest a more situational determined condition rather than a disorder with a clear familial risk. However, when adjustment was made for the first block of potential confounding variables, gender, age, household income and labour status, the interaction between history of any psychiatric disorders on G1 and G2 showed an almost 5-fold increased risk, $P<.02$, suggesting somekind of psychiatric familial liability and mostly on women probands. Only the lifetime history of psychiatric disorder in mothers was associated with the outcome in the offspring, when adjustment was made for the probands' psychosocial variables. In terms of the prevalence risk ratio, having -predominantly- a mother with a psychiatric disorder, employed, working as a couple more hours per week, and living in a low-income household, are risk factors associated with the outcome syndrome anxiety with inhibition in children and adolescents.

Based on these results, it is fair to ask: Is the anxiety with inhibition syndrome in descendants a gender-related parent disorder? Is it the result of different disadvantages, both individual and social?

3.2 Do the results on the screening anxiety syndromes in children and adolescents show sufficient evidence supporting an anxiety familial risk across generations?

With the preceding broad and encouraging panorama, the next inquire was on what kind of specific psychiatric familial antecedents are associated with the outcome of anxiety syndromes in children and adolescents. Results have shown that comorbid anxiety disorders in grandparents seems to interact with anxiety-only as well as with anxiety comorbid disorders in parents, determining a robust morbid risk for the generalized anxiety screening syndrome in descendants. Moreover, comorbid anxiety-depression followed by anxiety-only lifetime disorders in parents showed the highest attributable risk for this syndrome in the offspring, 15.4% and 10.2%, respectively. In contrast, the attributable risk of parents' depression-only for this syndrome is considerably low, from 1.9% to 3.3%.

These results are consistent with findings from a cohort longitudinal study over 32 years (Moffit et al. 2007) in which non-comorbid MDD involved lower levels of risk than comorbid MDD + Generalized Anxiety disorder (GAD).

Hale et al. (2009) in a prospective 5-year study in two cohorts of early and middle adolescents from the general population at The Netherlands, used a framework of structural equation modeling to investigate whether anxiety and depression disorder symptoms corresponds to one general factor or do they are two distinct disorders with parallel growth processes. The latter, was the best model and results also suggested that the development of one disorder may be affected by the initial symptom severity of the other disorder.

Weissman et al., (2005) found a 5-fold increased risk for an anxiety disorder in grandchildren when interaction between grandparental MDD and parental MDD was present. Our results are very similar, the PRR showed a 4.7-fold increase on parents with comorbid anxiety-depression having grandparents' psychiatric antecedents as separate covariables and a 5.1-fold increase when only parents' disorders were analyzed.

Considering exclusively the risk between parents' anxiety-only disorders and the generalized anxiety syndrome in descendants, our results have shown a 5.8-fold increased risk when grandparents' psychiatric antecedents were covariates and a 3.2-fold increased risk without them. Both results are higher than the relative risk reported on G1 MDD x G2 MDD interaction and offspring MDD, 2.08-fold increase, as well as for any mood disorder, 2.42-fold increase. As our results come from a general population sample rather than from a clinical setting, findings could suggest that familial risk for generalized anxiety across three generations is higher than the observed for MDD. However, this could be a mediation effect of the financial crisis.

On this, besides gender and familial antecedents as risk factors, offspring living in households with relative better income, and with parents reporting poor own's health perception were at increased risk for presenting generalized anxiety syndrome. The first variable indicates the struggle of mostly the middle class population, in order to face the economic crisis, while the second one also speaks about the concern on social support, a risk that is equally shared by parents with offspring showing anxiety with inhibition.

The presence of lifetime anxiety disorders in both grandparents and parents, as opposed to only one generation, may reflect higher genetic loadings for emotional disorders as observed for the generalized anxiety syndrome. In contrast, at a first glance, the anxiety with inhibition syndrome seemed not show the same pattern. However, following closely the results, in the first analysis, crude odds ratios showed that parent's comorbid anxiety-depression as well as anxiety-only, are significantly associated with the outcome. Adjusting for the first group of potential confounders, only history of comorbid anxiety-depression in parents' remains significantly associated, which indicates the more severe form of the disorder as discussed earlier. However, when psychosocial variables were introduced to the model, parents' history of anxiety-only became the single psychiatric antecedent significantly associated with this syndrome. Nonetheless, odds ratios and risk ratios indicated that the morbid risk is practically the same for parents' history of anxiety-only and for comorbid anxiety-depression (Tables 9 & 10). Moreover, the attributable risk is 5.4% for the first, while slightly higher, 7.7%, for comorbid anxiety-depression, and its noteworthy the 3.5% contribution from grandparents' comorbid anxiety-depression disorders. These results suggest that the anxiety with inhibition syndrome also has a familial anxiety risk across generations, although less pronounced as compared to the generalized anxiety syndrome.

4. Conclusion

The present study has shown consistent evidence that anxiety syndromes in children and adolescents from the general population, as screened with the CBTD, have a clear anxiety-related familial risk across generations. The morbid risk is more evident for the generalized anxiety syndrome, and possibly higher than what has been reported on MDD-only by other studies. However, this could be a mediation effect of the financial crisis that occurred at the time of the study. The morbid risk associated with comorbid anxiety-depression in precedent generations is higher than the obtained on anxiety-only disorders and almost the same as reported in multigeneration MDD studies.

The anxiety with inhibition syndrome has a less pronounced anxiety-related familial risk across generations and results suggest that it is a gender-related parent disorder where different disadvantages, both individual and social, may play a moderating role.

Findings have clinical implications; some of them have been already taken into practice. The Brief Screening and Diagnostic Questionnaire, CBTD, has been tested in primary care settings an incorporated as a basic tool for health services in Mexico City. Obtaining a screening family history of anxiety, depression and substance-abuse disorders as used in this study, as well as the assessment of impairment in children, evaluation of child-rearing practices, family style for solving problems at home, and report of domestic violence, have been tested as basic issues for the surveillance of mental health in childhood and andolescence.

5. Acknowledgment

This study was funded by The National Council of Science and Thechnology (CONACYT), award 2077-H9302.

6. References

Aguilar-Gaxiola, S., Alegría, M., Andrade, L., Bijl, R., Caraveo-Anduaga, J., Dewit, D.J., Kolody, B., Kessler, R.C., Ustun, T.B., Vega, W.A. & Wittchen H-U. (2000) The international consortium in psychiatric epidemiology. In: *Sociální psychiatrie v case zmen (Social Psychiatry in Changing Times)* pp. 86-96, Psychiatrické centrum; ISBN 80-85121-08-5, Praha

American Psychiatric Association. (1994) *Diagnostic and statistical manual of mental disorders,* (fourth edition), American Psychiatric Association, ISBN 0-89042-062-9, Washington D.C.

Andrade, L., Caraveo, A.J., Berglund, P., Bijl, R., De Graaf, R., Vollebergh, W. Dragomirecka, E., Kohn, R., Keller, M., Kessler, R.C., Kawakami, N., Orford, D., Ustun, T.B., & Wittchen, H.U. (2003) The epidemiology of major depressive episodes: results from the International Consortium of Psychiatric Epidemiology (ICPE) surveys. *International. Journal of Methods in Psychiatric Research,* 12, 1, pp.3-21, ISSN 1049-8931

Andreasen, N.C., Endicott, J., Spitzer, R. L. & Winokur, G. (1977) The family history method using diagnostic criteria. *Archives of General Psychiatry,* 34, pp. 1229-1235, ISSN 0003-990X.

Andreasen, N. C., Rice, J. Endicott, J., Reich, T., & Coryell W. (1986) The Family history approach to diagnosis: How useful is it? *Archives of General Psychiatry,* 43, pp. 421-429, ISSN 0003-990X

Ashman, S. B. Dawson, G., Panagiotides, H., Yamada, E., & Wilkinson C. W. (2002) Stress hormone levels of children of depressed mothers. *Development and Psychopathology;* 14, pp. 333-349, ISSN 0954-5794.

Biederman, J., Hirshfeld-Becker, D R., Rosenbaum, J. F., Hérot, C., Friedman, D., Snidman, N., Kagan, J., & Faraone S. V. (2001) Further evidence of association between behavioral inhibition and social anxiety in children. *American Journal of Psychiatry;* 158, pp. 1673-1679, ISSN 0002-953X

Caraveo, A. J., Medina-Mora, M. E., Tapia, C. R., Rascón, M. L., Gómez, M., & Villatoro, J. (1993) Trastornos psiquiátricos en niños de la República Mexicana. Resultados de una encuesta de hogares. *Psiquiatría*, 9, pp.137-151, ISSN 0187-4543

Caraveo, A. J., Medina-Mora, M. E., Villatoro, J., & Rascón M. L. (1994) La depresión en el adulto como factor de riesgo en la salud mental de los niños. *Salud Mental*, 17, 2, pp.56-60, ISSN 0185-3325

Caraveo A. J., Medina-Mora M. E. Villatoro J. Rascón M. L. & Martínez V. A. (1995) El consumo de alcohol como factor de riesgo asociado a desórdenes psíquicos en los niños. *Salud Mental*, 18, 2, pp.18-24, ISSN 0185-3325

Caraveo-Anduaga, J. (1996) Prevalencia de trastornos psiquiátricos en la población Mexicana. Estado actual y perspectivas. *Salud Mental*, 19,(Suppl. 1), pp.8-13, ISSN: 0185-3325.

Caraveo, A. J., Martínez, N., & Rivera, E. (1998) Un modelo para estudios epidemiológicos sobre la salud mental y la morbilidad psiquiátrica. *Salud Mental*; 21, 1, pp. 48-57, ISSN 0185-3325

Caraveo, A. J., Colmenares, B. E., & Saldívar, H. G. (1999) Morbilidad psiquiátrica en la Ciudad de México: prevalencia y comorbilidad en la vida. *Salud Mental*, 22 (especial), pp. 62-67, ISSN 0185-3325

Caraveo-Anduaga, J., Nicolini, S.H., Villa, R.A., & Wagner, E.F. (2005) Psicopatología en familiares de tres generaciones: un estudio epidemiológico en la Ciudad de México. *Salud Pública De México*, 47, 1, pp. 20-26, ISSN 0036-3634, ISSN 1606-7916.

Caraveo-Anduaga J. (2006). Cuestionario Breve de tamizaje y diagnóstico de problemas de salud mental en niños y adolescentes, CBTD: confiabilidad, estandarización y validez de construcción. *Salud Mental*, 29, 6, pp.65-72, ISSN 0185-3325

Caraveo-Anduaga J. (2007) Cuestionario Breve de tamizaje y diagnóstico de problemas de salud mental en niños y adolescentes: algoritmos para síndromes y su prevalencia en la Ciudad de México. *Salud Mental*, 30, 1, pp.48-55, ISSN 0185-3325

Caraveo-Anduaga, J. López J. J. L. Soriano R. A. López H. J. L. Contreras G. A. & Reyes M. A. Eficiencia y validez concurrente del CBTD para la vigilancia de la salud mental de niños y adolescentes en un centro de atención primaria de México. (Under revision, 2011) Revista De Investigación Clínica. ISSN: 0034-8376.

Caspi, A., Moffitt, T. E., Newman, D. L., & Silva, P. A. (1996) Behavioral observations at age 3 years predict adult psychiatric disorders. *Archives of General Psychiatry*, 53, pp. 1033-1039. ISSN 0003-990X

Fernández-Torres, J.E. (2005) *La crisis financiera de 1994-1995 y el TLCAN a diez años* [Web Page].; Accessed 2011 Apr 24. Available at: www.EUMED.NET/libros/2005/JEFT/.

Giel R., de Arango, M. V., Climent, C. E., Harding, T. W., Ibrahim, H. H. A., Ladrido-Ignacio, L., Srinivasa-Murthy, R., Salazar, M. C., Wig, N. N., & Younis Y. O. A. (1981) Childhood mental disorders in primary health care: results of observations in four developing countries. *Pediatrics*, 68, 5, pp. 677-683, .ISSN 0003-990X

Goldsmith, H. H., Buss, K. A.., & Lemery, K. S. (1997) Toddler and childhood temperament: Expanded content, stronger genetic evidence, new evidence for the importance of environment. *Developmental Psychology*, 33, pp. 891-905, ISSN 0031-4005

Hale III, W. W. Raaijmakers, Q. A. W., Muris, P., & van Hoof, A. (2009) One factor or two parallel processes? Comorbidity and development of adolescent anxiety and depressive disorder symptoms. *Journal of Child Psychology and Psychiatry*, 50, 10, pp. 1218-1226;. ISSN: 0021-9630.

Hammen, C., Shih, J. H., & Brennan, P. A. (2004) Intergenerational transmission of depression: Test of an interpersonal stress model in a community sample. *Journal of Consulting and Clinical Psychology*, 72, pp. 511-522, ISSN 0012-1649.

Hayward, C., Killen, J. D., Kraemer, H. C., & Taylor C. B. (1998) Linking self-reported childhood behavioral inhibition to adolescent social phobia. *Journal of the American Academy of Child and Adolescent Psychiatry*, 37, pp. 1308-1316, ISSN 0890-8567

Kagan, J., Reznick, J. S., Clarke, C., Snidman, N., & Garcia-Coll, C. (1984) Behavioral inhibition to the unfamiliar. *Child Development*, 55, pp. 2212-2225, ISSN 0009-3920.

Kendler, K., Davis, C. G., & Kessler, R. C. (1997) The familial aggregation of common psychiatric and substance use disorders in the National Comorbidity Survey: a family history study. *British Journal of Psychiatry*, 170, pp. 541-548, ISSN 0007-1250

Kendler, K. S., Walters, E. E., Neale, M. C., Kessler, R. C., Heath, A. C., & Eaves, L. J. (1995) The structure of the genetic and environmental risk factors for six major psychiatric disorders in women: Phobia, generalized anxiety disorder, panic disorder, bulimia, major depression, and alcoholism. *Archives of General Psychiatry*, 52, pp. 374-383, ISSN 0003-990X

Kessler, R.C., McGonagle, K. A., & Zhao, S., Nelson, C.B., Hughes, M., Eshelman, S., Wittchen, H-U., & Kendler, K.S. (1994) Lifetime and 12-month prevalence of DSM-III-R psychiatric disorders in the United States. *Archives of General Psychiatry*, 51, pp. 8-19, ISSN 0003-990X

Kessler, R. C., Nelson, C. B., McGonagle, K. A., Liu, J., Swartz, M., & Blazer, D. G. (1996) Co-morbidity of DSM-III-R major depressive disorder in the general population: results from the US National Co-morbidity Survey. *British Journal of Psychiatry*, 168, pp. 17-30, ISSN 0007-1250

Kessler, R.C., Aguilar-Gaxiola, S., Andrade, L., Bijl, R., Borges, G., Caraveo, A.J., De Witt, D.J., Kolody, B., Merikangas, K.R., Molnar, B.E., Vega, W.A., Walters, E.E., & Wittchen, H-U. (2003) Cross-national comparisons of comorbidities between substance use disorders and mental disorders: Results from the International Consortium in Psychiatric Epidemiology. In: *Handbook of Drug Abuse Prevention Theory, Science and Practice*, Zili Sloboda & William J. Bukoski., eds., pp. 447-472, Kluwer Academic/Plenum Publishers; ISBN 0-306-47342-9

Klein, R.G. & Pine D.S. (2002) Anxiety disorders. In: *Child and adolescent psychiatry*, Michael Rutter & Eric Taylor, (Eds.), fourth edition, pp. 486-509, Blackwell Science Ltd; ISBN 0-632-05361-5, Bath, Great Britain.

Kovacs, M. & Devlin, B. (1998) Internalizing Disorders in Childhood. *Journal of Child Psychology and Psychiatry*, 39, pp.47-63, ISSN 0021-9630

Malcarne, V., Hansdottir, I., & Merz, E. L. (2010) Vulnerability to anxiety disorders in childhood and adolescence. In: *Vulnerability to psychopathology*, Rick E. Ingram & Joseph M. Price, (Eds),. pp. 291-333, The Guilford Press, ISBN 978-1-60623-347-4, New York, N.Y.

McNutt, L. N. Wu Ch. Xue X. & Hafner J. P. (2003) Estimating the relative risk in cohort studies and clnical trials of common outcomes. *American Journal of Epidemiology*, 157, pp. 940-943, ISSN: 0002-9262.

Merikangas, K.R., Mehta, R. L., Molnar, B. E., Walters, E. E., Swendsen, J. D., Aguilar-Gaxiola, S., Bijl, R., Borges, G., Caraveo-Anduaga, J., Dewit, D. J., Kolody, B., Vega,

W. A., Wittchen, H-U., & Kessler, R. C. (1998) Comorbidity of susbtance use disorders with mood and anxiety disorders: results of the International Consortium in Psychiatric Epidemiology. *Addictive Behaviors*, 23, 6, pp. 893-907; ISSN 0306-4603.

Moffitt, T. E., Caspi, A., Harrington, H., Milne, B. J., Melchior, M., Goldberg, D., & Poulton, R. (2007) Generalized anxiety disorder and depression: childhood risk factors in a bith cohort followed to age 32. *Psychological Medicine*, 37, pp. 441-452, ISSN: 0033-2917.

Pettit, J. W., Olino, T. M., Robert, E. R., Seeley, J. R., & Lewinsohn, P. M. (2008) Intergenerational Transmission of Internalizing Problems: Effects of Parental and Grandparental Major Depressive Disorder on Child Behavior. *Journal of Clinical Child & Adolescent Psychology*, 37, pp. 640-650; ISSN 1537-4416.

Rapoport, J.L. (2000) *Childhood onset of "adult" psychopathology*. American Psychiatric Press, Inc., ISBN 0-88048-821-2, Washington D.C.

Schwartz, C. E. Snidman, N. & Kagan, J. (1999) Adolescent social anxiety as an outcome of inhibited temperament in childhood. *Journal of the American Academy of Child and Adolescent Psychiatry*, 38, pp. 1008-1015, ISSN 0890-8567.

Sheehan, D.V., Lecrubier, Y., Shytle, D., Milo, K., Hergueta, T., Colón-Soto, M., Díaz, V., & Soto, O. (2000, c1998) Mini International Neuropsychiatric Interview for children and adolescents [M.I.N.I. KID]. Version 1.1. Medical Outcome Systems, Inc.

Thornberry, T. P. Freeman-Gallant A. Lizotte A. J. Krohn M. D. & Smith C. A. (2003) Linked lives: The intergenerational transmission of antisocial behavior. *Journal of Abnormal Child Psychology*, 31, 2, pp.171-184, ISSN: 0091-0627.

Twisk J.W.R. (2003) *Applied longitudinal data analysis for epidemiology*. Cambridge University Press, ISBN 0-521-52580-2, Cambridge, UK

Vega, W.A., Kolody, B., Aguilar-Gaxiola, S., Alderte, E., Catalano, R., & Caraveo-Anduaga, J. (1998) Lifetime prevalence of DSM-III-R psychiatric disorders among urban and rural Mexican Americans in California. *Archives of General Psychiatry*, 55, pp. 771-778, ISSN 0003-990X

Warner, V., Wickramaratne, P., & Weissman, M. M. (2008) The role of fear and anxiety in the familial risk for major depression: a three-generation study. *Psychological Medicine*, 38, pp.1543-1556, ISSN 0033-2917.

Weissman, M.M., Warner, V., Wickramaratne, P., Moreau, D., & Olfson, M. (2000) Offspring at risk: Early-onset major depression and anxiety disorders over a decade. In: *Childhood onset of "adult" psychopathology*, Judith L..Rapoport (ed), pp. 245-258, American Psychiatric Press, Inc., ISBN 0-88048-821-2; Washington D.C.

Weissman, M. M., Wickramaratne, P., Nomura, Y., Warner, D., Verdeli, H., Pilowsky, D. J., Grillon C., & Bruder, G. (2005) Families at high and low risk for depression: A three generation study. *Archives of General Psychiatry*, 62, pp.29-36, ISSN 0003-990X

World Health Oragnization. (1993) *The ICD-10 Classification of Mental and Behavioural Disorders: Diagnostic criteria for research*. MEDITOR, ISBN 84-87548-13-X, Madrid, España.

Part 2

Primary Care and Prevention

4

Challenges and Opportunities in Diagnosis and Management of Generalized Anxiety Disorder in Primary Care

Mehtap Kartal
Dokuz Eylul University, Faculty of Medicine, Department of Family Medicine
Turkey

1. Introduction

It is known that General Anxiety Disorder (GAD), falling into the category of anxiety disorders with symptoms of anxiety, worry and apparent alertness, displays a fairly constant prevalence in the general population. Its lifelong prevalence in the general population is 5% according to the criteria of DSM and 6.5% according to broader criteria of ICD-10.

Among anxiety disorders, GAD patients often consult primary care physicians (PCPs) for their treatment. An international study conducted by the World Health Organization (WHO) found the frequency of GAD in primary health care at 14.9%, 3.7% and 0.9% in Greece, Italy and Turkey respectively. Despite these different figures among countries which are thought to emerge from structural differences of primary health care services, it was found out that the point prevalence of GAD in primary care was much higher (7.9%) than that of the general population. Through reanalysis of WHO's data, it was also shown that 25% of these patients have pure GAD without any comorbidity. In light of this data, it can be concluded that GAD is the most frequent mental disorder after depression in primary care, and that patients favour primary health care services for their treatment.

The comorbidity of GAD patients with other psychiatric disorders brings about an increase in the frequency of the health care system use, with longer periods of hospitalization, more frequent use of diagnostic tests and medication, and therefore, a heavy financial burden. This, in turn, implies more serious family problems and prolonged absence from work. There is abundant evidence showing that GAD decreases the quality of life considerably due to invalidity and disability.

It is reported that patients complain of physical symptoms more often than psychological, and worry is cited as the main problem for only 13% of GAD patients in primary care. The patients with GAD mostly consult primary care for aches, sleep problems and somatic problems. Somatic complaints of patients usually appear in the form of chronic medical conditions such as chest pain, chronic fatigue syndrome, irritable bowel syndrome and hypertension, diabetes and cardiac diseases. This is an important factor that complicates the accurate diagnosis of patients and also delays their treatment. The period between the time when the first symptoms of GAD appear and the time of the patient's consultation with the family physician or its equivalent can last for up to one year. Furthermore, it can take as long as seven years for the first consultation with the expert at an anxiety clinic. It was observed that about one third of GAD patients were not given a proper psychological diagnosis by family physicians.

Stigmatization is an important factor in insufficient diagnosis and this can account for why a significant number of patients do not express their emotional problems to their physicians. Patients with GAD are often unsuccessful at identifying that their symptoms as related to psychological disorders. People who minimize and normalize their symptoms are mostly young male patients and it is reported that they receive fewer correct diagnoses.

Along all these patient-related factors, it is clear that there are huge discrepancies in physicians' diagnostic skills, emerging from their knowledge, abilities and approaches. Longer consultation periods do not increase chance of correct diagnosis of diseases either. However, while empathy, interest in psychiatry and asking questions about family and domestic problems can increase the chance for an accurate diagnosis, coexisting organic diseases complicate it further. In a study conducted over a group of patients who mostly rely on using primary care services, GAD was found to be the disease which was most difficult to diagnose and caused most frustration for the physicians. It could be argued that this seriously affects physicians' skills to diagnose and treat their patients appropriately. It is apparent that physicians require tools to use for diagnosis.

The low rate of recognition and diagnosis of GAD in primary care presents a barrier for appropriate treatment and referrals needed for it. However, primary care physicians are the group with access to the largest body of patients.

The problems encountered in primary care diagnosis and management of anxiety in GAD are multifaceted and multiphase, which complicates the solutions as well. First of all, social interventions, including education campaigns which would improve society's approach to mental problems and decrease stigmatization, are required. Furthermore, increasing awareness of primary care physicians and equipping them with proper scanning tools is a necessity. Finally, developing national diagnosis and treatment guidelines, and promoting evidence based medical practice is also of great importance.

2. Epidemiology of GAD

Before the 1980s, Generalized Anxiety Disorder (GAD) was labelled as 'anxiety neurosis' characterized by excessive worrying and marked symptoms of hypervigilence and anxiety. GAD was first conceptualized in the Diagnostic and Statistical Manuel of Mental Disorders-III (DSM) in 1980 and its diagnostic criteria have changed since then. The current criteria in DSM-IV (Table 1) and the International Classification of Diseases-10 (ICD) (Table 2) for GAD differ considerably with ICD-10 listing a broader spectrum of symptoms. The differences in the understanding GAD between Europe and the United States predominantly based on the fact that ICD-10 is preferred in Europe, while DSM-IV is preferred in the United States (Wittchen & Hoyer, 2001; Lieb et al., 2005). These preferences have a substantial impact on the epidemiological results. The most likely lifetime prevalence for GAD in the general population is 5% (ranges between 0.8-21.7% with different assessment tools in different countries) with DSM criteria and slightly higher, 6.5%, with ICD-10 criteria (Bijl et al., 1998; Wittchen & Hoyer, 2001; Lieb et al., 2005; Mergl et al., 2007; Serrano-Blanco et al., 2010).

A. Excessive anxiety and worry (apprehensive expectation), occurring more days than not and for at least 6 months, about a number of events or activities (such as work or school performance)
B. The person finds it difficult to control the worry
C. The anxiety and worry are associated with three (or more) of the following six symptoms (with at least some symptoms present for more days than not for the past 6 months). Note: only one item is required in children
(1) restlessness or feeling keyed up or on edge
(2) being easily fatigued
(3) difficulty concentrating or mind going blank
(4) irritability
(5) muscle tension
(6) sleep disturbance (difficulty falling or staying asleep, or restless unsatisfying sleep)
D. The focus of the anxiety and worry is not confined to features of an Axis I disorder. E.g., the anxiety or worry is not about having a panic attack (as in panic disorder), being embarrassed in public (as in social phobia), being contaminated (as in obsessive compulsive disorder), being away from home or close relatives (as in separation anxiety disorder), gaining weight (as in anorexia nervosa), having multiple physical complaints (as in somatisation disorder), or having serious illness (as in hypochondriasis), and the anxiety and worry do not occur exclusively during posttraumatic stress disorder
E. The anxiety, worry, or physical symptoms cause clinically significant distress or impairment in social, occupational, or other important areas of functioning.
F. The disturbance is not due to the direct physiological effects of a substance (e.g, a drug of abuse, a medication) or general medical condition (e.g., hyperthyroidism) and does not occur exclusively during a mood disorder, a psychotic disorder or a pervasive developmental disorder

Table 1. DSM-IV criteria for generalized anxiety disorder

Anxiety that is generalized and persistent but not restricted to, or even strongly predominating in, any particular environmental circumstances (i.e. it is "free-floating"). The dominant symptoms are variable but include complaints of persistent nervousness, trembling, muscular tensions, sweating, light-headedness, palpitations, dizziness, and epigastric discomfort. Fears that the patient or a relative will shortly become ill or have an accident are often expressed.
Anxiety:
neurosis
reaction
state
Excludes: neurasthenia (F48.0)

Table 2. ICD-10 Criteria for Generalized anxiety disorder (F41.1)

The data, both European and non-European, suggests that GAD is most common among older age groups, unlike other anxiety disorders. It also shows that the likelihood of diagnosis of GAD increases with age: for women after the age of 35, and for men after the age of 45. It is relatively rare in the first two decades of life, with lower prevalence rates among adolescents and young adults. However, the age of onset has a bimodal distribution- GAD onset occurs earlier if it is the primary presentation and later if it is secondary (Culpepper, 2002; Lieb et al, 2005). GAD occurs twice as often in women as men, with total lifetime prevalence rates of 6.6% and 3.6%, respectively (Carter et al., 2001; Allgulander, 2006). Other factors significantly associated with GAD are determined to be: discontinued marriage (separated, widowed, or divorced), unemployed or being a house-wife while urbanicity, low income, fewer years of education, more life difficulties, and chronic medical disorders and religion showed limited associations (Wittchen & Hoyer, 2001; Young et al., 2001)

Similarly to patients that suffer of panic disorders, GAD patients often consult primary care physicians for their treatment. An international study conducted by the World Health Organization (WHO) found the frequency of GAD in primary health care at 14.9%, 3.7% and 0.9% in Greece, Italy and Turkey respectively. Despite these different figures among countries which are thought to emerge from structural differences in primary health care services, it was found out that the point prevalence of GAD in primary care was much higher (7.9%) than that of the general population (Ustun & Sartorius, 1995). Through reanalysis of WHO's data, it was also shown that 25% of these patients have pure GAD without any comorbidity (Lieb et al., 2005). The GADIS study determined the prevalence of pure GAD at 4.1%, and all GAD at 8.3% in primary care, while Kroenke et al. found the prevalence of GAD in primary care to be 7.6% (Ansseau et al., 2005; Kroenke et al., 2007). In light of this data, it can be concluded that GAD is the most frequent mental disorder after depression in primary care, and that patients favour primary health care services for their treatment.

3. Presentation and recognition of GAD in primary care

GAD symptoms wax and wane over time, with exacerbations of acute anxiety to response stress. Many patients with GAD readily report "I've been a worrier all my life". Studies support its episodic pattern with remission and recurrence periods evident for many years. (Wittchen & Hoyer, 2001; Allgulander, 2006).

GAD is a disabling condition and a social disability as severe as chronic somatic disorders such as arthritis, hypertension, asthma, and diabetes (Maier et al., 2000; Wittchen & Hoyer, 2001; Kessler et al., 2001; Roy-Byrne Wagner, 2004 ; Lieb, 2005). Wittchen et al. have shown that only 13% of GAD patients in primary care identify anxiety as the primary problem (Wittchen, 2002). Mostly, patients complain of somatic and sleeping problems (Wittchen & Hoyer, 2001). Accompanying symptoms include muscle tension, headache, muscle aches, restlessness, irritability, gastrointestinal symptoms, and difficulty in concentrating, fatigue, insomnia (Shearer, 2007). Patients are unlikely to directly and openly complain of anxiety symptoms. Cardiac and gastrointestinal symptoms of anxiety deserve special attention so as not to be misinterpreted in differential diagnosis and to avoid high costs of potential unnecessary screening for accurate diagnosis. GAD was determined to be primary diagnosis among 20% of patients with an atypical chest pain; 55% of patients with chest pain & normal coronary arteries; and 50% of patients seeking a cardiac evaluation (Roy-Byrne Wagner, 2004). Similarly, - in patients with inflammatory bowel syndrome GAD was showed to be in high prevalence (Roy-Byrne Wagner, 2004). A longitudinal study that determines the under-recognition of mental disorders showed that 18% of patients that had severe symptoms of depression or anxiety according to the general health questionnaire had never received a diagnosis from their general practitioners (GPs) (Kessler et al., 2002).

In another study, first three common reasons for the GP visit were listed as oto-rhino-laryngology (ORL), cardiovascular, and rheumatologic problems. However, a psychiatric problem was mentioned only in 5.4% of the cases. On the other hand, for the same sample, the prevalence of a psychiatric disorder was found 42.5%, and GAD prevalence was 10.3%, detected by PRIME-MD (Ansseau et al., 2004). A different study showed that 69.6% of the patients reporting anxiety/depression as a reason for consulting their GP had GAD (Ansseau et al., 2005).

Not only patients and primary care physicians' factors, but also the waxing and waning nature of GAD, leading to a "*discrepancy*" between primary reasons for visiting the GPs and actual diagnosis is important for recognizing GAD accurately (Ansseau et al., 2004; Tylee & Walters, 2007).

Chronic nature of GAD with remissions and recurrences, symptoms do not meet the criteria in periods of recovery between episodes and substantial overlap with other medical and psychological disorders may make it difficult to easily detect it (Kroenke et al., 1997, Roy-Byrne Wagner, 2004; Allgulander, 2006). Major depressive disorder is seen in at least one-third of primary care patients with GAD (Carter et al., 2001; Stein, 2003). Comorbidity with panic disorder, social phobia and specific phobia, and post-traumatic stress disorder is also common. Comorbidity is generally associated with increased severity and persistence of the disorders (Allgulander, 2006). However, GAD patients were found to be diagnosed with two or more comorbid disorders more often than any other disorder (Carter et al., 2001). Rodrigues et al. showed that primary care patients in the study population showed as much Axis I comorbidity as psychiatric treatment-seeking population. This is an important finding that questions previous assumptions about treatment-seeking in mental health settings as an indication of illness severity (Rodrigues et al.; 2004).

It is known that there is a wide variation in the ability of primary care physicians to diagnose GAD due to differences in knowledge, skills, and attitudes. Not only factual knowledge but also clinical skills, particularly communication skills and interview techniques, are important in the management of psychiatric disorder. Other obstacles have been mentioned: competing demands on PCPs time to interview patients within the limit of typical 15-min clinical encounters, frequent somatisation of mental disorders, underlying comorbidity, and preoccupation of an organic disease. However, empathy, an interest in psychiatry and asking about family and problems at home can help with the recognition (Ansseau et al., 2004; Rollman et al., 2005; Allgulander, 2006; Tylee & Walters, 2007). Harman et al. reported that vast majority of PCPs' diagnosis were branded "anxiety, unspecified". They concluded that this may reflect that the symptoms of primary care patients do not fulfil a specific diagnosis like GAD, or current description of anxiety disorders in commonly used classifications is too complicated to be easily applied by PCPs (Harman et al., 2002).

With regards to the patients, this discrepancy can be due to the considerable resistance to a psychiatric diagnosis and reluctance to discuss their psychiatric condition for the fear of stigmatization, and may account for 45% of people failing to share their emotional problems with their physicians (Cape & McCullech, 1999; Tylee & Walters, 2007). Another factor is that patients do not consider their psychiatric symptomatology as sufficiently unusual or troublesome to be mentioned until the underlying anxiety is identified (Harman et al., 2002; Ansseau et al., 2004). Kessler et al. found different styles of symptom attribution, and showed that patients who attribute a psychological cause are more likely to be recognized when compared to patients who normalize or minimize their symptoms. Normalisers were determined as younger and male patients (Kessler et al., 1999). Harman et al. argued that reimbursement issues or concerns over a patient's willingness to be diagnosed with an anxiety disorder could also be possible explanations (Harman et al., 2002). Besides these, a qualitative study had shown that patients were open to suggestions from their GPs or otherwise. Furthermore, several described their GPs as "marvellous" or "has never let me down". They believed it was helpful to talk to someone about their problem; however the search for this person was seen as difficult. Patients expressed the need for an easier access to professional help, suggesting their GPs should be more active in referrals, checking up on the patients' progress through phone calls, follow-up sessions, and home visits. Patients also expressed concern about interfering their GP's busy schedule, because of GP's involvement with more pressing medical cases. However some also conserve their hope for their GPs to do more than prescribe drugs, waiting for encouragement of to disclose their emotional or psychological problems. Another concern of theirs was the waiting time, since they wish to speak to someone at the moment they are feeling bad, instead of waiting for appointments (Kadam et al., 2001).

Since GAD is highly prevalent in the primary care setting, patients with the disorder are likely to be high users of primary care health services, both in terms of the frequency of visits and the sheer number of patients contacting primary care providers because of problems associated with the disorder (Wittchen & Hoyer, 2001). Young et al. showed that during a 1-year period, 84.3% of individuals with an anxiety disorder only visit PCPs (Young et al., 2001). Harman et al. found the proportion of visits to PCPs as 46.5-48.2%, which still holds true today. They also reported that anxiety disorder diagnose were recorded more often during visits where the physician had seen the patient before, and a depression diagnosis had also been recorded during that same visit (Harman et al., 2002). Patients with pure GAD are 1.6 times more likely to have four or more visits to PCPs than patients without GAD or major depressive episodes (MDE) (Wittchen, 2002). Bélanger et al. determined that patients with positive screening for GAD reported more annual medical visits (5.3 versus 3.4) than other patients, and 44.5% of the positive screening group reported consulting a family physician five times or more yearly, compared with 20.0% in the negative screening group. However, they did not report consulting other resources more often, suggesting that patients with GAD might mostly seek treatment from PCPs (Bélanger et al., 2005). Kronke et al. determined the self-reported 2.9 (2.2-3.6) physician visits in the preceding 3 months (Kroenke et al., 2007).

GAD patients have to be identified so they can be properly treated. Wagner et al. found that family physicians (FPs) diagnosed 39% of cases correctly while 29.3% left with no psychological diagnosis (Wagner et al., 2006).

There is an obvious need for tools that will help PCPs in diagnosing and monitoring GAD patients. There are several recommended specifically for GAD, such as Generalized Anxiety Disorder Inventory (GADI), GAD-7; tools for severity assessment such as Hamilton Anxiety Scale (HAM-A); and tools for measurement of functional impairment due to anxiety such as Overall Anxiety Severity and Impairment Scale (OASIS). Web-based screening can also be a choice as being cost-efficient (Allgulander, 2009; Katzman, 2009; Roy-Byrne, 2009). Ruiz et al. showed that GAD-7 highly correlated not only with specific anxiety measures but also with disability measures, which can be used for exploring the level of disability in GAD patients in primary care setting (Ruiz et al., 2011).

In the absence of systematic screening, 30-40% of anxiety and depression patients are identified in primary care setting. There are studies showing evidence for and against the screening. Some reviews point that screening alone does not improve patient's outcome. However, others concluded that screening has increased benefits when combined with effective treatment and follow up. A barrier for screening is that tools' length, specificity for a single disorder or both. Means-Christensen et al. recommended Anxiety and Depression Detector (ADD) as screening instrument for anxiety and depressive disorders in primary care. ADD's sensitivity and specificity ranges between 0.87-1.0 and 0.42-0.68, respectively (Means-Christensen et al.; 2001). Rollman et al. suggested that PRIME-MD can be used in identifying primary care patients with GAD as a part of broader strategy to improve quality of care for GAD patients (Rollman et al., 2005).

PCPs have to use their advantage of continuous contact and communication skills for efficient history taking. To aid accurate diagnosis and to rule out other possible diagnosis, both the patient's and the family's histories should be assessed carefully. Recent life events and other health problems including depression, substance or alcohol abuse and dependence should be noted. Multiple visits to PCPs, consultations with different specialists such as gastroenterologists, and consultations that end with no definite diagnosis should be carefully considered (Katzman, 2009).

4. Burden of GAD in primary care

There is abundant evidence not only on the impairment and disability but also the reduced quality of life in GAD patients. Hospitalization and loss of productivity were the two major components of costs both in patients with and without comorbidity. Health care utilization rates were higher among those with comorbid GAD patients compared to pure GAD (Lieb et al., 2005).

The burden of disability is clearly greater as the number of comorbidities increases (Wittchen et al., 2002; Kroenke et al., 2007; Löwe et al., 2008). Majority of pure GAD patients (66.7%) report impairment of occupational functioning, and selfreported disability days were 9.9 days in the preceding month. This was reported as 15.3 days for patients with pure MDE, and 16.5 days for comorbid GAD and MDE (Witthchen et al., 2002). Kroenke et al. reported in their study that self-reported disability days of the patients with pure GAD during the previous 3 months were 18.1 days (Kroenke et al., 2007). A recent study comparing the functional impact of different anxiety disorders and their combinations showed that disability in GAD was significantly less present in comparison with other anxiety disorders. However, all measures of functioning and disability, except for physical functioning, showed substantial impairment in the overall sample when compared to general population. (Sherborne et al., 2010). ESEMed study found that GAD is associated with substantial level of disability as well as a decrease in the quality of life (Alonso et al., 2004). Revicki et al. showed that anxiety symptoms of GAD patients in primary care settings were associated with impairments in generic health status, disability, disease-specific quality of life, and preference-based measures of health-related quality of life (Revicki et al., 2008). In the WHO Primary Care study, 27% of the patients with GAD reported moderate or severe social disability, with a mean loss of 4.6 work days due to disability in the month preceding the assessment. When GAD was accompanied by major depression, the mean number of lost work days increased to 8.0 days (Lieb et al., 2005).

Presence of GAD, especially comorbidity with major depression, leads substantial impairment of social, professional, and family conditions rated by Sheehan disability scale (Wittchen & Hoyer, 2001; Ansseau et al., 2005; Olfson and Gameroff, 2007). The most serious effects of GAD were observed in the subscales for emotional role limitations and physical health role limitations (Stein, 2003). In a study where Medical Outcomes Study Short Form-20 was used to determine functioning in GAD patients, all six domains of the scale were determined as impaired (Kroenke et al., 2007).
Andlin-Sobocki and Wittchen reported total direct medical costs at €1958 and €3194 and indirect costs at €969 and €1659 for GAD and GAD with comorbidity, respectively (Andlin-Sobocki and Wittchen, 2002). Olfson and Gameroff found that patients with GAD had a significantly higher median medical cost than patients without GAD ($2775 versus $1448), and patients with GAD and high pain interference had the highest mean predicted medical cost, $42.620. They also showed that GAD patients had a greater likelihood of making an emergency department visit (Olfson and Gameroff, 2007).

5. Management of GAD in primary care

The proper management of GAD in the primary care settings should not include only pharmacotherapy or psychotherapy but also education of patients and their families, counselling for lifestyle changes, as well as beneficial, continuous support, insomnia management, and development of coping strategies to manage their worries (Culpepper, 2002). There is no evidence-based approach for the combination of different treatment options for GAD patients so there is a need for further researches including large study populations targeted on current practice (Allgulander, 2009).
Education about GAD for both patients and their families must include its waxing and waning nature that can be managed by therapeutic interventions, compliance monitoring and feedback, and it should not reflect either moral weakness or character flaws leading to stigmatisation issue. Counseling; lifestyle changes like exercise, decreasing alcohol, caffeine, and tobacco consumption; regulating sleep; and controlling external stimuli for sleep improvement are encouraged. As insomnia, acute or chronic, is a norm among patients, PCPs have to understand and monitor its severity. Questions about "sleep hygiene", use of alcohol, daytime sleepiness and problems in functioning can be helpful. Although patients often require short-term pharmacological therapy for their insomnia at the time of initial diagnosis (especially if insomnia is the presenting symptom), or at times of acute exacerbations, the priority of the physician should be helping patients to develop appropriate lifestyle changes that will promote its long-term control. GAD patients often find themselves rehashing problems and unmet expectations, especially during exacerbations, which they find hard to cope with. Simple anxiety coping techniques that help in gaining improved sense of self-control in times of crises can be taught (Culpepper, 2002;Allgulander, 2009; Davidson et al., 2010).
GAD patients deserve effective medical treatment with short and long-term goals. The short-term goals of treatment include reduction in somatic and psychic symptoms, and resolution of insomnia. Long-term goals should include achieving fully functional status that is affected by anxiety, preventing relapses or recurrences, and treatment of comorbid disorders GAD patients suffer from, such as depression. PCPs need to be aware of short and long-term adverse effects of their treatment like worsening of insomnia and agitation, and weight gain and sexual dysfunction, respectively (Culpepper, 2002).

Pharmacotherapy is the most common treatment option chosen by the physicians that needs to be emphasized as an extended treatment option. There are several treatment guidelines and a general consensus among these guidelines is that the first-line pharmacotherapy for GAD patients should include selective serotonin reuptake inhibitors (SSRIs) or serotonin-norepinephrine reuptake inhibitors (SNRIs) (Katzman, 2009). The SSRIs such as paroxetine, first licensed SSRI for GAD, escitalopram; SNRIs such as venlafaxine, and duloxetine (recently approved in United States for GAD treatment) , buspirone, and benzodiazepins are commonly used agents in primary care (Katzman, 2009; Davidson et al., 2010). Tricyclic antidepressants and monoamine oxidase inhibitors should be reserved for patients not responding other regimens as they have potential for lethal overdose and serious adverse effects. Benzodiazepines are generally recommended for short-term use as they provide immediate relief of insomnia and somatic symptoms; however, those have less effect on psychological symptoms. Their long-term use causes problems of addiction and withdrawal leading conflicts with PCPs. Benzodiazepine use is also problematic for elderly due to the side effects like falling, memory impairment, and loss of coordination, drowsiness and confusion. PCPs have to be aware of adverse effects of these substances when used with other drugs like hypnotics, sedating antidepressants, opiate analgesics, anticonvulsants, anti histamines, and alcohol. (Culpepper, 2002; Davidson et al., 2010). Buspirone has disadvantages of delayed onset effect, short half-life , failure to treat comorbid anxiety or depressive disorders, and is generally less effective than the benzodiazepines, so it is not recommended as first-line treatment for GAD. Hydroxyzine, an antihistaminic, was also reported to be effective for GAD. Due to its sedating and anticholinergic effects, slow onset of action, and lack of efficacy for its comorbids, it is not preferred as first-line treatment (Davidson et al., 2010). SSRIs and an SNRI, venlafaxine are all equally efficient for treating GAD. When choosing between them, some parameters that need to be considered are cost and generic availability, the risk of breakthrough symptoms when a dose is missed, the ease of titration, the potential interaction with other drugs, and adverse effects. Venlafaxine, the first approved drug for GAD, is a valuable first-line treatment option for PCPs, indicated for long treatment of GAD, and also effective in comorbid depressive symptoms and depression. Its dosage should be titrated to minimise its adverse effects, such as nausea, dizziness, dry month, sleepiness. Patients should be monitored for a significant increase in blood pressure. Adverse effects include orthostatic hypotension, sweating, and urinary hesitancy (Culpepper, 2002; Davidson et al., 2010). Paroxetine has the disadvantages of long-term weight gain, and withdrawal symptoms in case of dose omission. Evidence is emerging for atypical antipsychotics that they are effective in the treatment of patients with anxiety disorders both as monotherapy and augmentation to the standard treatment (Katzman, 2009; Davidson et al., 2010).

There are different psychotherapy approaches and the most commonly used one is Cognitive-Behavioural Therapy (CBT). CBT includes psychoeducation, symptom management techniques, cognitive restructuring, exposure to anxiety producing events, relaxation training, and self-monitoring as important first-line treatment options in GAD with the advantage of patient preference and lack of adverse effects (Katzman, 2009). Although it was demonstrated that CBT is the most effective psychological treatment for GAD, clinical response for the treatment was found at less than 50% (Davidson et al., 2010). It is difficult to deliver the treatment adequately, as it needs extensive training of the therapist and time to take effect (van Boeijen et al., 2005). Although it is not possible for PCPs to provide CBT to their GAD patients they should act as guides in selection of experienced CBT therapists, prescribe and monitor pharmacotherapy in coordination with the patient's therapist, and help patients to use the therapeutic approaches of CBT following the conclusion of formal therapy, especially when they meet new stressors. Attempts have been made for CBT modifications such as 'self-help' approaches including 'bibliotherapy' (written format, self-help manuals), communication with peers, computerised systems, using a telephone and interactive voice response (Bower et al., 2001; van Boeijen et al., 2005a, Allgulander, 2009). Bower et al. provided some preliminary evidence about self-help packages may offer some clinical advantages over routine primary care for anxiety and depressive disorders and van Boeijen et al. concluded that with more time spent on guidance on the use of the self-help manual, positive results can be achieved for even the patients with longstanding anxiety symptoms (Bower et al., 2001; van Boeijen et al., 2005a). It was shown in the study that the primary care patients with GAD may be treated by their GPs as effectively as after their referral to a psychiatric outpatient clinic, and self-help manual usage is easier for GPs than less structured guidelines resulting in fewer referrals to specialized care (van Boeijen et al., 2005b). Principles of CBT can also be useful while counselling with "high utilisers" and patients suffering acute exacerbations. PCPs can help patients identify and correct their misconceptions about events they perceive as worrying and automatic thought processes that underline the misconceptions, and to develop self-regulation of these thoughts, feelings, and behaviours, namely cognitive restructuring (Culpepper, 2002). Another form of promising psychotherapy for GAD patients is the "well-being therapy" (Davidson et al., 2010).

A recent study published recommended a "unified approach" to the diagnosis, care management, and pharmacotherapy of primary care anxiety addressing the difficulty of assessing and managing multiple anxiety disorders in the primary care setting. The method emphasizes the identification of other medical or psychiatric comorbidities that can complicate the treatment, an approach for the initial education of the patient and discussion about treatment based on motivational interviewing, valid monitoring, an algorithmic approach for the selection of initial pharmacotherapy, and selection of alternative or adjunctive treatments (Roy-Byrne et al., 2009). This approach as a part of flexible treatment-delivery model, namely CALM ("Coordinated Anxiety Learning and Management"), was studied as a randomised controlled trial and compared with usual care in primary care settings. Roy-Byrne concluded that for patients with anxiety disorders treated by PCPs, a collaborative care resulted in greater improvement in managing anxiety symptoms and functional disability, and increasing quality of care over 18 months (Roy-Byrne et al., 2010).

6. Quality of care in primary care

Young et al., defining poor-quality care as no care or inappropriate care in their study, showed that 80.5% of individuals visiting only PCPs had a poor-quality of care. Patients receiving poor-quality care from PCPs were less likely to report evaluation of mental health, recommendation of psychiatric medication, or referral to a mental health specialist. Patients not receiving appropriate care were most often most often from the following groups: men, black, older adults, young adults, people with only primary or no education, and people of lower socioeconomic status (Young et al., 2001). Stein et al. found that the level of appropriate care for anxiety disorders was moderate to low in patients that attended a university affiliated primary care practice. Nearly one third of the patients had received counselling from their PCPs, with less than 10% receiving help from a mental health professional, including multiple elements of CBT. Approximately 40% of patients underwent appropriate pharmacotherapy in the preceding three months. However, only 25% received it at a minimally adequate dose and duration. Different studies determined different factors that had effects on receiving appropriate treatment. In one, the patients with comorbid depression and/or medical illnesses were more likely to receive appropriate treatment, while patients from ethnic minorities were less likely (Stein et al., 2004). Hyde et al., found that with greater severity of disease, measured by total score of GHQ-12, male patients had a significantly increased probability of receiving active treatment (Hyde et al, 2005). Weisberg et al. also emphasised in their study that racial/ethnic minority groups were less likely to be receiving treatments from psychiatrists (Weisberg et al., 2007).

Young et al. discussed that there are many factors that can contribute to improper care and management of depressive and anxiety disorders. These include the perceived need, willingness for care, insurance coverage, and detection by physicians, and knowledge and beliefs of health care providers regarding effective treatment (Young et al., 2001). In a study carried out with a subsample of ESEMeD, the percentage of patients receiving adequate treatment in specialised and general medical care were 31.8% and 30.5%, respectively. In this study factors associated with appropriate treatment were living in a large city, a high education level, and a good self-rated health state (Fernändes et al., 2006). Weisberg et al. pointed out that primary care patient who were not receiving pharmacotherapy for their anxiety disorder claimed two main reasons for this. One was that their doctor never recommended treatment and the other was that they did not believe in medication for emotional problems. In the same study the most commonly claimed reasons for not receiving psychotherapy were patients' lack of belief in psychotherapy, and their ignorance about the treatability of their emotional problems. Other barriers frequently mentioned for psychotherapy, but rarely for pharmacotherapy were cost, convenience, not knowing how to get into therapy (Weisberg et al., 2007). All of these seem to have a common base with barriers for accurate diagnosis.

In a study searching for the cause and length of delays in care of specific subcategories of anxiety disorders, it was found that GAD patients seek help from their family physician or his/her equivalent 10.3 months after showing symptoms and visit an anxiety clinic for 83.8 months after showing symptoms (Wagnet et al., 2006).

7. Interventions for primary care

It is obvious that problems encountered in diagnosis and management of GAD in PHC is multifaceted and multiphase and there is a need of integration of mental health in primary care. Primary care has the potential to reach the whole community as being the first point of contact and patient-centred interaction depending on long-lasting, trust based communication. This is also a support for the continuity of care, which is especially important for GAD patients having relapses and remissions. These advantages of primary care, along with all its handicaps can facilitate an integrated treatment approach (Rakel, 2007).

In a systematic review evaluating the effectiveness of interventions aimed to improve recognition, diagnosis and management of patients with anxiety disorders, it was concluded that the most promising choice of care in general practice is a combination of professional interventions with organisational interventions, including an education component where an external expert such as a nurse therapist or a psychologist is introduced (Heideman et al., 2005).

A report prepared by WHO and WONCA (World Organization of Family Doctors) put forward the principles for the integration of mental health into primary care that are, naturally, appropriate for GAD. Some of these principles are supported in this paper, especially for GAD. These include: adequate training of primary care workers, limited and doable tasks for mental care, support to primary care by specialist mental health professionals and facilities, access to essential psychotropic medications in primary care, and collaboration of PCPs with other government non-health sectors, nongovernmental organizations (WHO&WONCA, 2008).

8. Conclusions

GAD is the most prevalent anxiety disorder in primary care. Its comorbidity is well-documented, leading higher economic burden and a decrease in quality of life. Primary care settings are the best way of ensuring that GAD patients can get the care they need as they are accessible, affordable, acceptable, and cost-effective. Barriers for diagnosis and management of GAD in primary care include: nature of disease, patient- and physician-related factors, and societal factors such as stigmatisation. The proper management of GAD is also multifaceted, and multistage, which means that PCPs needs appropriate counselling with guidelines and screening tools. Primary care is the place that can ensure patients achieve care in a holistic manner, addressing both their physical and mental health needs. Advantages of primary care have to be taken into account for quality improvement programs that will be implemented to enhance awareness and utilization of appropriate treatment options.

9. Future research efforts

- Researches accurately reflecting, and modelling the complexities of recognition in primary care
- Models that increase patients' and society's awareness and physicians' recognition of GAD
- Effect of patients' attribution styles on the physician's recognition and recommendations needed to be studied for solutions to cope with the situation and achieving a more accurate diagnosis
- Development of reliable and easy to use screening tools/instruments, and increased frequency of their use in primary care setting
- Professional and organisational interventions for improvement of diagnosis and treatment of GAD need to be studied with a long-term follow up
- Evidence to support the therapeutic value of combined treatments for more complex cases
- Data showing the degree of unmet needs for treatment of GAD patients with economic burden, due to inappropriate treatment and inadequate inpatient and outpatient interventions
- Studies that provide a chance to understand the reasons underlying low rates of quality care, and implementation of measures to improve them.

10. References

Allgulander C. (2006). Generalized anxiety disorder: What are we missing? *European Neuropsychopharmacology*. Vol.16, Suppl No.2, (May 2006), pp. S101-108, ISSN: 0924-977X.

Allgulander C. (2009). Generalized anxiety disorder: between now and DSM-V. *Psychiatric Clinics of North America*. Vol.32, No.3, (September 2009), pp. 611-28, ISSN 0193-953X.

Alonso J, Angermeyer MC, Bernert S, Bruffaerts R, Brugha TS, Bryson H, de Girolamo G, Graaf R, Demyttenaere K, Gasquet I, Haro JM, Katz SJ, Kessler RC, Kovess V, Lépine JP, Ormel J, Polidori G, Russo LJ, Vilagut G, Almansa J, Arbabzadeh-Bouchez S, Autonell J, Bernal M, Buist-Bouwman MA, Codony M, Domingo-Salvany A, Ferrer M, Joo SS, Martínez-Alonso M, Matschinger H, Mazzi F, Morgan Z, Morosini P, Palacín C, Romera B, Taub N, Vollebergh WA; ESEMeD/MHEDEA 2000 Investigators, European Study of the Epidemiology of Mental Disorders (ESEMeD) Project. (2004). Disability and quality of life impact of mental disorders in Europe: results from the European Study of the Epidemiology of Mental Disorders (ESEMeD) project. *Acta Psychiatrica Scandinavica*. Suppl. 420, pp. 38-46, ISSN 0001-690X.

American Psychiatric Association. (2000). *Diagnostic and statistical manuel of mental disorders-TR, 4th ed.* American Psychiatric Association, Washington DC, ISBN: 0 89042 025 4

Andlin-Sobocki P, Wittchen HU. (2005). Cost of anxiety disorders in Europe. *European Journal of Neurology*. Vol.12, Supplement No. 1, (June 2005), pp.39-44, ISSN: 1468-1331.

Ansseau M, Dierick M, Buntinkx F, Cnockaert P, De Smedt J, Van Den Haute M, Vander Mijnsbrugge D. (2004). High prevalence of mental disorders in primary care. *Journal of Affective Disorders*. Vol.78, No.1, (January 2004), pp. 78.49-55, ISSN 0165-0327.

Ansseau M, Fischler B, Dierick M, Mignon A, Leyman S. Prevalance and impact of generalized anxiety disorder and major depression in primary care in Belgium and Luxemburg: the GADIS study care in Belgium and Luxemburg: the GADIS study. *European Psychiatry*. Vol.20, No.3, (May 2005), pp. 229-235, ISSN: 0924-9338.

Bijl RV, Ravelli A, van Zessen G. (1998). Prevalence of psychiatric disorder in the general population: results of The Netherlands Mental Health Survey and Incidence Study (NEMESIS). *Social Psychiatry and Psychiatric Epidemiology*. Vol. 33, No. 12, (December 1998), pp. 587-95, ISSN: 1433-9285.

Bélanger L, Ladouceur R, Morin CM. (2005). Generalized anxiety disorder and health care use. *Canadian Family Physician*. Vol.51, No.10, (October 2005), pp. 1362-3, ISSN: 1715-5258.

Bower P, Richards D, Lovell K. (2001). The clinical and cost-effectiveness of self-help treatments for anxiety and depressive disorders in primary care: a systematic review. *The British Journal of General Practice*. Vol. 51, No. 471, (October 2001), pp. 838-45, ISSN: 0960-1643.

Cape J, McCulloch Y. (1999). Patients' reasons for not presenting emotional problems in general practice consultations. The British Journal of General Practice. Vol.49, No.448, (November 1999), pp. 875-9, ISSN: 0960-1643.

Carter RM, Wittchen HU, Pfister H, Kessler RC. (2001). One-year prevalence of subthreshold and threshold DSM-IV generalized anxiety disorder in a nationally representative sample. *Depression and Anxiety*. Vol. 13, No. 2, (March 2001), pp. 78-88, ISSN: 1520-6394.

Culpepper L. (2002). Generalized anxiety disorder in primary care: emerging issues in management and treatment. *The Journal of Clinical Psychiatry*. Vol. 63, Suppl.8 (2002), pp. 35-42, ISSN: 1555-2101.

Davidson JR, Feltner DE, Dugar A. (2010). Management of generalized anxiety disorder in primary care: identifying the challenges and unmet needs. *The Primary Care Companion to the Journal of Clinical Psychiatry*. Vol.12, No.2, (2010).

Fernández A, Haro JM, Codony M, Vilagut G, Martínez-Alonso M, Autonell J, Salvador-Carulla L, Ayuso-Mateos JL, Fullana MA, Alonso J. (2006). Treatment adequacy of anxiety and depressive disorders: primary versus specialised care in Spain. *Journal of Affective Disorders*. Vol.96, No.1-2, (November 2006), pp. 9-20, ISSN 0165-0327.

Harman JS, Rollman BL, Hanusa BH, Lenze EJ, Shear MK. (2005). Physician office visits of adults for anxiety disorders in the United States, 1985-1998. *Journal of General Internal Medicine*. Vol.17, No.3, (March 2002), pp. 165-72, ISSN: 1525-1497.

Heideman J, van Rijswijk E, van Lin N, de Loos S, Laurant M, Wensing M, van de Lisdonk E, Grol R. (2005). Interventions to improve management of anxiety disorders in general practice: a systematic review. *The British Journal of General Practice*. Vol.55, No.520 (November 2005), pp. 867-74, ISSN: 0960-1643.

Hyde J, Evans J, Sharp D, Croudace T, Harrison G, Lewis G, Araya R. (2005). Deciding who gets treatment for depression and anxiety: a study of consecutive GP attenders. *The British Journal of General Practice*. Vol.55, No.520, (November 2005), pp.846-53, ISSN: 0960-1643.

Kadam UT, Croft P, McLeod J, Hutchinson M. (2001). A qualitative study of patients' views on anxiety and depression. *The British Journal of General Practice*. Vol.51, No. 466, (May 2001), pp. 375-80, ISSN: 0960-1643.

Katzman MA. Current considerations in the treatment of generalized anxiety disorder. (2009). *CNS Drugs*. Vol.23, No.2, (February 2009), pp. 103-20, ISSN: 1179-1934.

Kessler D, Bennewith O, Lewis G, Sharp D. (2002). Detection of depression and anxiety in primary care: follow up study. *The British Medical Journal*. Vol.235, No.7371, (November 2002), pp. 1016-7, ISSN: 1468-5833.

Kessler D, Lloyd K, Lewis G, Gray DP. (1999). Cross sectional study of symptom attribution and recognition of depression and anxiety in primary care. *The British Medical Journal*. Vol.318, No.7181 (February 1999), pp. 436-9, ISSN: 1468-5833.

Kroenke K, Jackson JL, Chamberlin J. (1997). Depressive and anxiety disorders in patients presenting with physical complaints: clinical predictors and outcome. *The American Journal of Medicine*. Vol.103, No.5, (November 1997), pp. 339-47, ISSN: 0002-9343.

Kroenke K, Spitzer RL, Williams JB, Monahan PO, Löwe B. (2007). Anxiety disorders in primary care: prevalence, impairment, comorbidity, and detection. *Annals of Internal Medicine*. Vol.146, No.5 (March 2007), pp. 317-325, ISSN: 1539-3704.

Lieb R, Becker E, Altamura C. (2005). The epidemiology of generalized anxiety disorder in Europe. *European Neuropsychopharmacology* Vol.15, No.4, (August 2005), pp. 445-452, ISSN: 0924-977X.

Löwe B, Spitzer RL, Williams JB, Mussell M, Schellberg D, Kroenke K. (2008). Depression, anxiety and somatization in primary care: syndrome overlap and functional impairment. *General Hospital Psychiatry*. Vol.30, No.3, (May 2008, pp. 191-9, ISSN: 0163-8343.

Maier W, Gänsicke M, Freyberger HJ, Linz M, Heun R, Lecrubier Y. (2000). Generalized anxiety disorder (ICD-10) in primary care from a cross-cultural perspective: a valid diagnostic entity? *Acta Psychiatrica Scandinavica*. Vol.101, No.1 (January 2000), pp. 29-36, ISSN: 1600-0447.

Means-Christensen AJ, Sherbourne CD, Roy-Byrne PP, Craske MG, Stein MB. (2006). Using five questions to screen for five common mental disorders in primary care: diagnostic accuracy of the Anxiety and Depression Detector. *General Hospital Psychiatry*. Vol.28, No.2, (March-April 2006), pp. 108-18, ISSN: 0163-8343.

Mergl R, Seidscheck I, Allgaier AK, Möller HJ, Hegerl U, Henkel V. (2007). Depressive, anxiety, and somatoform disorders in primary care: prevalence and recognition. *Depression and Anxiety*. Vol.24, No.3, (April 2007), pp. 185-95, ISSN: 1520-6394 .

Olfson M, Shea S, Feder A, Fuentes M, Nomura Y, Gameroff M, Weissman MM. (2000). Prevalance of anxiety, depression, and substance use disorders in an urban general medicine practice. *Archieves of Family Medicine*. Vol.9, No.9 (September-October 2000), pp. 876-883, ISSN: 1063-3987.

Olfson M, Gameroff MJ. (2007). Generalized anxiety disorder, somatic pain and health care costs. *General Hospital Psychiatry*. Vol.29, No.4, (July-August 2007), pp. 310-6, ISSN: 0163-8343.

Robert E Rakel. (2007). *Rakel Textbook of Family Medicine*. Printed in China, ISBN: 13 978 1 4160 2467 5

Revicki DA, Brandenburg N, Matza L, Hornbrook MC, Feeny D. (2008). Health-related quality of life and utilities in primary-care patients with generalized anxiety disorder. *Quality of Life Research*. Vol.17, No.10, (December 2008), pp. 1285-94, ISSN: 0962-9343.

Rodriguez BF, Weisberg RB, Pagano ME, Machan JT, Culpepper L, Keller MB. (2004). Frequency and patterns of psychiatric comorbidity in a sample of primary care patients with anxiety disorders. *Comprehensive Psychiatry*. Vol.45, No.2, (March-April 2004), pp. 129-37, ISSN: 0010-440X.

Rollman BL, Belnap BH, Mazumdar S, Zhu F, Kroenke K, Schulberg HC, Katherine Shear M. (2005). Symptomatic severity of PRIME-MD diagnosed episodes of panic and generalized anxiety disorder in primary care. *Journal of General Internal Medicine*. Vol.20, No.7, (July 2005), pp. 623-8, ISSN: 1525-1497.

Roy-Byrne PP, Wagner A. Primary care perspectives on generalized anxiety disorder. *Journal of Clinical Psychiatry*. Vol.65, No.13, (2004), pp. 20-6, ISSN: 1555-2101.

Roy-Byrne P, Veitengruber JP, Bystritsky A, Edlund MJ, Sullivan G, Craske MG, Welch SS, Rose R, Stein MB. (2009). Brief intervention for anxiety in primary care patients. *Journal of the American Board of Family Medicine*. Vol.22, No.2, (March-April 2009), pp. 175-86, ISSN: 1558-7118.

Roy-Byrne P, Craske MG, Sullivan G, Rose RD, Edlund MJ, Lang AJ, Bystritsky A, Welch SS, Chavira DA, Golinelli D, Campbell-Sills L, Sherbourne CD, Stein MB. (2010). Delivery of evidence-based treatment for multiple anxiety disorders in primary care: a randomized controlled trial. *JAMA*. Vol.303, No.19, (May 2010), pp. 1921-8, ISSN: 0098-7484.

Ruiz MA, Zamorano E, García-Campayo J, Pardo A, Freire O, Rejas J. Validity of the GAD-7 scale as an outcome measure of disability in patients with generalized anxiety disorders in primary care. *Journal of Affective Disorders*. Vol.128, No.3, (February 2011), pp. 277-86, ISSN 0165-0327.

Sherbourne CD, Sullivan G, Craske MG, Roy-Byrne P, Golinelli D, Rose RD, Chavira DA, Bystritsky A, Stein MB. Functioning and disability levels in primary care outpatients with one or more anxiety disorders. (2010). *Psychological Medicine*. Vol.40, No.12 (December 2010), pp. 2059-68, ISSN: 0033-2917.

Serrano-Blanco A, Palao DJ, Luciano JV, Pinto-Meza A, Luján L, Fernández A, Roura P, Bertsch J, Mercader M, Haro JM. (2010). Prevalence of mental disorders in primary care: results from the diagnosis and treatment of mental disorders in primary care study (DASMAP). *Social Psychiatry Psychiatric Epidemiology*. Vol.45, No.2 (February 2010), pp. 201-10, ISSN: 1433-9285.

Shearer SL. (2007). Recent advances in the understanding and treatment of anxiety disorders. *Primary Care*. Vol.34, No.3, (September 2007), pp. 475-504, ISSN: 1558-299X.

Stein MB. Attending to anxiety disorders in primary care. (2003). *Journal of Clinical Psychiatry*. Vol.64, Supplement 15, (2003), pp. 35-9, ISSN: 1555-2101.

Stein MB, Sherbourne CD, Craske MG, Means-Christensen A, Bystritsky A, Katon W, Sullivan G, Roy-Byrne PP. (2004). Quality of care for primary care patients with anxiety disorders. *The American Journal of Psychiatry*. Vol.161, No.12 (December 2004), pp. 2230-7, ISSN: 0002-953X.

Tylee A, Walters P. (2007). Underrecognition of anxiety and mood disorders in primary care: why does the problem exist and what can be done? *Journal of Clinical Psychiatry*. Vol.68, Supplement 2, (2007), pp. 27-30, ISSN 0165-0327.

Ustun TB, Sartorius N. *Mental Illness in General Health Care, An International Study*. England: Wiley; 1995. pp. 39-55, ISBN: 0 471 95491 8.

van Boeijen CA, van Balkom AJ, van Oppen P, Blankenstein N, Cherpanath A, van Dyck R. (2005a). Efficacy of self-help manuals for anxiety disorders in primary care: a systematic review. *Family Practice*. Vol.22, No.2, (April 2005), pp. 192-6, ISSN: 0263-2136.

van Boeijen CA, van Oppen P, van Balkom AJ, Visser S, Kempe PT, Blankenstein N, van Dyck R. (2005b). Treatment of anxiety disorders in primary care practice: a randomised controlled trial. *The British Journal of General Practice*. Vol.55, No.519, (October 2005), pp. 763-9, ISSN: 0960-1643.

Wagner R, Silove D, Marnane C, Rouen D. (2006). Delays in referral of patients with social phobia, panic disorder and generalized anxiety disorder attending a specialist anxiety clinic. *Journal of Anxiety Disorders*. Vol.20, No.3, (2006), pp. 363-71, ISSN: 0887-6185.

Weisberg RB, Dyck I, Culpepper L, Keller MB. (2007). Psychiatric treatment in primary care patients with anxiety disorders: a comparison of care received from primary care providers and psychiatrists. *The American Journal of Psychiatry*. Vol.164, No.2, (February 2007), pp. 276-82, ISSN: 0002-953X.

Wittchen H-U, Hoyer J. Generalized Anxiety Disorder: Nature and Course. (2001). *Journal of Clinical Psychiatry* Vol.62, No.11, (2001), pp. 15-18, ISSN: 1555-2101.

Wittchen HU, Kessler RC, Beesdo K, Krause P, Höfler M, Hoyer J. (2002). Generalized anxiety and depression in primary care: prevalence, recognition, and management. *Journal of Clinical Psychiatry*. Vol.63, Supplement No. 8 (2002), pp.24-34, ISSN: 0887-6185.

World Health Organization: ICD-10, Version 2007. http://apps.who.int/classifications/apps/icd/icd10online/.

World Health Organization and World Organization of Family Doctors (WONCA) 2008. *Integrating Mental Health into Primary Care: A Global Perspective*. Printed in Singapore, ISBN: 978 92 4 156368 0.

Young AS, Klap R, Sherbourne CD, Wells KB. (2001). The quality of care for depressive and anxiety disorders in the United States. *Archieves of General Psychiatry*. Vol.58, No.1, (January 2001), pp. 55-61, ISSN: 0003-990X.

5

Prevention of Childhood Anxiety Disorders

Sarosh Khalid-Khan
Dept of Psychiatry
Division of Child and adolescent Psychaitry
Queen's University, Kingston, Ontario
Canada

1. Introduction

Anxiety disorders consist of excessive and frequent worrying which causes physical and mental distress and impairment in overall functioning (NIH&SAMHSA, 1999). Anxiety disorders are the most common mental health problems reported by children, adolescents and adults (Costello, Angold, & Burns, 1996; Goodman, Ford, Richards, Gatward, & Melzer, 2000; Kessler et al., 2005; Muris, Merckelbach, Mayer, & Prins, 2000). The prevalence of childhood anxiety disorders ranges from 10% to 22% (Dadds, Spence, Holland, Barrett, & Laurens, 1997.) with lifetime prevalence estimated to be about 28.8% (Kessler et al., 2005) with ages of onset between 10 to 12 years (Kessler et al, 2005). About one in 6 children have anxiety that causes impairment in their daily lives (Dadds, Spence, Holland, Barrett, & Laurens, 1997). There are many sequelae of anxiety disorders including an elevated risk for later development of mood disorders, other anxiety disorders, substance use as well as physical health concerns (Kessler et al., 2005). In addition, anxiety disorders can result in much psychosocial suffering including higher rates of dropping out of school, lower income levels, difficulties in intimate relationships and difficulty keeping one's employment (Beidel & Turner, 1998; LeFauve et al., 2004; Lewinsohn & Clarke, 1999; Pine, Cohen, Gurley, Brook, & Ma, 1998; Schatzberg, Samson, & Rothschild, 1998; Woodward & Fergusson, 2001).

In addition to the impairment and suffering experienced by children and adolescents, there is a significant cost associated with anxiety disorders. It is estimated that the United States spends more than $42 billion a year on anxiety disorders (Greenberg et al, 1999). In a 2009 Status Report, the Canadian Pediatric Society indicated that mental health problems continue to grow among children and youth and are predicted to increase by 50% by the year 2020 (Children's Mental Health Ontario Pre-Budget Submission 2010). However, three out of four children who need specialized services do not receive them as access to mental health services continues to be insufficient and in some cases declining (Children's Mental Health Ontario Pre-Budget Submission, 2010). In clinics, waiting lists are long and no-show and attrition rates sometimes are over 50% (Weist et al,1999). Many children who do receive clinical intervention fail to respond (Barrett, Dadds, & Rapee, 1996; Donovan & Spence, 2000; Weisz et al., 1997) or experience recurrence of symptoms despite receiving treatment (Last et al., 1996). Yet, treating mental health issues in children and youth in a timely way prevent excessive health care costs and ensure productive lives (Children's Mental Health Ontario Pre-Budget Submission, 2010).

Anxiety disorders are diagnosed in children and adolescents if they begin to interfere in normal daily functioning in three domains i.e. home, school and with peers. Anxiety disorders are listed under the following headings: generalized anxiety disorder, separation anxiety disorder, social anxiety disorder, specific phobia, panic disorder, obsessive-compulsive disorder and post-traumatic stress disorder (DSM-IV, 2000). There are no definitive biological or psychological tests for anxiety disorders and diagnoses are made clinically based on information from multiple sources i.e.teachers, parents or other caregivers in other settings. Anxiety disorders in children often first manifest as physiological symptoms and are misinterpreted as physical illness. Stomach aches are a common physical manifestation of anxiety in younger children. Some young children may manifest temper tantrums when in fact they are having panic attacks. In adolescents headaches mixed in with nausea and stomach aches are more common. These physical symptoms often result in avoidance behavior which often manifests as school refusal. Behaviors resulting from anxiety such as school refusal and temper tantrums are viewed as oppositionality. Due to the avoidance as the end result of anxiety disorders, they are often unrecognized and hence untreated in children. Moreover, these children are usually perfectionistic and want to please so they further go unnoticed especially in a classroom setting. On the other hand, children with disruptive behavior disorders are noticed more and thus are more frequently referred for treatment (Compton et al, 2004, In-Albon & Schneider, 2007).

Currently, the most effective treatment available for anxiety disorders are cognitive-behavioral therapy (CBT) and antidepressant medications specifically the serotonin reuptake inhibitors (SSRIs). Both treatments alone are empirically supported options. For mild to moderate symptoms, usually CBT is offered first. For moderate to severe symptoms, a combination of CBT and SSRI is often helpful. Families, in general, prefer non-medical or psychosocial interventions at initial evaluation (Walker et al, 2001). However, often CBT therapists are in short supply (Andrews et al, 2002).

2. Prevention

Due to these concerns, it seems logical to move toward services that provide prevention of anxiety disorders. The benefits of prevention are that a large number of people can be targeted over a short period of time, it is more cost effective and there is reduced distress for children due to earlier intervention (Lowry-Webster, 2001). Preventive mental health programs serve two purposes. From a health care perspective, they address and identify risk and protective factors in individuals, providing for better long-term prognoses. In addition, these programs accrue economic benefits because prevention is often less expensive than the economic and societal costs once an illness has manifested (Beardslee et al, 2011).

For implementation of prevention programs, it is important to consider the risk factors, protective factors and strategies for prevention. There is a complex interplay of biological, psychological and environmental factors in the development of childhood anxiety disorders (Donovan et al, 2000). In the development of childhood anxiety the following risk factors have been implicated.

3. Risks and protective factors in childhood anxiety disorders

Puberty results in maturational changes not only physically but also emotionally. Puberty may increase risk factors for many psychiatric disorders including anxiety disorders.

According to Leen-Feldner et al, adolescents with advanced pubertal status and greater reactivity to a hyperventilation challenge were at increased risk for panic symptoms (Leen-Feldner et al, 2007).

Fear conditioning is known to be linked to the genesis of anxiety. In a study by Otto et al, 2007), risk factors for fear conditioning were examined in a nonclinical sample. Those in the sample that had higher levels of anxiety sensitivity (increased anxiety symptoms) predicted increased tendency towards fear conditioning (Otto et al,2007).

The quality of attachment between an infant and the primary caregiver is an important indicator of future development of anxiety disorders (Erickson et al, 1985; Lewis et al, 1984; Sroufe et al, 1990). In a study by Warren et al,1997, the role of attachment style on the later development of anxiety disorders was studied in 172 children at 12 months and then later at 17.5 years of age. At 12 months a pattern of anxious resistant attachment predicted later anxiety disorders, even after controlling for infant temperament and maternal anxiety.

Parental anxiety is a risk factor for childhood anxiety disorders both through the mechanism of heritability and parent's modeling of anxious behaviors (Rosenbaum et al., 1988; Turner et al, 1987; Weissman et al, 1984). It is estimated that heritability accounts for about 40-50% of anxiety symptoms in children (Thapar et al, 1995).

Behavioral inhibition has been identified by Kagan et al(Kagan et al, 1989; Kagan et al, 1991)as a stable temperament style consisting of shyness and elevated physiological arousal having a strong genetic component (DiLalla et al, 1994; Plomin et al, 1989). Children with behavior inhibition are more likely to develop an anxiety disorder (Biederman et al, 1993; Kagan, 1997; Rosenbaum et al, 1993).

Other risk factors for childhood anxiety disorders are traumatic and stressful life events following which children have higher levels of fears. Higher rates of anxiety disorders are present in children following major natural disasters (Dollinger et al, 1984). Moreover, parenting behaviors have been identified to interact with other risk factors in the development of childhood anxiety. Parents of anxious children often model, prompt, and reinforce anxious behavior in their children (Barrett et al, 1996). Other parental characteristics that contribute to risk factors for childhood anxiety are being overly controlling, critical and, overprotective (Krohne et al, 1991).

Protective factors either promote positive development or protect against risk factors. A person's temperament, cognitive ability and social competence can all serve as protective factors against developing anxiety disorders (Farrell et al, 2007). Other protective factors include parental monitoring of child's behaviors (Jessor et al., 1995), peers and adults in a child's life who are good role models (Hawkins et al, 1992) and acceptance and support by peers (Jessor et al, 1991; Quinton et al., 1993). In addition, a positive connection with the school with parental monitoring in both school and home setting and parents' having a positive relationship with the school (Greenberg et al, 2001) all contribute towards protection from risks of anxiety disorders. Lastly, the type of responses children use to cope with stressful experiences influence how much anxiety and distress they experience (Spence et al, 2001).

4. Prevention strategies

In the past few years school personnel have become interested in programming to address the social and emotional needs of children due to the resultant deleterious effects of difficulties in these areas on their academic and social functioning. In this regard, there has been a shift to implement evidence-based psychosocial treatments in schools in a preventative fashion (Miller et al, 2010). Recent governmental policy initiatives are requiring the implementation of evidence-based treatments in schools (Robertson, David & Rao, 2003). Schools are an important and dominant component of children's environment both for their academic and social learning. Having a classroom intervention by teachers and school counselors makes it easier to identify children suffering from anxiety. Teachers have unlimited access to children in their classroom and know their strengths and weaknesses well. It is not only cost-effective for teachers to provide the intervention to students but students can learn from peers and share their experiences with them thus providing support (Miller et al, 2010).

Individual cognitive behavioral therapy has been studied for childhood anxiety disorders and is effective for 70% for clinically referred children (In-Albon & Schneider, 2007). Group-based CBT has been adapted recently and researched as a school-based intervention (Barrett & Turner, 2001; Masia, Klein, Storch & Corda, 2001; Stallard, Simpson, Anderson, Hibbert & Osborn, 2007). The recent challenge for many researchers has been to study the successful implementation of these studies into a community or school setting. These studies have the challenge of following the treatment but being flexible to a real-world setting.

The Committee on Prevention of Mental Disorders (Mrazek et al, 1994) describes a continuum of interventions going from prevention at one end and treatment at the other end. The following are three main forms of prevention: universal, targeted or selective, and indicated. A *universal* preventive approaches are either designed to enhance resilience in all children (i.e. an entire grade or school population) or improve mental health regardless of risk and avoids the need for screening. Other universal programs are targeted at a specific disorder. These programs are more readily accepted because they are proactive, emphasizing positive coping skills and provided to everyone thus avoiding any possibility of stigmatization though labeling. Under the *targeted* programs, *selective* programs are for children who are at increased risk of developing disorders and involves screening. *Indicated* programs also require screening and are for individuals with minimal symptoms who do not meet diagnostic criteria for any disorder. Treatment programs target children with a diagnosed condition (Lowry-Webster et al, 2001). In this paper both the universal and targeted school-based anxiety prevention programs will be reviewed.

5. Universal prevention strategies

A study by Hains (Hains et al, 1992) examined the effectiveness of two cognitive-behavioral interventions to help adolescent boys cope with stress and other negative emotions. The project was described to all sophomores and juniors and those who were interested were invited to attend an orientation meeting. Twenty-five adolescent boys ages 15-16 year old were randomly assigned to either a group receiving cognitive restructuring or to a second group receiving anxiety management training. Both these groups were compared to a wait-list control group on measures of anxiety, anger, self-esteem, depression, and reports of anxious self-statements. Both the intervention groups showed significant decline in levels of anxiety, expression of anger, and depression. These treatment gains were maintained at an 11-week follow-up.

The FRIENDS program (Barrett et al, 2004) is a universal preventive program for both anxiety and depression with increasing evidence base and support from World Health Organization (World Health Organization, 2004). The FRIENDS program (acronym for

F=Feelings; R=Relax and feel good; I=I can do it! I can try my best!; E=Explore solutions and coping step plans; N=Now reward yourself! You've done your best!; D=Don't forget to practice; S=Smile! Stay calm for life!) consists of 10 weekly session and 2 booster sessions. This program is tailored for different developmental levels with a CBT protocol adapted from Phil Kendall's "The Coping Cat" (Kendall, 1994).. There are 2-4 parent sessions teaching parents coping strategies for their own anxiety, reinforcement strategies, contingency management and problem-solving and communications skills. The FRIENDS program has been validated as an effective prevention program for child and youth anxiety and depression (Dadds et al, 1997; Barrett et al, 2000; Lowry-Webster et al, 2001; Lowry-Webster et al, 2003; Lock et al, 2003).

Barrett et al (2000, 2001) evaluated a "train-the-trainer" model of intervention in children ages 9-10 years in grade 6. Children with internalizing symptoms were assigned to either an intervention led by a psychologist, a teacher or a control condition with a standard curriculum. The FRIENDS 12-session program was implemented as a curriculum in the classroom by training the teachers and psychologists. There were four sessions for parents. At the end, children reported considerable decrease in anxiety symptoms in either intervention by a psychologist or a teacher.

Lowry-Webster et al (2001) studied the effectiveness of the FRIENDS universal program for prevention of anxiety in 594 students aged 10-13 years randomized to either a control or an intervention condition. Both groups reported significant decrease in anxiety and the decline was significantly greater in the intervention group regardless of their risk status. A follow up study after one year by Lowry-Webster et al (2003) showed that results were maintained with the intervention group having lower scores on anxiety self-report measures. Eighty-five per cent of children in the intervention group who were scoring above the clinical cut-off for anxiety and depression were symptom free in the intervention condition compared to 31.2% in the control group.

In a study of universal prevention with 733 children enrolled in grade 6 (ages 9-10) and grade 9 (ages 14-16), Lock et al, 2003 studied children from 7 different socioeconomic school settings. The children were assigned randomly to a FRIENDS intervention program or a control condition of a standard curriculum. Students completed self-rating measures. Students who were "high risk" based on high scores on anxiety measures were given a structured diagnostic interview. Results showed a general decrease in anxiety scores which were significant for students in the intervention group at the end of the program and at 1 year follow up. This study also showed that children in Grade 6 had higher levels of anxiety before intervention but post-intervention had greater reductions in anxiety and depression at 12 month follow up compared to grade 9 children. In addition, there was a delayed effect in improvement of depression symptoms that was apparent only at the 1 year follow up. In addition, girls tended to have higher levels of anxiety than boys and girls in Grade 6 were more responsive to the intervention than Grade 9 girls.

Barrett et al (2006) evaluated the above mentioned study by Lock et al for its long term effectiveness at 36 months. The decrease in scores due to the intervention were maintained in grade 6 but not for children in grade 9 emphasizing the fact that intervention in grade 6 might be an optimal time for decreasing risk for anxiety. There were significantly fewer high-risk students at 36-month follow-up in the intervention condition than in the control condition proving the durability of prevention effects for children in Grade 6. The outcomes were noticeable for up to 3years following a brief cognitive behavioral intervention delivered by teachers within the school. For girls who had the highest anxiety and showed the biggest decline after one year, the preventive effect lasted for only 24 months.

The FRIENDS program was implemented in the UK in a school setting by Stallard et al (2007) and its effectiveness was examined. The program was delivered by school nurses to 10-11 year olds in one urban and 2 rural schools. The school nurses were supported by teachers and teacher's assistants. This was non-randomized study in which 106 children received the program. The children were assessed 6 months before the program, at the start of the program and 3 months after the program. Results showed that the levels of anxiety and self-esteem were stable 6 months before the program. Three months after the completion of the program, anxiety had significantly decreased and self-esteem had increased. Children with the most severe emotional problems benefited from the program. The study is limited by its small sample size, short follow-up and the single cohort design.

The study by Miller et al (2010) modified a locally developed CBT intervention program, Taming Worry Dragons (TWD; Garland & Clark, 2000). In a public elementary school, 118 children were randomly assigned either to an 8-week intervention or to a wait-list control. Teachers were trained in a full-day workshop by a licensed psychologist. The teachers then implemented the TWD program to all the children in the randomized treatment arm. The results showed no significant differences between the two groups and that the manualized CBT intervention did not reduce symptoms of anxiety in either self-reports or parent reports of anxiety symptoms in the general school population. The study cited its limitations as having a small sample size, absence of screening for co-morbid disorders and lack of follow-up.

6. Targeted prevention strategies

Early intervention and prevention programs can be more cost-effective in reducing the burden of illness of childhood disorders. To effectively conduct an early intervention program there should be a reliable way to screen children at risk, an access point to identify these at-risk children., and a cost-effective intervention program (Dadds, Spence, 1997).

The Queensland Early Intervention and Prevention of Anxiety Project (Dadds et al, 1997), an indicated prevention program in Australia, targeted 1,786 children ages 7-14 years to evaluate the effectiveness of a cognitive-behavioral and family-based group intervention (using the Coping Koala: Prevention Manual) for preventing the onset and development of anxiety problems in children. All the children were screened for anxiety symptoms using children self-reports and asking teachers to nominate children in their class who displayed the most anxiety. After screening, 128 children were assigned to a 10-week school-based child and parent-focused psychosocial intervention or a control group. The children received weekly 1-2 hour cognitive-behavioral sessions delivered by psychologists. The parents attended 3 child management training sessions. After completion of the program, both groups showed improvements. At six-month follow-up, the improvement in the intervention group was maintained. This group received follow up at 12 months and at 2 years (Dadds et al, 1999). At 12 months, both the intervention and the control group converged, however, at 2-year follow-up the group receiving the intervention was again superior to the control group. This study is an example of an indicated intervention targeted towards individuals who already show early signs or low levels of a disorder. Because the interventions are targeted only towards those at greatest risk, (Offord et al, 1998) they are more cost-effective and can be provided to only those who need it.

The above study was conducted by psychologists. To assess the effectiveness of an indicated early intervention and prevention program for anxiety disorders when conducted by school staff, Hunt et al, (2009) conducted a randomized controlled trial. A total of 1120 children in their first year of high school were recruited from 19 schools. Students who were at risk for the development of an anxiety disorder (1 standard deviation above the average score based on an age-related normative sample) were screened and identified. Teachers were asked to nominate 3 students with increased anxiety and subsequently 24 students were added to the study. Nine schools were randomly assigned to the control condition (n=137), and 10 to the intervention condition (n=260). A total of 260 students were entered in the study. The FRIENDS program was implemented in each school by a school counselor assisted by a support teacher both of whom attended a 2-day training workshop. The program was run within school hours. The students completed assessments at 2- and at 4-year follow-up. No differences in outcomes were found between intervention and control groups. There was little difference between conditions at the 2 year and 4 year follow up on self-reported symptoms. This study replicated the Queensland Early Intervention and Prevention Project (Dadds et al, 1997) with a few changes. The intervention was delivered by school counselors and teachers instead of psychologist, there was assessment of treatment fidelity and a long-term follow-up was added. This study highlights the challenges of delivering a school-based program effectively by school staff.

Because of the potential role of withdrawn or inhibited temperament as an important risk factor for later development of anxiety disorders, some researchers have focused on very young age groups. It is difficult to differentiate in this age group between temperament and disorder since these can be overlapping but are also distinct constructs (Rapee & Spence, 2004; Turner et al., 1996). It is possible that some of these children with inhibited temperament already meet criteria for an anxiety disorder and thus could qualify for assignment to either selective or indicated intervention (Mrazek & Haggerty, 1994). The following studies highlight the selective treatment programs.

LaFreniere & Capuano (1997) identified 43 anxious and withdrawn preschoolers, ages 31-70 months. These preschoolers were randomly assigned to either intervention or control condition. Over the next 6 months, the intervention group received 11 home visits which included child interaction skills, providing parent education and improving parenting skills and improving social support. The study showed significant difference between the intervention group and the control group with the intervention group showing improved social competence and less maternal control. In this study, however, levels of anxiety or withdrawn behavior, which was the main variable, did not differ significantly between the groups.

Rapee et al (2005) conducted an early intervention program to prevent the development of anxiety in preschool children. Withdrawn or inhibited behavior, which is one of the best identified risk factors for later anxiety disorders, was the main selection criteria for children in the program after a lab assessment. The participants who were 146 inhibited children (ages 3-5 years) and their parents were randomly assigned to either a parent-education group (n=73) or a control group (n=73). Parent education was conducted in groups of 6 sets of parents with mothers more frequently attending the groups. Parents received a total of 6 sessions which were 90 minutes each and were weekly for the first four sessions, then one session 2 weeks later and the last session one month after that. This program was group based and brief for ease of applicability and transportability. Results showed that children with parents in the intervention group at 12 months showed a significantly greater decrease in anxiety compared to the waitlist control group but no significant changes were seen on measures of inhibition/withdrawal. In fact, both groups showed decreases in measures of inhibition so the effects of parent intervention on inhibition could not be demonstrated.

The same group of children and their parents were assessed by Rapee et al (2010) at 3 years (n=121) as they were entering middle childhood. Diagnostic interviews and questionnaires were repeated at 12, 24 and 36 months. Laboratory observations were repeated only at 12 and 24 months. Results showed that children whose parents received the intervention had lower levels of anxiety symptoms according to parents' and child reports. No significant changes were noted on levels of inhibition.

Contrary to the above two studies, the study by Kennedy et al (2009) not only showed greater reductions in anxiety disorders but also showed greater reductions in parent and laboratory observed measures of behavioral inhibition. Participants in this study were 71 children aged 36-58 months and their parents who were randomly assigned to either a parent intervention (n=35) or a 6-month waitlist (n=36). Children were included if they met the following two criteria: they had a high score for behavioral inhibition on lab assessment and one of their parent met DSM-IV criteria for an anxiety disorder. The parent intervention was delivered in a group format with sets of 6 parents in the group. The program consisted of 8 sessions lasting 90 minutes each with a phone call after a month of the last session. Sessions consisted of psychoeducation, parent management strategies for anxious children, development of graded hierarchies, cognitive restructuring for both parents and children, exposure for parents' fears, coping plans, maintenance and relapse prevention, reinforcement of progress and trouble shooting.

An example of a selective prevention trial is the one by Balle et al (2010). This study focuses on Anxiety Sensitivity as an early risk factor for the development of anxiety disorders. The aim of this study was to assess the efficacy of a brief school-based selective prevention program for anxiety in children and adolescents with high levels of anxiety sensitivity. Children and adolescents n= 613 aged 11 -17 years of age from 4 schools were screened. Children with over 80th percentile in the Children Anxiety Sensitivity Index but with no current psychiatric disorder or treatment (n=130) were offered the study but 105 accepted participation in the study. Out of the 105 participants, 92 entered the trial. The rest were excluded on the basis of meeting criteria for a psychiatric disorder. These 92 participants were randomly assigned to either the prevention group (n=47), waitlist control (n=45) and a third normal control group. Both groups showed a significant decrease in all outcome variables but there was no differences between the prevention or the waitlist group. Differences emerged in the six-month follow-up with greater anxiety sensitivity reductions in the prevention group compared to the waitlist control. Also, the participants in the waitlist control began to get worse. This study showcases that brief interventions for a population with a risk factor (anxiety sensitivity) are effective.

The efficacy of a school-based intervention for social anxiety disorder was examined in a randomized wait-list control trial of 35 adolescents (Masia-Warner, Klein, Dent , 2005). Participants were drawn from 1,521 adolescents of grades 9 through 11 in New York City. They were screened for social anxiety disorder and classroom teachers were asked to nominate up to five students in their class who appeared shy. The nominated students and students who scored in the top 15% on self-rating instruments were selected for further screening. Parents of these adolescents were called and interviewed over the phone and adolescents whom had impairment in functioning were invited to participate in a diagnostic evaluation. Out of the 80 that were interviewed 42 met study criteria. Students were randomly assigned to either SASS (Skills for Social and Academic Success) (n=21) or wait-list control condtion (n=21). The SASS intervention consisted of 12 weekly group school sessions, two brief individual meetings and two group booster sessions. Additionally, four weekend social events which provided "real world exposures and opportunities for skills generalization were conducted. Parents attended two group meetings at school consisting of psychoeducation. All groups were led by psychologists. Participants were evaluated at the end of treatment and 9 months later. Adolescents in the intervention group had significantly greater reduction than the control group in social anxiety and avoidance as well as significantly improved overall functioning. In addition, 67% of treated subjects compared to 6% of wait-list control no longer met criteria for social anxiety disorder following treatment.

Masia-Warner, Fisher, Shrout et al (2007) conducted another study similar to the one above but this time compared it to a credible alternate treatment: Educational Supportive Group Function (ESGF). Participants (1789) from grades 9 through 11 were recruited. Out of these 1593 completed and returned screening questionnaires and teachers were asked to nominate shy students. Finally, 36 subjects agreed to participate. Nineteen adolescents were randomized to the SASS (Skills for Social and Academic Success) described above and 17 to the attention control group (ESGF) led by psychologists. The ESGF was designed to be identical to SASS in amount of professional attention and format, however, it omits any therapeutic elements considered specific to reversing social anxiety disorder but includes instructions on relaxation training. The study demonstrated significant reductions in social anxiety for SASS compared to the control group. Parent reports of their children's anxiety did not discriminate between groups. In the SASS group 59% compared to 0% in the control group no longer met criteria for social anxiety disorder. At 6-month follow-up, the gains from SASS were maintained.

7. Conclusion

In this review, universal prevention strategies are discussed with the beneficial effects of these programs on minimizing risk factors and enhancing protective factors in children. Given the high prevalence rates of childhood anxiety disorders, the distress and impairment associated with them and the high costs of treatment, preventive strategies implemented in the school setting seem to be the most sensible approach. Although anxiety disorders are amongst the most treatable psychiatric disorders, many children fail to receive treatment. Utilizing universal prevention strategies target the greatest number of children in a cost effective manner without stigmatizing or labeling them. By teaching coping skills to students, their anxiety is reduced. These effects have proven to be durable over the course of a few years.

The FRIENDS program (Barrett et al, 2004, 2005) has shown promise as a school based program to decrease anxiety and is being implemented in many different countries. Implementation of the program should be done in a way that fidelity is maintained but the program is still valid within the context of its implementation. It is important that outcome research is done post implementation to study effectiveness of the program and the long term gains.

Prevention and treatment exist on a spectrum and both are required to reduce the distress and impairment associated with anxiety disorders in children. Historically, however, most public investments have been made in treatment services (Waddell et al, 2004) whereas prevention efforts are often neglected. In the future, the availability of a balance between both prevention and treatment services would be ideal. Both risk and protective factors should be targeted by prevention programs to be more effective.

8. References

American Psychiatric Association. (2000). *Diagnostic and statistical manual of mental disorder* (4th ed., text revision). Washington, DC: American Psychiatric Association.

Andrews, G., & Wilkinson, D. D. (2002). Preventing depression: The prevention of mental issorders in young people. *Medical Journal of Australia,* 177, S97-S100.

Balle, M. & Tortella-Feliu, M. (2010). Efficacy of a brief school-based program for selective prevention of childhood anxiety. *Anxiety, Stress & Coping,* 23:1, 71.

Barrett, P.M., Dadds, M.R., & Rapee, R. (1996). Family treatment of childhood anxiety: A controlled trial. *Journal of Consulting and Clinical Psychology,* 64, 333-342.

Barrett, P. M. (2004). *Friends for Life! For children.* Participant workbook and leader's Manual. Brisbane, Australia: Australian Academic Press.

Barrett, P. M. (2005). Friends for Life! For youth. Participant workbook and leader's manual. Brisbane, Australia: Australian Academic Press.

Barrett, P. M., & Turner, C. M. (2000). Childhood anxiety in ethnic families: Current status and future directions. *Behavior Change,* 17, 113-123.

Barrett, P. M., & Turner, C. M. (2001). Prevention of anxiety symptoms in primary school children: Preliminary results from a universal school-based trial. *British Journal of Clinical Psychology,* 40, 399-410.

Barrett, P. M., Farrell, L. J., Ollendick, T. H., & Dadds, M. (2006). Long term outcomes of an Australian universal prevention trial of anxiety and depression symptoms in children and youth: An evaluation of the FRIENDS Program. *Journal of Clinical Child and Adolescent Psychology,* 35, 403-411.

Beardslee W., Chien, P., Bell, C., (2011). Prevention of mental disorders, substance abuse and problem behaviors: A Developmental Perspective, *Psychiatric News,*

Beidel, D. C., & Turner, S. M. (1998). Clinical presentation of social phobia in children and adolescents. In D. C. Beidel, & S. M. Turner (Eds.), *Shy children, phobic adults: Nature and treatment of social phobia* (pp. 33057) Washington DC; American Psychological Association, p. 6.

Beiderman, J., Rosenbaum, J.F., Bolduc-Murphy, e. A., Faraone, S. V., Chaloff, J., Hirshfeld, D.R., & Kagan, J. (1993). A 3-year follow-up of children with and without behavioral inhibition. *Journal of the American Academy of Child and Adolescent Psychiatry,* 32, 814-821.

Children's Mental Health Ontario Pre-Budget Submission 2010 [On-line]. Available: http://www.kidsmentalhealth.ca.

Compton, S. N., March, J. S., Brent, D., Albano, A. M., Weersing, V. R. & Curry, J. (2004). Cognitive-behavioral psychotherapy for anxiety and depressive disorders in children and adolescents: An evidence-based medicine review. *Journal of the American Academy of Child nd Adolescent Psychiatry,* 43, 930-959.

Costello, E. J., Angold, A., & Burns, B. J. (1996). The Great Smoky Mountains study of youth: Goals, design, methods, and the prevalence of DSM-III-R disorders. *Archives of General Psychiatry*, 53, 1129-1136.

Dadds, M. R., Spence, S., Holland, D. E., Barrett, P. M., & Laurens, K. R. (1997). Prevention and early intervention for anxiety disorders: A controlled trial. *Journal of Consulting and Clinical Psychology*, 65, 627-635.

Dadds, M. R., Holland, D. E., Laurens, K, Mullins, M., Barrett, P. M. Spence, S. H. (1999). Early ntervention and Prevention of Anxiety Disorders in Children: Results at 2-year Follow-up. *Journal of Consulting and Clinical Psychology*, 67:1,145-150.

DiLalla, L. F., Kagan, J., & Reznick, J. S. (1994). Genetic etiology of behavioral inhibition among 2-year-old children. *Infant Behavior and Development*, 17, 412-415.

Dollinger, S. J., O'Donnell, J. P., & Staley, A. A. (1984). Lightening-strike disaster: Effects on children's fears and worries. Journal of Consulting and Clinical Psychology, 52, 1028-1038.

Donovan, C.L., & Spence, S. H. (2000). Prvention of childhood anxiety disorders. *Clinical Psychology Review*, 20, 509-531.

Dubow, E. F., Schmidt, D., McBride, J., Edwards, S., & Merk, F. L. (1993). Teaching children to cope with stressful experiences: Implementation and evaluation of a primary prevention program. *Journal of Clinical Child Psychology*, 22, 428-440.

Erickson, M. F., Sroufe, L. A., & Egeland, B. (1985). The relationship between quality of attachment and behavior problems in preschool and a high-risk sample. *Monographs of the Society for Research in Child Development*, 50, 147-166.

Farrell, L. J. & Barrett, P.M. (2007). Prevention of Childhood Emotional Disorders: Reducing the Burden of Suffering Associated with Anxiety and Depression. *Child and Adolescent Mental Health*, 12; 2, 58-65.

Garland, J., & Clark, S. (2000). *Taming Worry Dragons: A manual for children, parents and other Coaches* (Rev.). Vancouver, Canada: British Columbia Children's Hospital.

Goodman, R., ford, T., Richards, H., Gatward, R., & Meltzer, H. (2000). The development and well-being assessment: Description and initial validation of an integrated asessessment of child and adolescent psychopathology. *Journal of Child Psychiatry*, 41, 645-655.

Greenberg, M. T., Domitrovich, C., Bumbarger, B. (1999). *Preventing mental disorders in school age children: A review of the effectiveness of prevention programs* (US Department of Health and Human Services, Centre for Mental Health Services report). [On-line]. Available: http:/www.psu.edu/dept/prevention/CMHS.html.

Haines, A. A., (1992). Comparison of Cognitive-Behavioral Stress Management Techniques with Adolescent Boys. *Journal of Counseling & Development*, 70, 600- 605.

Hawkins, D. J., & Catalano, R. F. (1992). *Communities that care: Action for drug abuse Prevention*. San Francisco, CA; Jossey-Bass.

Hunt, C., Andrews, G., Crino, R., Erskine, A., Sakashita, C. (2009). Randomized controlled trial of an Early Intervention programme for adolescent Anxiety Disorders. *Australian and New Zealand Journal of Psychiatry*, 2009: 43:300-304.

In-Albon, T., & Schneider, S. (2007). Psychotherapy of childhood anxiety disorders: A meta-analysis. *Psychotherapy and Psychosomatics*, 76, 15-24.

Jessor, R. (1991). Risk behavior in adolescence: A psychosocial framework for understanding and action. *Journal of Adolescent Health Special Issue: Adolescents at Risk*, 12, 597-605.

Jessor, R., Van Den Bos, J., Vanderryn, J., Costa, F. M., &Turbin, M. S. (1995). Protective factors in adolescent problem behavior: Moderator effects and developmental change. *Developmental Psychology*, 31, 923-933.

Kagan, J., Reznick, J. S., & Gibbons, J. (1989). Inhibited and uninhibited types of children. *Child Development*, 60, 838-845.

Kagan, J., & Snidman, N. (1991). Infant predictors of inhibited and uninhibited profiles. *Psychological Science*, 2, 40-43.

Kagan, J. (1997). Temperament and the reactions to unfamiliarity. *Child Development*, 68, 139-143.

Kendall, P.C. (1994). Treating anxiety disorders in youth; Results of a randomized clinical trial. *Journal of Consulting and Clinical Psychology*, 62, 100-101.

Kennedy, S. J., Rapee, R. M., Edwards, S. (2009). A Selective Intervention Program of Inhibited Preschool-Aged Children of Parents with an Anxiety Disorder: Effects on Current Anxiety Disorders and Temperament. *Journal of Am Acad of Child and Adol. Psychiatry*, 48:6, 602-609.

Kessler, R. C., Berglund, P., Demler, O., Jin, R., Merikangas, K., & Walters, E. (2005). Lifetime prevalence and age-of-onset distributions of DSM-IV disorders in the National Comorbidity Survey Replication. *Archives of General Psychiatry*, 62, 593-602.

Krohne, H.W., & Hock, M. (1991). Relationships between restrictive mother-child interactions and anxiety of the child, *Anxiety Research*, 4, 109-124.

Last, C. G., Perrin, S., Hersen, M., & Kazdin, A. E. (1996). A prospective study of childhood anxiety disorders. *Journal of the American Academy of Child and Adolescent Psychiatry*, 35, 1502-1510.

Lefeuve, C.E., Litten, R. Z., Randall, C. L., Moak, D. H., Salloum, I. M., & Green, A I. (2004). Pharmacological treatment of alcohol abuse/dependence with psychiatric comorbidity. *Alcoholism, Clinical and Experimental Research*, 28, 302-312.

LaFreniere, P.J., & Capuano, F. (1997). Preventive intervention as a means of clarifying direction of effects in socialization: Anxious-withdrawn preschoolers case. *Development and Psychopathology*, 9, 551-564.

Lewinsohn, P. M., & Clarke, G. N. (1999). Psychosocial treatment for adolescent depression. *Clinical Psychology Review*, 19, 329-342.

Lewis, M., Feiring, C., McGafey, C., & Jaskir, J. (1984). Predicting psychopathology in six-year- olds from early social relations. *Child Development*, 55, 123-136.

Leen-Feldner, E. W., Reardon, L.E., & Zvolensky, M.J. (2007). Pubertal status and emotional reactivity to a voluntary hyperventilation challenge predicting panic symptoms and somatic complaints: A laboratory-based multi-informant test. *Behavior Modification*, 21, 8-31.

Lock, S., & Barrett, P. M. (2003). A longitudinal study of developmental differences in Universal preventative ntervention for child anxiety. *Behavior Change*, 20, 183-99.

Lowry-Webster, H. M., Barrett, P. M., Dadds, M. R. (2001). A Universal Prevention Trial of Anxiety and Depressive Symptomatology in Childhood: Preliminary data from an Australian Study. *Behaviour Change*, 18:1, 36-50.

Lowry-Webster, H. M., Barrett, P. M., & Lock, S. (2003). A universal prevention trial of anxiety symptomatology during childhood: Results at 1-year follow-up. *Behavior Change*, 20, 25-43.

Masia-Warner, C, Klein, R. G., Dent, H. C., Fisher, P. H. Alvir, J, Albano, A. M., Guardino, M. (2005). School-based interventions for adolescents with social anxiety disorder: Results of a controlled study, *Journal of Abnormal Child Psychology*, 33:6, 707-722.

Masia-Warner, C, Fisher, P. H., Shrout, P. E., Rathor, S., Klein, R. G.. (2007). Treating Adolesents with social anxiety disorder in school: an attention control trial. *Journal of Child Psychology and Psychiatry*, 48:7, 676-686.

Miller, L. D., Short, C, Garland, E. J. Clark, S., (2010). The ABCs of CBT (Cognitive Behavior Therapy): Evidence-Based Approaches to Child Anxiety in Public School Settings, *Journal of Counseling & Development*, 88, 432-439.

Mrazek, P. J., & Haggerty, R. J. (1994). Reducing risks for mental disorders. Washington, DC: National Academy Press.

Muris, P., Merckelbach, H., Mayer, B., & Prins, E. (2000). How serious are common childhood fears? *Behaviour Research and Therapy*, 38, 217-228.

National Institutes of Health & Substance Abuse and Mental Health Services Administration (1999). Mental health and mental disorders {pp. 18(1)-18(32)}. In National Institutes of Mental Health (Ed.) *Healthy People 2010: Conference Edition.* Washington, DC: National Institutes of Health.

Otto, M. W., Leyro, T. M., Christian, K., Deveney, C. M., Reese, H., Pollack, M. Hl, et al. (2007). Prediction of "fear"acquisition in health control participants in a de novo fear-conditioning paradigm. *Behavior Modification*, 31, 32-51.

Offord, D. R., Chmura Kraemer, H., Kazdin, A. E., Jensen, P. S., & Harrington, R. 1998). Lowering the burden of suffering from child psychiatric disorder: Trade-offs among clinical, targeted, and universal interventions. *Journal of American Academy of Child and Adolescent Psychiatry*, 37, 686-694.

Pine, D. S., Cohen, P., Gurley, D., Brook, J., & Ma, Y. (1998). The risk for early adulthood anxiety and depressive disorders in adolescents with anxiety and depressive disorders. *Archives of General Psychiatry*, 55, 56-64.

Quinton, D., Pickles, A., Maughan, B., & Rutter, M. (1993). Partners, peers, and pathways: Assortative pairing and continuities in conduct disorder. *Development and Psychopathology Special Issue: Milestones in the development of resilience*, 5, 763-783.

Rapee , R. M., & Spence, S. H. (2004). The etiology of social phobia: Empirical evidence and an initial model. *Clinical Psychology Review*, 24, 737-767.

Rapee, R. M., Kennedy, S., Ingram, M., Edwards, S., and Sweeney, L. (2005). Prevention and Early Intervention of Anxiety Disorders in Inhibited Preschool Children. *Journal of Consulting and Clinical Psychology*, 73:3, 488-497.

Rapee, R. M., Kennedy, S., Ingram, M, Edwards, S., and Sweeney, L. (2010). Altering the Trajectory of Anxiety in At-Risk Young Children. *Amerian Journal of Psychiatry*, 167:12, 1518- 1525.

Robertson, E. B., David, S. L., & Rao, S. A., (2003). *Preventing drug use among children and adolescents: A research-based guide for parents, educators, and community leaders, second edition* [NIH Publication No, 04-421 (A)]. Retrieved from the National Institute on Drug Abuse website: http://www.drugabuse.gov/prevention/prevopen.html

Rosenbaum, J.F., Biederman, J., Gerten, M., Hirshfeld, D. R., Meminger, S. R., Herman, J. B., Kagan, J., Reznick, J.S. & Snidman, N. (1988). Behavioral inhibition in children of parents with panic disorder and agoraphobia: A controlled study. *Archives of General Psychiatry*, 45, 463-470.

Rosenbaum, J.F., Biederman, J., Bolduc-Murphy, E. A., Faraone, S.V., Chaloff, J., Hirshfeld, D. R. & Kagan, J. (1993). Behavioral inhibition in childhood: A risk factor for anxiety disorders. *Harvard Review of Psychiatry*, 1 (1), 2-16.

Schatzberg, A. F., Samson, J. A., & Rothschild, A. J. (1998). McLean Hospital Depression Facility: Early-onset phobic disorders and adult onset major depression. *British Journal of Psychiatry*, 173, 29-34.

Spence, S. H. (2001). Prevention strategies. In m. W. Vasey & M. R. Dadds (Eds.). *The developmental psychopathology of anxiety*, 101-132. New York: Oxford University Press.

Sroufe, L.A., Egeland, B., & Kreutzer, T. (1990). The fate of early experience following developmental change: Longitudinal approaches to individual adaptation in childhood. *Child Development*, 61, 1363-1373.

Stallard, P, Simpson, N. Anderson, S. Hibbert, S., Osborn C. (2007). The FRIENDS emotional health programme: Initial findings from a school based project. *Child and Adolescent Mental Health*, 12:1, 32-37.

Thapar, A., & McGuffin, P. (1995). Are anxiety symptoms in childhood heritable? *Journal of Child Psychology and Psychiatry*, 36, 439-447.

Turner, S. M., Beidel, D. C., & Costello, A. (1987). Psychopathology in the offspring of anxiety disorders patients. *Journal of Consulting and Clinical Psychology*, 55, 229-235.

Turner, S. M., Beidel, D. C., & Wolff, P.L. (1996). Is behavioral inhibition related to the anxiety disorders? *Clinical Psychology Review*, 16, 157-172.

Waddell, C., Godderis, R., Hua, J., McEwan, K., Wong, W. (2004) Preventing and treating Anxiety Disorders in Children and Youth: A Research report prepared for the British Columbia Ministry f Children and Family Development. *Children's Mental Health Policy Research Program*, University of BC Walker, J. R., Ediger, J., Joyce, B., Furer, P., Vincent, N., & Kjernisted, K. D. (2001). *A survey of preference for pharmacological and psychological treatment for anxiety problems in an anxiety disorders clinic*. Poster session presented at the Anxiety Disorders Association of America, 21st National Conference, Atlanta, GA.

Warren, S. L., Huston, L., Egeland, B., & Sroufe, L. A. (1997). Child and adolescent anxiety disorder and early attachment. Journal of the American Academy of Child and Adolescent Psychiatry, 36, 637-644.

Weissman, M. M., Leckman, J.F., Merikangas, K. R., Gammon, g. D., & Prusoff, B. (1984). Depression and anxiety disorders in parents and children: Results from the Yale Family Study. *Archives of General Psychiatry*, 41, 845-852.

Weist, M. D. (1999). Challenges and opportunities in expanded school mental health. *Clinical Psychology Review*, 19(2), 131-135.

Weisz, J. R., Thurber, C. a., Sweeney L., Proffitt V. D. & LeGagnoux G. L. (1997). Brief treatment of mild-to-moderate child depression using primary and secondary control enhancement training. Journal of Consulting and Clinical psychology, 65, 703-707.

World Health Organization (2004). Prevention of Mental Disorders: Effective interventions and policy options. Geneva. Retrieved October 1, 2004, from http://www.who.int/entity/mental/health/evidence/en/prevention_of_mental_disorders.sr.pdf

Part 3

Co-Morbidity and Somatic Symptoms of Anxiety Disorders

6

Somatic Conditions Intrinsic to Anxiety Disorders

Antonio Bulbena and Guillem Pailhez
Anxiety Disorders Unit – INAD, Barcelona
Spain

1. Introduction

Although Johann Christian August Heinroth (1773-1843) introduced the term 'psychosomatic' into medical literature, up to the present day his contributions to the development of medicine and psychosomatics have been little acknowledged. The relationship between somatic and psychiatric conditions is assumed to be fluent; however, the concept "psychosomatic" brings with it a heavy semantic burden that has its roots in the philosophical dualism, accentuated in the Cartesian proposal, which has spread through modern rationality, and, with it, the conception of the disease in the medical field.
The modern notion of health and illness make necessary to review dualistic positions, but often the everyday clinical practice still shows separated approaches for the mental and the somatic parts of the patient's illness. A clear example of this useless but very spread dualistic approach is the group of anxiety disorders, which have been included alternatively among the somatic and among the mental conditions when, in fact, anxiety disorders include both strong somatic and mental dimensions which need to be dealt with. In this chapter we shall review the link of the joint hypermobility syndrome (JHS) and several anxiety conditions. This relationship is probably one of the strongest available evidences of the somatic components of anxiety disorders.

2. Somatic conditions related with anxiety disorders

Anxiety disorders are related with other medical illness and have also been associated with high rates of medically unexplained symptoms and increased utilization of healthcare resources (McLauglin et al., 2006) and poor quality of life and disability (Sareen et al., 2006). Patients with anxiety disorders often complain of somatic features, especially cardiac (tachycardia, chest pain), gastrointestinal (epigastric pain), and neurological complaints (headaches, dizziness, or presyncope), in emergencies and primary services (Muller et al., 2005; Wells et al., 1989; Zaubler & Katon, 1998). This clinical phenomenon helped to deepen into the study of differential diagnoses between somatic symptoms of anxiety and somatic symptoms of comorbid conditions (Katon & Roy-Byrne, 1989; Stein, 1986; Wise & Taylor, 1990). More recent research suggests a strong association between anxiety disorders and somatic conditions, although some authors emphasize the huge amount of published research about somatic conditions and depression in contrast to the few studies about the same relationship with anxiety disorders (Harter et al., 2003; Roy Byrne et al., 2008;

Sareen et al., 2005). Furthermore, results from the National Comorbidity Survey-Replication (NCS-R) showed that various anxiety disorders had equal or greater association than depression with four chronic physical disorders (hypertension, arthritis, asthma, and ulcers) (Kessler et al., 2003).

The more recent review articles about this relationship are organized according to medical illness specifically associated to anxiety disorders in several descriptive and analytic studies with clinical samples (Katon, 1996; Muller et al., 2005; Roy Byrne et al., 2008; Simon & Fischmann, 2005; Wells et al., 1989). These reviews often include the following somatic conditions: irritable bowel syndrome, asthma, cardiovascular disease, cancer, chronic pain, vestibular and thyroid dysfunction, chronic obstructive pulmonary disease, and mitral valve prolapse. Some of the main general conclusions of these reviews are the following: 1) emerging evidence about the bi-directional relationship between anxiety disorders and medical illness suggests that they may be as important as depression (Roy Byrne et al., 2008); 2) such associations provide important clues for understanding the neurobiology of anxiety disorders (Muller et al., 2005); and 3) such associations are greater for panic disorder (Katon, 1996; Wells et al., 1989), worsening its identification, presentation and treatment (Simon & Fischmann, 2005).

Along this way, there are four studies relying on clinical samples that have shown higher rates of somatic conditions among patients with anxiety disorders. The first one was published in 1994. Rogers et al. examined the prevalence and characteristics of medical illness in 711 patients with present or past index anxiety disorders (Rogers et al., 1994). Patients were assessed using structured diagnostic interviews and the Medical History Form II. The rates of medical illness for all subjects were later compared with data extracted from an epidemiological sample. Results showed that patients with panic disorder had more reported medical problems than the general population, in particular, more ulcer disease, angina, and thyroid disease.

In 2003, Härter et al. studied the associations between anxiety disorders and medical illnesses in a total of 262 probands (169 cases with an anxiety disorder and 93 controls with no evidence of an anxiety disorder according to DSM-III-R criteria) (Härter et al., 2003). Diagnoses were obtained based on direct interview (SADS) or family history information, and lifetime history of numerous medical illnesses was obtained. Results showed that patients with a lifetime anxiety disorder reported higher rates of several medical illnesses than did persons without anxiety. After controlling for the effects of gender, comorbid substance abuse/dependence and/or depression, significant associations were found between anxiety disorders and cardiac disorders (OR = 4.6), hypertension (OR = 2.4), gastrointestinal problems (OR = 2.4), genitourinary disorders (OR = 3.5), and migraine (OR = 5.0). A similar pattern was observed for probands with panic or generalized anxiety disorder.

Sareen et al. examined the relationship between anxiety disorders and a wide range of physical conditions in a nationally representative sample. Data came from the National Comorbidity Survey (N=5,877). Physical disorders were assessed based on a list of several conditions shown to respondents. Results showed that anxiety disorders were positively associated with physical conditions even after adjusting for mood disorders, substance-use disorders, and sociodemographics. Among specific anxiety disorders, panic disorder and agoraphobia were more likely to be associated with cardiovascular disease and bone and joint diseases (Sareen et al., 2005).

In 2008, in a case-control study carried out by our group (Pascual et al., 2008) using retrospective data extracted from clinical records, patients with anxiety disorders showed higher risk of medical illnesses than patients without anxiety disorders. The aim of the study was to investigate the comorbidity between anxiety disorders and somatic conditions in three groups: patients with anxiety disorders (n=130) including panic disorder with/without agoraphobia and agoraphobia without panic attacks, patients from a primary care unit without any psychiatric disorder (n=150), and patients from a psychiatric service without anxiety disorders (n=130). Multivariate statistical logistic regression analysis showed that patients with anxiety disorders presented 4.2-fold increase in the risk of cephalea, 3.9 of cardiopathy, 3.8 of osteomuscular disorder and 2-fold increase in the risk of digestive diseases.

There are various hypotheses on how anxiety disorders and medical conditions may be related (Rogers et al., 1994). Medical illness may sometimes directly trigger the development of anxiety symptoms (e.g., cardiomyopathy or anxiety as a psychological reaction towards an illness), or mimic anxiety symptoms (e.g. pheochromocytoma). Conversely, anxiety disorders may sometimes directly trigger the development of somatic symptoms (e.g., angina in cardiovascular disease), mimic symptoms of a medical illness (leading to high costly procedures or inadequate treatment), or may contribute to the onset or exacerbation of certain somatic conditions (e.g., hypertension or gastric ulcer).

However, there is evidence that some medical conditions that are often comorbid with anxiety disorders could share a common genetic etiology (Collier, 2002; Gratacos et al., 2001; Pailhez et al., 2009). For example, a recent family study found that panic or social anxiety patients and their first-degree relatives were more likely to have interstitial cystitis, mitral valve prolapse and headaches, and this was hypothesized to be linked to a common genetic susceptibility. Talati et al. studied probands with diagnosis and family history of panic disorder (n=219), social anxiety disorder (n=199), or both (n=173), and 102 control subjects with no personal/family history of anxiety. Subjects were blindly interviewed with a diagnostic instrument and medical history was obtained via medical checklist and the family history screen (Talati et al., 2001).

3. Anxiety disorders and the role of collagen tissue

According to this hypothesis, several studies have shown a noticeable association between anxiety disorders (particularly panic/phobic cluster) and the joint hypermobility syndrome (JHS) (Bulbena et al., 1993; Bulbena et al., 2004; Bulbena et al. 2007). JHS is an inherited connective tissue disorder associated with a generalized collagen laxity and characterized by an increase of active or passive joint mobility. The condition was not described for the first time until fifty years ago, when it was properly identified and associated to pathology of the musculoskeletal system (Rotés & Argany, 1957). In 1973, after an epidemiological study by Beighton et al., the syndrome gained general interest in the rheumatological field and began to be studied in a broader way, as a separate entity (Beighton et al., 1973) (see Fig.1).

In 1992, the Hospital del Mar criteria (table 1) compiled all the items included in the most clinically used criteria. This new scale showed consistent indicators of reliability, internal consistency and predictive validity, and provided evidence for using different scores according to age and gender (Bulbena et al., 1992).

JHS has an estimated prevalence in the general population ranging between 10% - 15%, it is more frequent among females (3:1) and is one of the hereditary disorders of the connective tissue, which include other conditions such as Ehlers-Danlos syndrome, Marfan syndrome and ostogenesis imperfecta (Beighton et al., 1999). Clinical features in JHS can be articular or

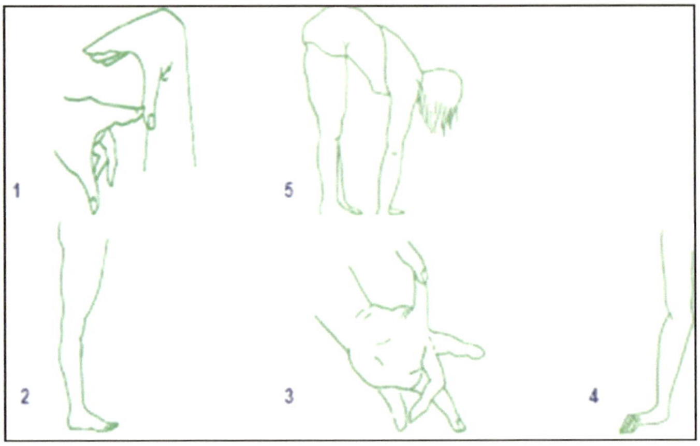

1. Passive apposition of the thumbs to the flexor aspects of the forearm (one point for each thumb).
2. Hyperextension of the knee beyond 10º (one point for each knee).
3. Passive dorsiflexion of the little fingers beyond 90º (one point for each hand).
4. Hyperextension of the elbows beyond 10º (one point for each elbow).
5. Forward flexion of the trunk with knees fully extended so that the palms of the hands rest flat on the floor (one point).

Fig. 1. Joint Hypermobility criteria (Beighton et al., 1973)

Upper extremities	
1.	Passive apposition of the thumb to the flexor aspect of the forearm at a distance of less than 21 mm.
2.	The passive dorsiflexion of the fifth finger is 90º or more.
3.	The active hyperextension of the elbow is 10º or more.
4.	External rotation of the shoulder up to more than 85º.
Lower extremities. Supine position	
5.	The passive hip abduction can be taken to an angle of 85º or more.
6.	Hypermobility of the rotula.
7.	Hypermobility of the ankle and foot.
8.	Dorsal flexion of the toe of 90º or more.
Lower extremities. Prone position	
9.	Hyperflexion of the knee.
10.	Ecchymoses.

Table 1. Hospital del Mar criteria (Bulbena et al., 1992) for JHS. Male patients scoring 4 or more are considered cases; female patients are considered cases with scores 5 or over.

extra-articular and are always related to the connective tissue. Among the best known articular features of JHS are arthralgia, lumbalgia, soft-tissue rheumatism (e.g., epicondilytis, tenosynovitis, bursitis), recurrent dislocations, childhood scoliosis, or rheumatoid arthritis (Bravo, 2009; Keer & Grahame, 2003). Among the best-known extra-articular features of JHS are hernias, varicose veins, "easy bruising", keloids, uterine or rectal prolapse, spontaneous pneumothorax, fibromyalgia, dysautonomia and some other conditions also linked to panic disorder as asthma, mitral valve prolapse, thyroid dysfunction or irritable bowel syndrome (Keer & Grahame, 2003; Mishra et al., 1996). Therefore, most of the conditions linked to anxiety disorders can be explained as clinical features of JHS. Unfortunately, the relationship between anxiety disorders and JHS is often neglected.

The clinical relationship between anxiety disorders and JHS was found 50 years ago. In 1957, the rheumatologist J. Rotés Querol pointed out for the first time the remarkable degree of nervous tension suffered by patients with hypermobility (Rotés & Argany 1957). To a certain extent, there are some indirect references about the relationship between "hypotonia" and anxiety/phobias in the classical psychosomatic literature (Flanders, 1950). On the other hand, Carlsson and Rundgren in 1980 (Carlsson & Rundgren 1980) found a higher score in hypermobility among alcoholic patients than among controls. Although not mentioned, the percentage of anxiety patients among the case group might have been high.

Empirical history of the clinical relationship between anxiety disorders and JHS starts in the case-control study conducted by our group in 1993, with rheumatologic outpatients affected by JHS (Bulbena et al., 1993). Diagnoses of panic disorder, agoraphobia and simple phobia were significantly more frequent among hypermobile patients. There were no significant differences in the diagnoses of generalized anxiety disorder, dysthymia, or major depressive disorder. Around 70% of rheumatological patients with JHS had some kind of anxiety disorder. However, this only occurred in 22% of controls, a usual figure in chronic patient samples. Cases were 10 times more likely to suffer from anxiety than controls. Specifically, agoraphobia and panic disorders were, respectively, 5 and 7 times more likely (table 2).

	% JHS	% Non-JHS	Age-Sex Adjust. Odds Ratio	95 % C. I.
Any Anxiety D.	69,3	22,0	**10.69**	4.80-23.81
Panic D.	34.2	6.8	**6.96**	2.31-20.91
Panic & Agora.	24.6	5.1	**6.40**	1.82-22.43
Simple Phobia	29.8	8.5	**5.77**	2.05-16.24
Agoraphobia	37.7	11.9	**5.08**	2.06-12.49
General.Anx.	10.5	5.1	**2.49**	0.65-9.45
Major Depress.	14.9	3.4	**4.51**	0.99-20.56
Dysthymic D.	7.9	5.1	**2.15**	0.53-8.65

Table 2. Lifetime psychiatric disorders in JHS cases (n=114) and non-JHS controls (n=59) seen at an outpatient rheumatological unit (Bulbena et al., 1993).

For a subsequent second study, conducted to support this hypermobility-anxiety association, outpatients with new diagnoses of panic disorder and/or agoraphobia were examined, as well as non-anxious psychiatric and non-psychiatric outpatients as control groups (Martín-Santos et al., 1998). Results showed that JHS was present in almost 70% of anxiety cases, versus slightly over 10% of controls. This meant that cases with panic disorders and/or agoraphobia were 17 times more likely to suffer from JHS. Conclusions were valid particularly for women, but also for men (figure 2).

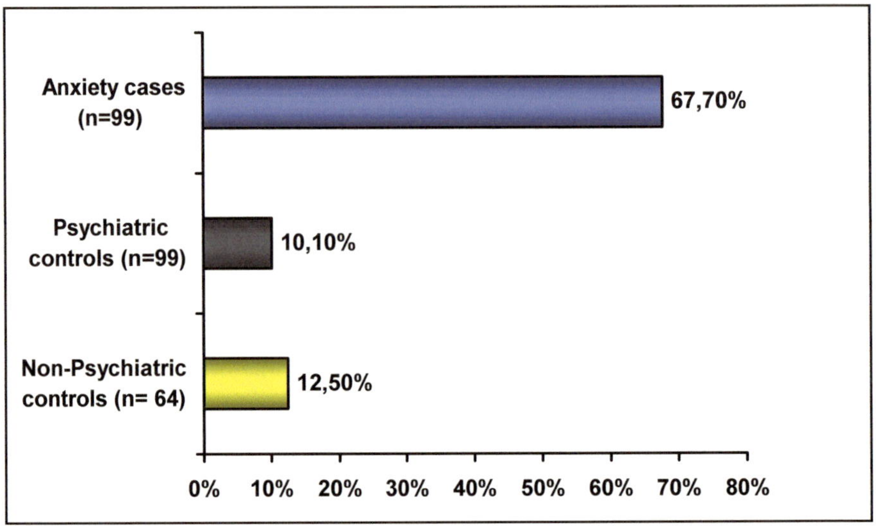

Fig. 2. Frequency of JHS diagnoses in anxiety cases (n=99), psychiatric (n=99) and non-psychiatric controls (n=64) (Martín-Santos et al., 1998). [O.R. = 16.9; CI 95% 8.8 to 32.2].

Later on, it was suggested that this association needed to be studied in the general population. To that end, a two-phase cross-sectional epidemiological study was carried out in a rural town in order to establish lifetime risk for anxiety and affective disorders in subjects with JHS. A sample of 1,300 individuals were examined at baseline and over 500 were subsequently subjected to follow-up in a two-stage epidemiological study. Hypermobile patients were eight times more likely to suffer from panic disorder (OR 8.2, CI 95% 3.4 to 19.7), eight times more likely to suffer from social phobia (OR 7.8; CI 95% 2.4 to 24.8) and six times more likely to suffer from agoraphobia (OR 5.9; CI 95% 3 to 11.7) than non-JHS patients. Results were valid for both genders. No differences were found for other anxiety disorders or mood disorders (Bulbena et al., 2004a).

In the same sample of general population it was also reported that hypermobiles had significantly higher scores in fear and phobia scales, reinforcing the hypothesis that intensity of fears is greater in subjects with JHS (Bulbena et al., 2006). We assessed fear intensity and frequency using a modified version of the Fear Survey Schedule (FSS-III). When we compared the groups with and without joint hypermobility, the mean total scores for both genders were significantly higher for the hypermobile group (figure 3). These results showed that the association of JHS and phobic anxiety is sustained for intense fears and might represent a susceptibility factor for these anxiety conditions.

In 2005, we studied schizophrenic outpatients (N=124) with the hypothesis that anxiety disorders mediated by JHS were not symptoms, but an independent comorbid entity in schizophrenic patients (Bulbena et al., 2005; Bulbena et al., 2007). Joint Hypermobility was noticeably more likely among panic disorder/phobia-clustered schizophrenic patients, than among the non-comorbid group (OR = 9.35; IC = 95% [3.85-22.73]; $p<0.0001$). The cluster panic disorder/phobia had higher scores in fear scales and schizophrenia positive symptom scales.

After several significant cross-sectional studies we sought to conduct a prospective incidence analysis that assesses whether JHS could be a risk factor in developing anxiety conditions (Bulbena et al., 2011).

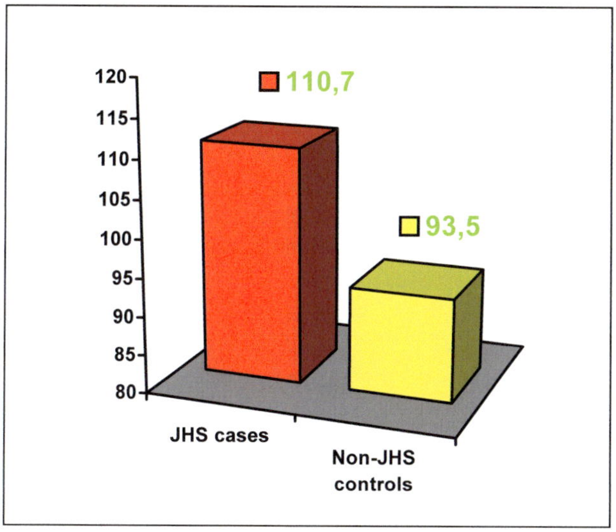

Fig. 3. Mean total scores of the Fear Survey Schedule (FSS-III) in JHS cases (n=182) and non-JHS controls (n=1,123) (Bulbena et al., 2006).

In 2004, our group also assessed a non-clinical sample of subjects working in the same company (N=526) (Bulbena et al., 2004b). Subjects with JHS had significantly higher scores in STAI trait anxiety [female average: 16.5 vs. 11, $p<0.001$] [male average: 13 vs. 11, $p<0.03$]. STAI state anxiety scores were also higher among hypermobile subjects, although not significantly (figure 4).

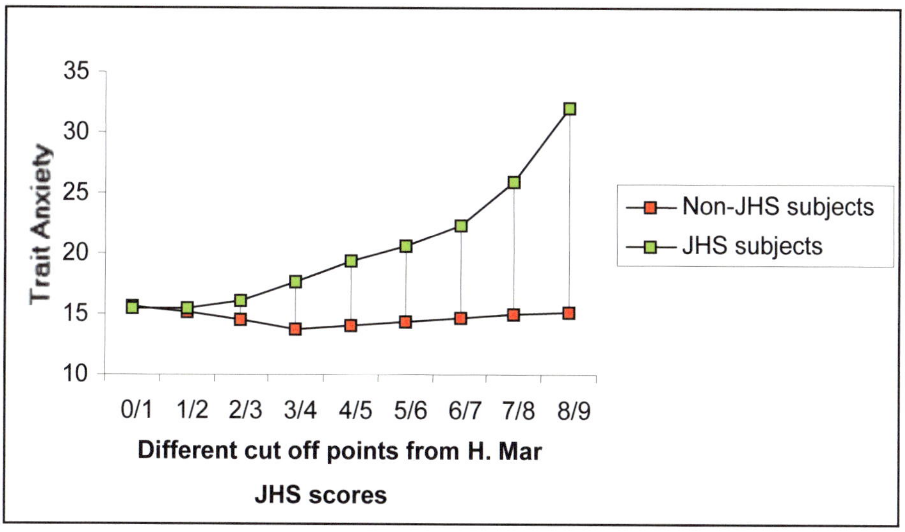

Fig. 4. Trait anxiety in 203 women with or without joint hypermobility according to all possible cutoff scores on the Hospital del Mar hypermobility criteria (Bulbena et al., 2004b).

The main objective was to determine the cumulative incidence of anxiety disorders in a cohort of young subjects recruited from the general population who had not developed any type of anxiety condition up to then; consequently we planned a scheduled 15-year follow-up covering subjects from late adolescence to adulthood. The total population sample was 1,305 subjects, and in order to observe the development of anxiety disorders during the 15-year study period, only the lower age segment (at that time subjects aged between 16 and 20) included in the town's municipal registry was invited to participate. We sought to describe the occurrence of new cases of anxiety disorders during the study period, therefore the exclusion criterion for the study was having already had an anxiety disorder at baseline examination. At baseline, 158 subjects were screened for participation in the study, and after the 15-year follow-up the final sample comprised 137 subjects (86.7% retention rate). Results showed that cumulative incidence of panic/agoraphobia at follow-up was significantly higher for the JHS group (41.4%) than for the control group (1.9%) with relative risk of 22.3 (CI 95% 4.6-108.7), p<0.0001, (NNT 3, CI 95% 2.9-2.3). Incidence of social phobia and simple phobia was also significantly higher for the JHS group at (RR=6.52; CI 95% 1.7-24.2) p<0.001 and (RR=3.31; CI 95% 1.1-9.6) p=0.02, respectively. Moreover, anxiolytic drug use was nearly fourfold higher among JHS subjects compared to non-JHS.

Total Sample n = 137	**JHS Status**						
	JHS present *n* = 29		JHS absent *n* = 108				
	n	%	*n*	%	*RR*	95% CI	*P*
Anxiety Disorders							
Panic/Agoraphobia	12	41.4	2	1.9	22.3	(4.6 to 108.7)	0.0001***
Social Phobia	7	24.1	4	3.7	6.5	(1.7 to 24.2)	0.001*
Simple Phobia	8	27.6	9	8.3	3.3	(1.1 to 9.6)	0.02*
GAD	7	24.1	9	8.3	2.9	(0.97 to 8.62)	0.14 ns
Other Disorders							
Depression/Dysthymia	7	24.1	7	6.48	3.7	(1.2 to 11.7)	0.15 ns

JHS, Joint Hypermobility Syndrome according to Beighton criteria assessed at baseline.
GAD, Generalized Anxiety Disorder
Statistical significance: * p<0.05, ** p<0.001, *** p<0.0001, ns: non significant.

Table 3. Incident cases and relative risk after 15 years of follow-up according to JHS status (Bulbena et al., 2011).

Recent work from another Spanish group, (García-Campayo et al., 2010) has shown again a high prevalence of JHS (61.8%) among panic subjects compared with 10.9% in the healthy control group and 9% in the psychiatric control group. Interestingly these authors found an intermediate figure among subjects suffering from fibromyalgia (25.4%). A paper from a Turkish group, albeit declaring no significant association, also found JHS in 59.5% of panic disorder patients with mitral valve prolapse, in 42.9% of patients without mitral valve prolapse but also in 52.6% of control subjects (Gulpek et al., 2004). Gülsün et al., studying subjects with thorax deformities, found that the anxiety level of males with thorax deformity and JHS is higher than males with thorax deformity without JHS (Gülsün et al., 2007). And finally, Baeza-Velasco and Bulbena also found high prevalence of social anxiety and joint hypermobility among subjects of high stature (Baeza-Velasco & Bulbena 2009).

	Type	Popul.	N groups	Sex	Age	JHS ass.	Association tendencies
Bulbena et al., 1993	CC	Spain	114 JHS 59 CTL	Matched	Matched	Beighton	JHS cases: 5 x Aph and 7 x PD
Martin-Santos et al., 1998	CC	Spain	99 PD & APh 99 Psychiatric CTL 64 Medical CTL	Matched	Matched	Beighton	PD cases: 17 x JHS
Benjamin et al., 2001	CC	Israel	101 PD 39 Healthy CTL	35 / 65 64 / 36	39.3 (11) 23.4 (3)	Beighton	No statistically significant relationship
Bulbena et al., 2004a	E	Spain	1305 subjects	45.7 / 54.3	43.4 (18.3)	Beighton	JHS cases: 6 x Aph, 8 x SPh and 8 x PD
Gulpek et al., 2004	CC	Turkey	42 PD & MVP 35 PD 38 MVP CTL	Matched	Matched	Beighton	No statistically significant relationship
Bulbena et al., 2004b	D	Spain	526 subjects	61.4 / 38.6	25.4 (3)	H. Mar	JHS cases: higher scores in STAI trait anxiety
Bulbena et al., 2005 & 2007	D	Spain	124 SCHZ	54 / 46	33.6 (10)	Beighton & H. Mar	Schizophrenic & PD cases: 9 x JHS and higher positive symptoms
Bulbena et al., 2006	D	Spain	1305 subjects	45.7 / 54.3	43.4 (18.3)	Beighton	JHS cases: higher scores in fear and phobia scales
Gülsün et al., 2007	CC	Turkey	52 thorax deformity 40 CTL	Males	21.9 (1.3)	Beighton	JHS cases: higher scores in HAM-A
Baeza-Velasco & Bulbena 2009	D	Several countries	158 high stature	46.8 / 53.2	25.7 (8.1)	Hakim & Grahame	JHS cases: higher scores in LSAS
García-Campayo et al., 2010	CC	Spain	55 PD 55 Psychiatric CTL 55 Fibromyalgia 55 Healthy CTL	Matched	Matched	Beighton	PD cases: 13 x JHS
Bulbena et al., 2011	C	Spain	137 subjects	53.3 / 46.7	31.9 (2.4)	Beighton & H. Mar	JHS cases: 22 x PD, 6.5 x SPh and 3.3 x Ph

Table 4. Relationship between JHS and anxiety disorders. Basic features of studies reviewed. D, descriptive study; CC, case-control study; C, cohort study; E, epidemiological study; CTL, controls; PD, Panic disorder; Aph, Agoraphobia; MVP, Mitral valve prolapse; SCHZ, Schizophrenia; SPh, Social phobia; Ph, Specific phobia. Sex expressed in percentage (%) male/female. Age expressed in mean (SD).

4. Perspectives

There is enough evidence showing that comorbidity of anxiety disorders and some medical conditions share a similar physiopathological mechanism mediated by the clinical features of JHS. Having arrived at this point, it might be relevant to remind the high association of JHS and the so called dysautonomia. In this way, significant research by Gazit and colleagues (Gazit et al., 2003) found that symptoms related to anxiety such as palpitations, light-headedness, nausea, shortness of breath, hyperventilation, tremulousness, chest discomfort, fatigue, etc., were significantly more common among patients with JHS. Moreover, they found that orthostatic hypotension, postural orthostatic tachycardia syndrome and uncategorized orthostatic intolerance were present in 78% of the studied patients with JHS compared to 10% of control subjects. Thus, they suggested that dysautonomia could be an extra-articular related feature of JHS.

However, under the "modern" name dysautonomia not only anxiety features can be found (Bulbena et al, 2004c) but also many symptoms described for more than two centuries in the present group of anxiety disorders (Berrios, 1999). Anxiety manifestations are among the most difficult to identify in the clinical practice even in patients suffering from generalized anxiety disorder, in which only 13% present anxiety as main complaint. Although dysautonomia and anxiety disorders are not in the same spectrum, they probably overlap. Therefore, the link between JHS and dysautonomia provide an interesting physiological connection to interpret this unexpected association between a "somatic" and a "psychiatric" condition.

Our results address the biological basis of anxiety and a common source of this condition with other constitutional disturbances in relation to connective tissue and the autonomic nervous system. Patients with a diagnosis of JHS provide a highly valuable opportunity for an in-depth study of the genetic basis of anxiety. Anxiety is also a comorbidity and a risk factor in itself for a poor prognosis in several psychiatric diseases, as is the case with schizophrenia and bipolar disorders. These diseases also provide opportunities to further explore the connection between joint hypermobility and the development of anxiety in these conditions.

It is also important to point out a possible application of this evidence; as patients with JHS are at greater risk of suffering from anxiety conditions, it would be desirable to prevent the development of anxiety disorders by means of community programs at the very early stages of development. We strongly recommend screening for joint hypermobility in routine health assessment protocols in teenagers and early adulthood subjects. Even though the clinical evaluation of JHS is not extremely difficult, it does inevitably require formal training and an external validation of the procedure. In this context, some anamnestic questions might be useful for detecting positive cases at risk of suffering from anxiety disorders.

5. Conclusions

Finally, several conclusions can be made after more than 30 years of active research and clinical work in that field.

First, the association between anxiety (clinical and non clinical) and JHS is strong and replicated in several setting and samples.

Second, both conditions carry high genetic and heritable load. This is clinically very well established, but at the genetic level, there is no clear conclusion yet. Our finding of both conditions in the chromosome 15 is now actively revisited.

Third, according to the type and number of somatic conditions found in the otherwise named "endogenous" anxiety disorders (panic, agoraphobia and social phobia), it seems that these patients tend to suffer from a particular cluster of disorders, particularly, osteomuscular, irritable bowel, hypo/hyperthyroid, migraine, asthma, etc. It might well be that all these conditions share some common abnormalities in the autonomic nervous system as well as in the collagen structure as found in JHS. This may be a diathesis not yet identified, but worthy to investigate.

And fourth, the autonomic disregulation, although very difficult to assess at that level, may be one of the clues to understand the association, and also to develop appropriate treatments.

In summary, this intriguing relationship gives rise to several physio-pathological questions and prevention-related issues. JHS is a risk factor for anxiety disorders, worthy of evidence-based identification in the context of preventive psychiatry not only among adults but also among at-risk pediatric populations.

6. References

Baeza-Velasco, C. & Bulbena, A. (2009). Ansiedad social y alteración del colágeno en personas de gran estatura. *Cuadernos Psicosomática y Psiquiatria de Enlace*. Vol.89/90, pp.40-46.

Beighton, P.; Solomon, L. & Soskolne, C. (1973). Articular mobility in an African population. *Ann Rheum Dis*. Vol.32, pp.413-8.

Beighton, P.; Grahame, R. & Bird, H. (1999). Hypermobility of joints, Springer, London, UK.

Benjamin, J.; Ben-Zion, IZ.; Dannon, P.; Schreiber, S.; Meiri, G.; Ofek, A. & Palatnik, A. (2001). Lack of association between joint hyperlaxity and, I: panic disorder, and II: reactivity to carbon dioxide in healthy volunteers. *Hum Psychopharmacol*. Vol.16, No.2, pp.189-192.

Berrios, GE. (1999). Anxiety disorders: a conceptual history. *J Affect Disord*. Vol.56, pp.83-94.

Bravo, JF. (2009). Síndrome de Ehlers-Danlos con especial énfasis en el síndrome de hiperlaxitud articular. *Rev Med Chile*. Vol.137, pp.1488-97.

Bulbena, A.; Duró, JC.; Porta, M.; Faus, S.; Vallescar, R. & Martín-Santos, R. (1992). Clinical assessment of Hypermobility of joints: Assembling criteria. *J Rheumatol*. Vol.19, pp.115-22.

Bulbena, A.; Duró, JC.; Porta, M.; Martín-Santos, R.; Mateo, A.; Molina, L.; Vallescar, R. & Vallejo, J. (1993). Anxiety disorder in the joint hypermobility syndrome. Psychiatric Res. Vol.43, pp.59-68.

Bulbena, A.; Gago, J.; Martín-Santos, R.; Porta, M.; Dasquens, J. & Berrios, GE. (2004). Anxiety disorder & joint laxity a definitive link. *Neurology, Psychiatry and Brain Research*. Vol.11, pp.137-40.

Bulbena, A.; Agullo, A.; Pailhez, G.; Martin-Santos, R.; Porta, M.; Guitart, J. & Gago, J. (2004). Is joint hypermobility related to anxiety in a nonclinical population also? *Psychosomatics*. Vol.45, pp.432-7.

Bulbena, A.; Pailhez, G. & Gago, J. (2004). "Connective tissue" between panic disorder and dysautonomia. *Am J Med*. Vol.116, No.11, pp.783.

Bulbena, A.; Anguiano, JB.; Gago, J.; Basterreche, E.; Ballesteros, J.; Eguiluz, I.; González Torres, ME.; Reddy, DP.; Coplan, JD. & Berrios, GE. (2005) Panic/phobic anxiety in schizophrenia: a positive association with joint hypermobility syndrome. *Neurology, Psychiatry and Brain Research*. Vol.12, pp.1-6.

Bulbena, A.; Gago, J.; Sperry, L. & Berge, D. (2006). The relationship between frequency and intensity of fears and a collagen condition. *Depress Anxiety*. Vol.23, No.7, pp.412-7.

Bulbena, A.; Sperry, L.; Anguinano, B.; Pailhez, G. & Gago, J. (2007). Joint hypermobility in schizophrenia: a potential marker for co-morbid anxiety. *The open psychiatry journal*. Vol.1, pp.31-3.

Bulbena, A.; Gago, J.; Pailhez, G.; Sperry, L.; Fullana, MA. & Vilarroya, O. (2011). Joint Hypermobility Syndrome is a Risk Factor Trait for Anxiety Disorders: a 15-year follow-up cohort study. *General Hospital Psychiatry*. Accepted for publication.

Carlsson, C. & Rundgren, A. (1980) Hypermobility of the joints in women alcoholics. *J Stud Alcohol*. Vol.41, No.1, pp.78-81.

Collier, DA. (2002). FISH, flexible joints and panic: are anxiety disorders really expressions of instability in the human genome? *Br J Psychiatry*. Vol.181, pp.457-9.

Flanders, H. (1950) *Diagnóstico y tratamiento psicosomáticos*. José Janés, Buenos Aires, Argentina.

García-Campayo, J.; Asso, E.; Alda, M.; Andres, EM. & Sobradiel, N. (2010). Association between joint hypermobility syndrome and panic disorder: a case-control study. *Psychosomatics*. Vol.51, No.1, pp.55-61.

Gazit, Y.; Nahir, AM.; Grahame, R. & Jacob, G. (2003). Dysautonomia in the joint hypermobility syndrome. *Am J Med*. Vol.115, No.1, pp.33-40.

Gratacos, M.; Nadal, M.; Martín-Santos, R.; Pujana, M.; Gago, J.; Peral, B.; Armengol, L.; Ponsa, I.; Miró, R.; Bulbena, A. & Estivill, X. (2001). A polymorphic genomic duplication on human chromosome 15 is a susceptibility factor for panic and phobic disorders. *Cell*. Vol.106, pp.367-79.

Gulpek, D.; Bayraktar, E.; Akbay, SP.; Capaci, K.; Kayikcioglu, M.;, Aliyev, E. & Soydas, C. (2004). Joint hypermobility syndrome and mitral valve prolapse in panic disorder. *Prog Neuropsychopharmacol Biol Psychiatry*. Vol.28, No.6, pp.969-73.

Gulsun, M.; Yilmaz, MB.; Pinar, M.; Tonbul, M.; Celik, C.; Ozdemir, B.; Dumlu, K. & Erbas, M. (2007). Thorax deformity, joint hypermobility, and anxiety disorders. *Saudi Med J*. Vol.28, No.12, pp.1840-4.

Härter, MC.; Conway, KP. & Merikangas, KR. (2003). Associations between anxiety disorders and physical illness. *Eur Arch Psychiatry Clin Neurosci*. Vol.253, No.6, pp.313-20.

Katon, W. & Roy-Byrne, P. (1989). Panic disorder in the medically ill. *J Clin Psychiatry*. Vol.50, pp.299-302.

Katon, W. (1996). Panic disorder: Relationship to high medical utilization, unexplained physical symptoms, and medical costs. *J Clin Psychiatry*. Vol.57, pp.11-18.

Keer, R. & Grahame, R. (2003). *Hypermobility Syndrome: Recognition and Management for Physiotherapists,* Butterworth - Heinemann, London, UK.

Kessler, RC.; Ormel, J.; Demler, O. & Stang, PE. (2003). Comorbid mental disorders account for the role impairment of commonly occurring chronic physical disorders: results from the National Comorbidity Survey. *J Occup Environ Med.* Vol. 45, No.12, pp.1257-66.

Martín-Santos, R.; Bulbena, A.; Porta, M.; Gago, J.; Molina, L. & Duró, JC. (1998). Association between the joint hypermobility syndrome and panic disorder. *Am J Psychiatry.* Vol.155, pp.1578-83.

McLaughlin, TP.; Khandker, RK.; Kruzikas, DT. & Tummala, R. (2006). Overlap of anxiety and depression in a managed care population: Prevalence and association with resource utilization. *J Clin Psychiatry,* Vol.67, No.8, pp.1187-93.

Mishra, MB.; Ryan, P.; Atkinson, P.; Taylor, H.; Bell, J.; Calver, D.; Fogelman, I.; Child, A.; Jackson, G.; Chambers, JB. & Grahame, R. (1996). Extra-articular features of benign joint hypermobility syndrome. *Br J Rheumatol.* Vol.35, No.9, pp.861-6.

Muller, JE.; Koen, L & Stein, DJ. (2005). Anxiety and medical disorders. *Curr Psychiatry Rep.* Vol.7, No.4, pp.245-51.

Pailhez, G.; Bulbena, A.; Fullana, MA. & Castaño, J. (2009). Anxiety disorders and joint hypermobility syndrome: the role of collagen tissue. *Gen Hosp Psychiatry.* Vol.31, No.3, pp.299.

Pascual, JC.; Castaño, J. ; Espluga, N.; Diaz, B.; Garcia-Ribera, C. & Bulbena, A. (2008). Medical conditions in patients suffering from anxiety disorders. *Med Clin (Barc).* Vol.130, No.8, pp.281-5.

Rogers, MP., White, K., Warshaw, MG., Yonkers, KA., Rodriguez-Villa, F., Chang, G., & Keller, MB. (1994). Prevalence of medical illness in patients with anxiety disorders. *Int'l. J. Psychiatry in Medicine.* Vol.24, No.1, pp.83-96.

Rotés, J. & Argany, A. (1957). La laxitud articular como factor de alteraciones del aparato locomotor. *Rev Esp Reumatol.* Vol. 1, pp.59-62.

Roy-Byrne, PP.; Davidson, KW.; Kessler, RC.; Asmundson, GJ.; Goodwin, RD.; Kubzansky, L.; Lydiard, RB.; Massie, MJ.; Katon, W.; Laden, SK. & Stein, MB. (2008). Anxiety disorders and comorbid medical illness. *Gen Hosp Psychiatry.* Vol.30, No.3, pp.208-25.

Sareen, J.; Jacobi, F.; Cox, BJ.; Belik, SL.; Clara, I. & Stein MB. (2006). Disability and poor quality of life associated with comorbid anxiety disorders and physical conditions. *Arch Intern Med.* Vol.166, No.19, pp.2109-16.

Sareen, J.; Cox, BJ.; Clara, I. & Asmundson, GJ. (2005). The relationship between anxiety disorders and physical disorders in the U.S. National Comorbidity Survey. *Depress Anxiety.* Vol.21, No.4, pp.193-202.

Simon, NM. & Fischmann, D. (2005). The implications of medical and psychiatric comorbidity with panic disorder. *J Clin Psychiatry.* Vol.66, pp.8-15.

Stein, MB. (1986). Panic disorder and medical illness. *Psychosomatics.* Vol.27, pp.833-40.

Talati, A.; Ponniah, K.; Strug, LJ.; Hodge, SE.; Fyer, AJ. & Weissman, MM. (2001). Panic disorder, social anxiety disorder, and a possible medical syndrome previously linked to chromosome 13. *Biol Psychiatry.* Vol.63, No.6, pp.594-601.

Wells, KB.; Golding, JM. & Burnam, MA. (1989). Chronic medical conditions in a sample of the general population with anxiety, affective, and substance use disorders. *Am J Psychiatry*. Vol.146, No.11, pp.1440-6.

Wise, MG. & Taylor, SE. (1990). Anxiety and mood disorders in medically ill patients. *J Clin Psychiatry*. Vol.51, pp.27-32.

Zaubler, TS. & Katon, W. (1998). Panic disorder in the general medical setting. *Journal of Psychosomatic Research*. Vol.44, No.1, pp.25-42.

7

Generalised Anxiety Disorder, Mortality and Disease: A Stronger Predictor than Major Depressive Disorder

Anna C. Phillips
University of Birmingham, School of Sport & Exercise Sciences
UK

1. Introduction

This chapter will examine the associations between Generalised Anxiety Disorder (GAD) and key health outcomes, including mortality, the metabolic syndrome, and hypertension, citing relevant research and recent findings from the Vietnam Experience Study. It aims to show that GAD is as strong a determinant of such health outcomes, if not a stronger one than MDD. It also aims to illustrate the importance of considering the comorbidity of GAD with other psychiatric diagnoses when predicting mortality and other health outcomes.

2. GAD and mortality

Mental health disorders in the general population are relatively common (Kessler et al., 2005; Kessler, Chiu, Demler, Merikangas, & Walters, 2005). In fact, an estimated 14% of the global disease burden has been attributed to mental health disorders (World Health Organisation, 1992-1994), and this figure is likely to be an underestimate as it fails to take into consideration the association between mental health and other health conditions (Prince et al., 2007). Populations who have been exposed to traumatic events, such as war veterans, have an even higher prevalence of Generalised Anxiety Disorder (GAD) and Major Depressive Disorder (MDD) (Gaylord, 2006; Hoge, Auchterlonie, & Milliken, 2006; Reeves, Parker, & Konkle-Parker, 2005). For example, soldiers assessed a few months after returning from deployment to Afghanistan and Iraq had a GAD prevalence of around 14% and 15%, respectively, and prevalence of MDD of around 17% and 16% (Hoge et al., 2004). Others have reported depressive symptom rates as high as 19% in veterans based on prior diagnosis records (Kinder et al., 2008), and 31% using self-report measures (Hankin, Spiro, Miller, & Kazis, 1999), although some studies have shown lower rates of 6.9% and 1.7% for MDD and GAD, respectively (Sareen et al., 2007). Little has been reported about the consequences for survival of these mental health disorders in veterans.

In the general population, MDD has been associated with increased mortality rates (see e.g. O'Leary & Lee, 1996; Surtees & Barkley, 1994). Although much of this excess is attributable to non-medical causes of death such as injury and suicide, it is becoming clear that MDD also increases the risk of death from common chronic diseases such as cardiovascular disease (CVD) (Osby, Brandt, Correia, Ekbom, & Sparen, 2001). There is now substantial evidence linking depression with CVD morbidity and mortality (see e.g. Musselman, Evans,

& Nemeroff, 1998; Wulsin, Vaillant, & Wells, 1999). However, much of this research has examined the impact of depressed mood rather than a diagnosis of MDD. In a recent meta-analysis of 11 studies of coronary heart disease (CHD), MDD, which had been measured in only three studies, was a much stronger predictor of CHD outcomes than depressed mood (Rugulies, 2002). Few studies have examined GAD as a risk factor for all-cause mortality, although two population studies suggest that, for causes of death other than suicide, GAD does not present a significant risk (Holwerda et al., 2007; Murphy, Monson, Olivier, Sobol, & Leighton, 1987). However, other manifestations of anxiety have been associated with an increased risk of CVD morbidity and/or mortality (see e.g. Eaker, Sullivan, Kelly-Hayes, D'Agostino, & Benjamin, 2005; Haines, Imeson, & Meade, 1987; Weissman, Markowitz, Ouellette, Greenwald, & Kahn, 1990). It would appear that no studies have measured the relationship between diagnosed GAD and CVD mortality.

The bulk of research examining the consequences of mental health disorders for chronic disease in veterans has concentrated on post-traumatic stress disorder (PTSD). For example, lifetime prevalence of PTSD was linked with an increased mortality rate (Boscarino, 2006a, 2006b). In addition, PTSD in veterans has also been associated with cardiovascular, digestive, musculoskeletal, endocrine-nutritional-metabolic, nervous system, respiratory, and nonsexually transmitted infectious diseases (J.A. Boscarino, 1997), chronic changes in immunity (Boscarino & Chang, 1999), and markers of inflammatory disorders (Boscarino, 2004). However, there appear to be few studies examining the influence of other major mental health disorders on mortality risk in veterans. In a study of PTSD and MDD in veterans, MDD was related to increased mortality following adjustment for age, demographic variables, health behaviours, and medical co-morbidities (Kinder, et al., 2008). The association between GAD and mortality in veterans does not appear to have been studied.

Given the reported high prevalence of GAD and MDD in army veterans and the significant prevalence of these disorders in the general population, their individual and combined impact merits research attention. Recently, it was possible to address this issue in the Vietnam Experience Study.

2.1 The Vietnam experience study

The Vietnam Experience Study is an epidemiological study commissioned by the US congress to investigate the health consequences of the military experiences of Vietnam veterans. The participants were male military personnel drawn from approximately five million US Vietnam-era army veterans whose service files were stored at the National Personnel Records Center (Vietnam Experience Study, 1987). The Centers for Disease Control, Atlanta, had access to U.S. Veteran Administration records and provided a fully anonymised dataset. Those who entered military service between January 1, 1965 and December 31, 1971; served only one term of enlistment; served at least 16 weeks of active duty; earned a military specialty other than "trainee" or "duty soldier"; at discharge from active duty had a military pay grade no higher than sergeant; and had not died during military duties were eligible for inclusion. On reviewing a random sample of 48 513 records, 1355 were found to be incomplete, 28 577 did not meet study entry criteria and 268 men died during military duties, so the final cohort included 18,313 former military personnel. Of those included in the original cohort, 17,867 were considered to be alive on December 31st 1983 and therefore eligible for active follow-up.

Information pertaining to place of service, military rank, ethnicity, and cognitive ability scores from the Army General Technical Test (hereafter referred to as "IQ") was extracted from the military archives. Participants were designated as being Vietnam veterans if they had served at least one tour of duty in Vietnam, and as non-Vietnam veterans if they did not (this group included men who served one or more tours of duty in Korea, Germany or the US). The ethnic origin of the study members were classified as 'white', 'black', or 'other'; the latter group comprising Hispanics, Asians, Pacific Islanders, American Indians, and Alaskan Natives.

In 1985 these participants were invited to participate in a telephone interview. Telephone directories, credit bureau searches, driver's license and motor vehicle registration records, city directories, local records and personal field visits were all utilized to locate the whereabouts of apparently surviving men. Of those traced (N = 16 349), an interview was not possible for reasons of incarceration (N = 63), physical or mental disability (N = 20), refusal (N = 949), death during the tracing process (N = 53), or 'other' (N = 6). This resulted in a sample of 15,288 men (85.6% of those alive on December 31st 1983) who participated in the 1985 telephone survey (Batty et al., 2008). During the telephone survey, enquiries were made about the study participants' socio-economic characteristics, health behaviours, and health. Socio-economic position was measured using household income in midlife. Frequency of alcohol consumption was classified as number of units consumed per week. Smoking habits and marital status were ascertained using standard questions. Participants were also asked whether or not they had a range of somatic physician-diagnosed health problems which included hypertension, cancer, diabetes and coronary heart disease (The Centers for Disease Control Vietnam Experience Study., 1988a, 1988b).

In 1986, a random sample of telephone interview respondents (N=6443) were invited to attend a three day medical examination with orientation at a single facility in Albuquerque, New Mexico, for which travel expenses and a nominal stipend were met; 4462 attended (69.3% of those invited). The mean age at medical examination was 38.3 years (range: 31.1 to 49.0). Of those invited, medical examination was not possible for reasons of incarceration (N = 26), physical or mental disability (N = 10), refusal (N = 949), death before invitation (N = 10), or 'refusal' (N = 372). The main reasons for refusing to participate at this stage of data collection were: work related, e.g. unable to get leave with pay; a lack of interest in the study, e.g. unable to see how it would benefit them; or personal, e.g. did not like to travel. The final number of participants with complete data after the medical examination was 4256. This group represents 23.3% of persons originally enrolled in the study. Sampling in the study is shown in Figure 1, below. For the medical examination, all men were requested to fast from 19.00 the evening before medical testing. Following the drawing of blood the following morning, cholesterol level was ascertained using a Kodak Ektachem 700 autoanalyzer (The Centers for Disease Control Vietnam Experience Study., 1988a, 1988b). Serum glucose level was determined with a standard adaptation of the glucose oxidase-peroxidase-chromogen-coupled system for glucose determination in biologic fluids (The Centers for Disease Control Vietnam Experience Study., 1988a, 1988b). Blood pressure, while seated, was measured twice in the right arm using a standard mercury sphygmomanometer; for the purposes of analyses, an average was computed. Height and weight, measured using standard protocols, were used to calculate body mass index (BMI) (kg/m^2).

2.1.1 Psychological morbidity

Psychological morbidity was assessed using the Diagnostic Interview Schedule (version 3A) as administered by a trained psychological technician. The Diagnostic Interview Schedule is

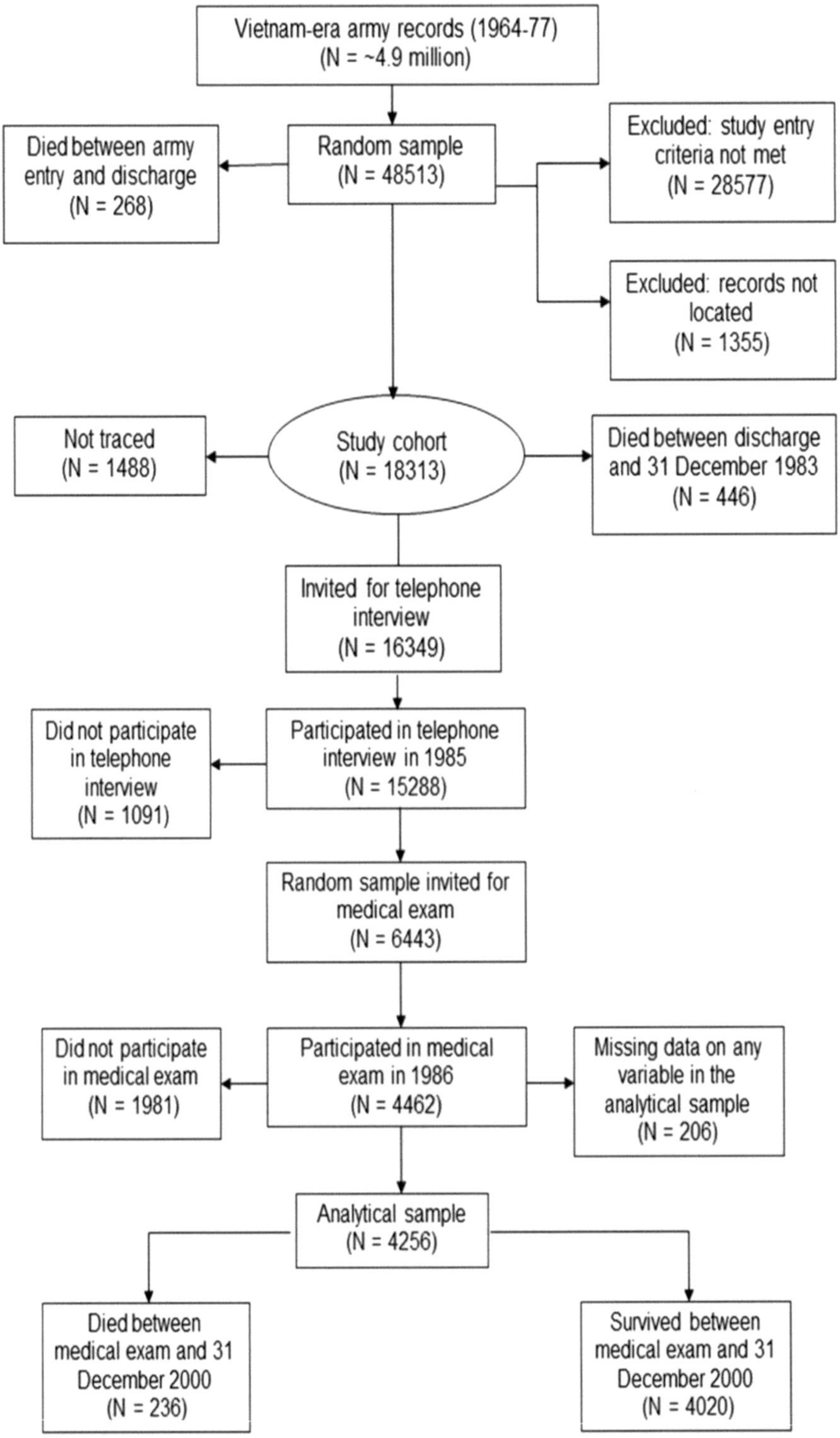

Fig. 1. Sampling in the Vietnam Experience Study

a standardized questionnaire that is designed to assess the prevalence of certain psychiatric conditions according to the Diagnostic and Statistical Manual of Mental Disorders (version III) criteria of the American Psychiatric Association (APA, 1980; Robins, Helzer, & Cottler, 1987). Study participants were considered positive for GAD and MDD if they reported a pattern of symptoms in the previous 12 months that satisfied full Diagnostic and Statistical Manual of Mental Disorders (version III) criteria. Characteristics of those with and without a diagnosis of GAD are shown in Table 1.

		Generalised Anxiety Disorder (N = 411)		No Generalised Anxiety Disorder (N = 3845)		*p*
		Mean	SD	Mean	SD	
Standardised IQ score from enlistment		96.5	16.18	101.9	14.99	<.001
Units of alcohol per week		10.6	22.87	6.7	13.15	<.001
Age at medical examination (years)		38.0	2.65	38.4	2.50	.003
Total cholesterol (mmol/l)		5.5	1.01	5.5	1.09	.42
Blood glucose (mg/dL)		95.6	20.44	94.2	16.66	.10
SBP (mmHg)		123.8	13.06	122.9	11.93	.17
BMI (kg/m2)		25.9	3.70	25.9	4.12	.88
		N (%)		N (%)		*p*
Place of service	Ever in Vietnam	267 (65)		2082 (54)		<.001
	Other overseas	85 (21)		1010 (26)		
	US only	59 (14)		753 (20)		
Ethnicity:	White	311 (76)		3179 (83)		.001
	Black	61 (15)		435 (11)		
	Other	39 (9)		231 (6)		
Household income in midlife	<$20,000	184 (45)		1018 (26)		<.001
	-$40,000	171 (42)		1958 (51)		
	>$40,000	56 (13)		869 (23)		
Smoking Status:	Non smoker	79 (19)		1006 (26)		<.001
	Ex smoker	90 (22)		1119 (29)		
	Current smoker	242 (59)		1720 (45)		
Marital Status:	Married	244 (59)		2887 (75)		<.001
	Divorced/separated/widowed	116 (28)		651 (17)		
	Never married	51 (12)		307 (8)		
Physical Illness	No	335 (82)		3349 (87)		.002
diabetes/hypertension/cancer or CHD	Yes	76 (18)		496 (13)		

Table 1. Characteristics of those with and without a diagnosis of GAD

2.1.2 Mortality status

The vital status of men between army discharge and December 31st 1983 (the date the cohort was established) was ascertained by cross-checking against a variety of mortality databases supplied by the US army, the Veterans Administration (Beneficiary Identification and Records Locator Subsystem), the Social Security Administration, the Internal Revenue Service, and the National Center for Health Statistics (National Death Index). Vital status post-medical exam continued to be ascertained until 31st December 2000 using the same mortality databases. Mortality due to major CVD was classified using the International Classification of Diseases (ICD) (World Health Organisation, 1992) codes: ICD-9: 390–434,436–448, and ICD-10: I00–I78 which comprised: acute rheumatic fever; chronic rheumatic heart diseases; hypertensive diseases; ischaemic heart diseases; pulmonary heart disease and diseases of pulmonary circulation; other forms of heart disease; cerebrovascular diseases; diseases of arteries, arterioles and capillaries. The CVD mortality variable thus encompasses death from a variety of disorders.

2.2 Characteristics of those with GAD and who were deceased

Of the 4256 participants, 9.7% for GAD and 6.5% met diagnostic criteria for MDD. GAD was significantly associated with serving in Vietnam, younger age at the time of the medical examination, being non-white, and equally likely to be divorced/separated/widowed as never married. These individuals also had lower IQ scores, and lower household income in mid life. Finally, they were more likely to be a current smoker and to drink more units of alcohol per week; and were more likely to have a physical illness. During the 15 years of follow-up there were 236 deaths. Higher mortality was associated with service in Vietnam, not being married, being non-white, having lower household income in midlife, higher blood pressure and blood glucose level, smoking; higher alcohol consumption, and reported physical illness at examination. The characteristics of those who were and were not deceased are shown in Table 2.

2.3 Associations with mortality

Following adjustment for age and the other covariates measured, described above in section 2.1 and shown in Table 1, it was found that both those with GAD and those with MDD were at an increased risk of death during follow-up. This risk of all-cause mortality was roughly 1.6 times greater than that of those with no diagnosis. However, the effect for GAD was stronger than that for MDD. In analyses using cardiovascular disease mortality as the outcome, adjusting for confounding variables, neither GAD nor MDD were related increased risk of death, although the associations were in the same direction as for all-cause mortality.

Interestingly, 153 (3.6%) of participants had a diagnosis of both MDD and GAD in the past year. In fully adjusted analyses, simultaneously using comorbidity as a predictor variable as well as MDD or GAD alone, only comorbidity was significantly related to both all-cause and cardiovascular disease mortality. These differences between the diagnoses groups and risk of death are shown in Figure 2.

The prevalence of GAD and MDD are higher than general population estimates (Kessler, Chiu, et al., 2005). However, even higher prevalence has been observed in other veteran groups when mental disorders were measured more proximally to combat exposure (Hoge, et al., 2004). Undoubtedly the most compelling and robust associations with mortality, both all-cause and CVD, emerged for MDD and GAD comorbidity. The present results regarding GAD contrast with those from the two previous studies on GAD and all-cause mortality, which suggest that GAD does not present a significant risk (Holwerda, et al., 2007; Murphy, et al., 1987). However, this discrepancy might be due to the difference in populations

		Died: All-cause (N = 236)		Surviving (N = 4020)		p
		Mean	SD	Mean	SD	
Standardised IQ score from enlistment		96.5	15.2	101.6	15.14	< .001
Units of alcohol per week		11.9	23.00	6.8	13.7	< .001
Age at medical examination (years)		38.6	2.68	38.3	2.51	.15
Total cholesterol (mmol/l)		5.6	1.35	5.5	1.06	.45
Blood glucose (mg/dL)		102.6	40.75	93.8	14.38	< .001
SBP (mmHg)		125.4	15.65	122.9	11.79	.001
BMI (kg/m²)		25.9	3.69	26.2	4.50	.20
		N (%)		N (%)		p
Place of service	Ever in Vietnam Other overseas US only	148 (63) 49 (21) 39 (17)		2201 (55) 1046 (26) 773 (19)		.06
Ethnicity:	White Black Other	162 (69) 51 (21) 23 (10)		3328 (83) 445 (11) 247 (6)		< .001
Household income in midlife	<$20,000 -$40,000 >$40,000	110 (47) 105 (44) 21 (9)		1092 (27) 2024 (50) 904 (23)		<.001
Smoking Status: smoker	Non Ex smoker Current smoker	42 (18) 44 (19) 150 (64)		1043 (26) 1165 (29) 1812 (45)		< .001
Marital Status:	Married Divorced/separated/widowed Never married	129 (55) 71 (30) 36 (15)		3002 (75) 696 (17) 322 (8)		< .001
Physical Illness diabetes/hypertension/cancer or CHD	No Yes	62 (26) 174 (74)		3510 (87) 510 (13)		< .001

Table 2. Characteristics of those who were and were not deceased

examined: older adults (Holwerda, et al., 2007) and the general population (Murphy, et al., 1987). It is also possible that anxiety may only predict mortality in men, as in one previous study where an association between anxiety disorders and mortality was found for men but not women (van Hout et al., 2004). GAD has not been previously studied in terms of CVD mortality in the general population, or in the context of mortality per se in veterans. This seems unfortunate given that it is a strong predictor of all-cause mortality in the present analyses. The present findings are consistent with the results of previous research linking MDD with all-cause mortality in the general population (e.g. O'Leary & Lee, 1996; Surtees & Barkley, 1994) and in veterans (Kinder, et al., 2008). Although many studies have considered depression as a predictor of CVD mortality, surprisingly few have examined diagnosed MDD. Of those available, both positive (Osby, et al., 2001) and null (Hallstrom, Lapidus, Bengtsson, & Edstrom, 1986; Vogt, Pope, Mullooly, & Hollis, 1994) findings have been reported. Although little attention has been paid to MDD and all-cause mortality in veterans, our findings are consistent with those of one recent study in which individuals with a diagnosis of depression were at increased risk of death over an average of two years (Kinder, et al., 2008).

Some studies have examined the prognostic importance of both symptoms of anxiety and depression and mortality in cardiac patient groups. In a review of 25 studies of chronic heart failure patients, anxiety symptoms were measured along with depression in just three studies (Pelle, Gidron, Szabo, & Denollet, 2008). Anxiety symptoms were not associated with mortality, whereas depressive symptoms significantly predicted death (Pelle, et al., 2008). A number of studies have examined both anxiety and depression symptoms and mortality in myocardial infarction patients. High depression and anxiety scores have both been found to predict all-cause mortality (Herrmann et al., 1998), and cardiac death (Denollet & Brutsaert, 1998). However, in three studies, symptoms of depression but not anxiety in multivariate models predicted all-cause or cardiac mortality (Ahern et al., 1990; Frasure-Smith & Lesperance, 2003; Frasure-Smith, Lesperance, & Talajic, 1995). Finally, neither depression nor anxiety symptoms were found to predict mortality in myocardial infarction patients (Lane, Carroll, Ring, Beevers, & Lip, 2001). Thus, in prognostic studies, it would appear that depressive symptoms may be a more stable predictor of mortality than anxiety. However, it is unclear the extent to which the results of these studies of patients with chronic inflammatory disease relate to the present aetiological study where only 1% had a diagnosis of coronary heart disease at the medical examination. It is possible that the effects of depression on mortality and the underlying mechanisms may not be identical in patient versus population-based studies. Further, none of the prognostic studies that we know of have examined psychiatric comorbidity effects on mortality.

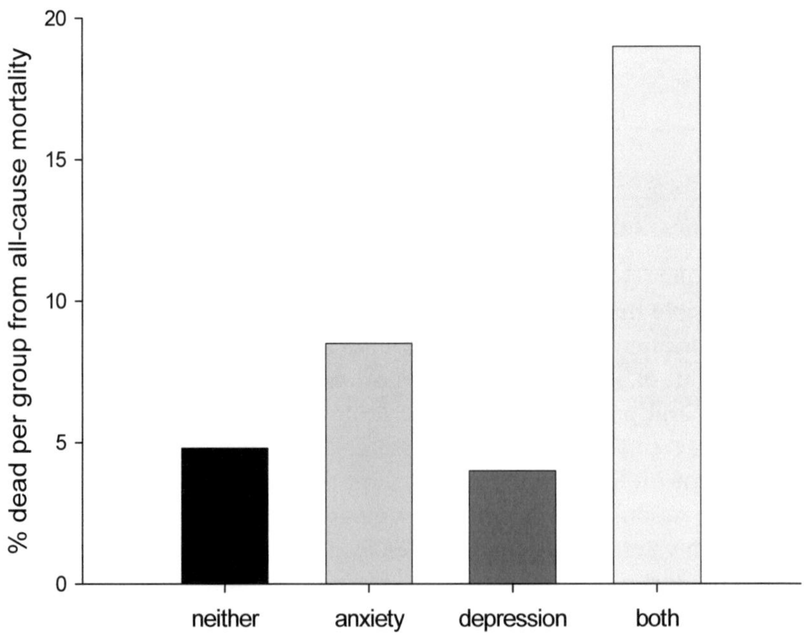

Fig. 2. Percentage deceased in each diagnosis category

GAD and MDD are highly comorbid psychiatric conditions (Kessler, Chiu, et al., 2005). In the present study, 3.6% of participants had a diagnosis of both MDD and GAD. More strikingly, 55% of those with a diagnosis of MDD also had GAD. Patients with comorbid MDD and GAD have been found to have poorer functional status than those with either condition alone (Kessler, DuPont, Berglund, & Wittchen, 1999) and it has been proposed that they are at increased risk for CVD (Sevincok, Buyukozturk, & Dereboy, 2001). However, we know of no previous studies that have examined the mortality risk associated with this comorbidity. The present analysis indicates that comorbid MDD and GAD confers a stronger mortality risk than either condition alone. The importance of comorbidity was further demonstrated in the supplementary analyses of the effects of comorbidity with PTSD where it was the comorbidity of MDD and GAD, and of PTSD, MDD, and GAD that emerged as the most consistent predictors of mortality. Consequently, this argues that comorbidity should receive considerably more attention in future research on mental disorders and health outcomes, at least in studies of non-patient groups. Further, clinical interventions have tended to concentrate on single mental health diagnoses; these findings suggest that targeting comorbidity might be a fruitful new approach.

2.4 Limitations

It should be conceded that there are a number of limitations to this analysis and its interpretation. First, the weaker effects for CVD in comparison to all-cause mortality may reflect the small number of deaths due to CVD in this sample resulting in lower power to detect significant associations, particularly when adjusting for a large number of covariates. Support for this assertion can be found in the hazard ratios which were of comparable size in the fully adjusted models for both all-cause and CVD mortality, but only attained significance when all-cause mortality was the outcome. Second, residual confounding as a consequence of un-measured variables cannot be wholly discounted. The present analysis, however, did adjust for a large number of potential confounding variables. Third, as this sample was exclusively male, there is the issue of generalisation. It should be noted that the previous studies with null results tested women only in one case (Hallstrom et al., 1986) and both sexes in the other (Vogt et al., 1994). It is also worth noting, though, that these studies had much smaller samples, reducing their power to detect effects on mortality. In addition, it is possible that veterans differ in other ways from the broader population. For example, one study of stable coronary heart disease that included veterans found no evidence that depression was associated with elevated levels of inflammation (Whooley et al., 2007); a finding opposite to that of many studies in non-cardiac disease patients. However, not all the patients in this study were veterans (Whooley et al., 2007). Fourth, it has been suggested that the prevalence of mental health disorders in the Vietnam Experience Study are underestimated (Dohrenwend et al., 2006, 2007). However, this criticism has mainly been levelled at estimations of PTSD prevalence. Nevertheless, it is possible that severely depressed veterans were less likely to participate in the medical examination, which may have accounted for the attenuated associations for major depression in the present analyses. However, this seems unlikely given that only 10 (<2%) veterans were unable to attend on the basis of physical/mental disability, and only 372 (<6%) refused to attend, with the main reasons being a lack of interest or unwillingness to travel. Moreover, underestimation in the present study would make the associations demonstrated between MDD, GAD, their comorbidity and mortality more compelling. Fifth, given that a diagnosis of MDD only requires two weeks of symptoms, whereas GAD requires symptoms for at least six months, it is possible that MDD diagnoses were less trustworthy. However, evidence indicates that the DSM-III criteria for diagnosis of both MDD and GAD are highly reliable (Riskind et al., 1987).

In conclusion, the present analysis in Vietnam veterans showed that MDD and GAD were positively associated with all-cause and CVD mortality. However, in the fully adjusted analyses reported, the relationships with CVD mortality were non-significant, possibly due to low statistical power. A diagnosis of both MDD and GAD proved much the strongest predictor of all-cause and CVD mortality. The effects of comorbidity of MDD and GAD, and with PTSD would suggest that future research on mental health disorders and physical health outcomes, as well as future clinical interventions, should pay more attention to comorbidity. In addition, future studies should attempt to measure and take account of a full range of factors likely to be associated with both mental and physical health.

3. GAD and the metabolic syndrome

The metabolic syndrome (MetS) is a prevalent cluster of symptoms (obesity, high triglyceride levels, low levels of HDL cholesterol, raised blood pressure, and high levels of fasting blood glucose or a diagnosis of diabetes) (Isomaa et al., 2001; Lakka et al., 2002; Thomas et al., 2007; Trevisan, Liu, Bahsas, & Menotti, 1998). As the metabolic syndrome increases risk for cardiovascular and all-cause mortality (Isomaa, et al., 2001; Lakka, et al., 2002; Thomas, et al., 2007; Trevisan, et al., 1998), recently there has been interest in the relationship between it and various mental health disorders.

The bulk of this research has focused on depression and although contrary indications exist (Herva et al., 2006), there is evidence of a positive association between depression and the metabolic syndrome (Dunbar et al., 2008; Heiskanen et al., 2006; Kinder, Carnethon, Palaniappan, King, & Fortmann, 2004; Koponen, Jokelainen, Keinanen-Kiukaanniemi, Kumpusalo, & Vanhala, 2008; McCaffery, Niaura, Todaro, Swan, & Carmelli, 2003; Raikkonen, Matthews, & Kuller, 2002; Skilton, Moulin, Terra, & Bonnet, 2007; Vaccarino et al., 2008). However, the vast majority of these studies were concerned with depressive symptoms; a recent review (Goldbacher & Matthews, 2007) identified only two studies examining MDD in this context. In a small study of outpatients, those who still had a diagnosis at 6-year follow-up showed a higher prevalence of the metabolic syndrome (Heiskanen, et al., 2006). In a larger scale study, a history of MDD was associated with the metabolic syndrome in women but not men (Kinder, et al., 2004). Much less attention has been paid to anxiety and the metabolic syndrome and the three most recent studies reported null findings (Herva, et al., 2006; Raikkonen, Matthews, & Kuller, 2007; Skilton, et al., 2007). However, an earlier study of women found an association between the metabolic syndrome and increased anxiety seven years later (Raikkonen, et al., 2002). These studies have all been concerned with anxiety symptoms; no study has tested the association with GAD. We were able to utilise the Vietnam Experience Study dataset in order to examine the potential links between GAD and the metabolic syndrome. In this dataset, the metabolic syndrome was defined as having at least three of: BMI > 30 kg/m^2 (in the absence of waist circumference data, BMI at this threshold is regarded by World Health Organization as an acceptable substitute in defining MetS); triglycerides ≥ 1.7 mmol/l (150 mg/dl); HDL cholesterol < 1.036 mmol/l (40 mg/dl); blood pressure ≥ 130/85 mmHg or taking antihypertensive medication; fasting glucose ≥ 6.1 mmol/l (110 mg/dl) or taking diabetes medication.

3.1 Associations with the metabolic syndrome

Seven hundred and seventy-three (18%) of the men in the Vietnam Experience Study were identified as having the metabolic syndrome. Aside from differing on all the components of the metabolic syndrome, participants with it were slightly older, had lower IQ scores and a briefer education, were less likely to be divorced, widowed or separated and more likely to come from ethnic groups other than white or black, i.e. Hispanic. Full details of the characteristics of those with and without the metabolic syndrome are shown in Table 3.

		Metabolic syndrome (N = 773)		No metabolic syndrome (N = 3483)		*p*
		Mean	SD	Mean	SD	
Metabolic Syndrome Markers:						
BMI (kg/m2)		30.00	4.16	25.03	2.96	<.001
Triglycerides (mg/dL)		214.20	151.22	91.97	56.70	<.001
HDL cholesterol (mg/dL)		34.85	7.78	46.85	12.24	<.001
SBP (mmHg)		131.46	11.87	121.13	11.25	<.001
DBP (mmHg)		91.16	8.64	82.56	8.88	<.001
Blood glucose (mg/dL)		104.57	28.06	92.04	12.35	<.001
Covariates:						
Age at medical examination (years)		38.67	2.51	38.25	2.51	<.001
Units of alcohol per week		6.69	15.46	7.17	14.18	.40
Standardised IQ score from enlistment		99.63	15.03	101.75	15.20	<.001
Grade achieved in education		13.04	2.26	13.35	2.31	.001
		N (%)		N (%)		*p*
Metabolic Syndrome Markers:						
Obese		396 (51)		154 (4)		<.001
Hypertension Diagnosis		189 (24)		252 (7)		<.001
Diabetes Diagnosis		27 (4)		22 (1)		<.001
Predictor variables:						
MDD		57 (7)		220 (6)		.28
GAD		94 (12)		317 (9)		.009
Covariates:						
Place of service	Ever in Vietnam	444 (63)		1905 (55)		.29
	Other overseas	195 (21)		900 (26)		
	US only	134 (17)		678 (19)		
Ethnicity:	White	633 (82)		2857 (82)		.005
	Black	74 (10)		422 (12)		
	Other	66 (8)		204 (6)		
Household income in midlife	<$20,000	234 (30)		968 (28)		.35
	-$40,000	380 (49)		1749 (50)		
	>$40,000	159 (21)		766 (22)		
Smoking Status:	Non smoker	194 (25)		891 (26)		.85
	Ex smoker	226 (29)		983 (28)		
	Current smoker	353 (46)		1609 (46)		
Marital Status:	Married	612 (79)		2519 (72)		< .001
	Divorced/separated/widowed	99 (13)		668 (19)		
	Never married	62 (8)		296 (9)		

Table 3. Characteristics of those with and without the metabolic syndrome

In this sample, MDD was not significantly associated with the metabolic syndrome in either age-adjusted analyses or those adjusting for other confounding variables described above. However, there was a positive association between GAD and the metabolic syndrome, such that those with GAD were 1.36 times more likely to have the metabolic syndrome than those without GAD diagnosis. Depression and anxiety are highly co-morbid conditions, and in the present sample, MDD and GAD were significantly correlated, $C(1) = .38$, $p < .001$, and 153 (4%) were diagnosed with both conditions. Consequently, in competitive models, entering MMD alone, GAD alone, and their co-morbidity simultaneously, only GAD was associated with metabolic syndrome incidence.

These findings contrast with the results of previous studies, however, these have been concerned with symptoms of anxiety and the analysis reported above is the first to examine GAD in the context of the metabolic syndrome. Further, only two studies, to date, have explored the links between MDD and the metabolic syndrome (5,7). The much larger of these two studies reported an association with MDD in women, but not men (Kinder, et al., 2004). Thus, the apparent discrepancy between the present findings and those of others may be more illusory than real. Of the components of the metabolic syndrome, it was hypertension, obesity, and triglycerides that differentiated those with and without GAD. There was no association with diabetes.

3.2 Limitations and potential mechanisms

Unfortunately, with cross-sectional analyses it is impossible to determine the direction of the association and whether it is causal. If anxiety precedes metabolic syndrome, there are at least two pathways through which it might contribute to its aetiology. First, anxiety has been associated with unhealthy behaviour, such as smoking, binge drinking, physical inactivity, and unhealthy diet (Strine et al., 2008). However, despite the fact that participants with GAD consumed more units of alcohol per week and were more likely to be current smokers, the present association between GAD and metabolic syndrome was unaffected by adjustment for smoking and alcohol consumption. Second, it has been postulated that hypothalamic-pituitary-adrenocortical dysregulation associated with affective disorders, including anxiety, may contribute over time to the metabolic syndrome (Raikkonen, et al., 2002). There is evidence linking anxiety with altered cortisol activity; high levels of anxiety symptoms were found to be associated with a less pronounced cortisol awakening response (Therrien et al., 2008). However, it remains possible that the causal pathway is from the metabolic syndrome to GAD. The metabolic syndrome has been shown to predict symptoms of anxiety seven years later (Raikkonen, et al., 2002), whereas the reverse was not found (Raikkonen, et al., 2002, 2007). Further, it is reasonable to presume that diagnosis of some of the components of the metabolic syndrome may be anxiolytic. For example, irrespective of actual blood pressure levels, perceived hypertensive status was positively associated with anxiety (Spruill et al., 2007). Whatever the underlying mechanism of the association with GAD, it remains true that depression has been the main focus for studies of mental health and physical health outcomes. The current data suggest that future research should perhaps pay equal attention to GAD.

The present analyses may have other limitations. The generalisability of the sample, being wholly male was raised above. A recent review concluded that evidence relating depression to the metabolic syndrome was stronger for women than men (Goldbacher & Matthews, 2007). Our failure to find an association for depression might also reflect lower power, since there were fewer participants with MDD than GAD, as discussed above. Finally, although we adjusted for many possible confounders, residual confounding as a consequence of poorly measured or unmeasured variables cannot be wholly discounted. For example, both GAD and MetS are associated with poor sleep quality (Tyrer & Baldwin, 2006; Jennings et al., 2007). Future studies should not only pay more attention to GAD as a serious predictor of health outcomes, but also take into account health behaviours such as sleep quality.

4. GAD and hypertension

Despite the health risks associated with hypertension (Chiong, 2008), few studies have examined whether mental health disorders can contribute to hypertension risk. Nothing is known about the association between GAD and hypertension, although three studies have examined the association between hypertension and symptoms of anxiety. Whereas the National Health and Nutrition Examination Survey (NHANES) (Jonas, Franks, & Ingram, 1997) and the Framingham study (Markovitz, Matthews, Kannel, Cobb, & D'Agostino, 1993) both observed a positive prospective association between symptoms of anxiety and hypertension, the Coronary Artery Risk Development in Young Adults (CARDIA) study reported no consistent relationship between the two (Yan et al., 2003). However, the measures of anxiety used in these studies were not synonymous with a clinical diagnosis of GAD. Similarly, few studies have examined the relationship between MDD and hypertension. However, there is at least some cross-sectional and prospective evidence of a positive association (Patten et al., 2005; Patten et al., 2009). GAD and MDD are highly co-morbid, and as outlined above, both GAD and its co-morbidity with MDD predicted both all-cause and cardiovascular disease mortality, and GAD was also related to metabolic syndrome incidence. Using the Vietnam Experience Study again, it was hypothesised that both GAD and MDD would be linked to hypertension. It was also hypothesised that hypertension would be particularly prevalent among those with co-morbid MDD and GAD. At the medical examination in 1986, with the participant in a sitting position, a registered nurse, using a standard mercury sphygmomanometer to blood pressure measured, twice consecutively, from both arms. For analysis, an average of the two right arm values was computed. Measurements from the left arm were used to verify individual results. Hypertension was defined by having one of the following: a reported physician-diagnosis at interview; reported taking antihypertensive medication; an average systolic blood pressure ≥ 140 mmHg; an average diastolic blood pressure ≥ 90 mmHg at the medical examination. There were 441 participants who indicated during the telephone interview that they had a physician diagnosis of hypertension and a further 98 who, although not reporting a diagnosis of hypertension, indicated that they were taking antihypertensive medication. Others have encountered individuals without an acknowledged diagnosis of hypertension who report taking antihypertensive medication and have designated them as hypertensive (Patten et al., 2009). The remainder and majority (N = 842) of those classified as hypertensive was as a result of the blood pressure assessment at the medical examination. This suggests that there was substantial undiagnosed and/or untreated hypertension. As our outcome measure is hypertension, it is essential to include participants with a physician diagnosis of hypertension in that outcome. Of the participants with a diagnosis of hypertension, 292 (66%) were taking anti-hypertensive medication. The effect of this would be to lower blood pressure, such that some of these participants (N = 108) no longer met a criterion solely based on measured blood pressure. Nevertheless, they are still rightly regarded as suffering from hypertension.

4.1 Associations with hypertension

One thousand, three hundred, and eighty-one (33%) of the veterans were classified as hypertensive. Veterans who were older, black, had served in Vietnam, were non smokers, had a relatively high BMI, and consumed more units of alcohol per week, and had lower household income in midlife were more likely to be hypertensive. The characteristics of those with and without hypertension are shown in Table 4.

		Hypertensive (N = 1381)		Normotensive (N = 2801)		*p*
		Mean	SD	Mean	SD	
SBP (mmHg)		132.80	12.01	118.07	8.69	<.001
DBP (mmHg)		93.42	8.19	79.40	6.05	<.001
Age at medical examination (years)		38.57	2.48	38.20	2.54	<.001
BMI (kg/m^2)		27.64	4.28	25.07	3.13	<.001
Alcohol consumption (units/week)		8.89	18.42	6.26	12.03	<.001
		N (%)		N (%)		*p*
Place of service	Ever in Vietnam	818 (59)		1491 (53)		<.001
	Other overseas	342 (25)		732 (26)		
	US only	221 (16)		578 (21)		
Ethnicity	White	1056 (76)		2375 (85)		<.001
	Black	236 (17)		252 (9)		
	Other	89 (7)		174 (6)		
Education grade	≤ 11	179 (13)		326 (12)		.08
	= 12	529 (38)		1007 (36)		
	< 12	673 (49)		1468 (52)		
Household income in midlife	<$20,000	428 (31)		752 (27)		.01
	-$40,000	676 (49)		1420 (51)		
	>$40,000	277 (20)		629 (22)		
Smoking status	Non smoker	393 (28)		670 (24)		.001
	Ex smoker	400 (29)		793 (28)		
	Current smoker	588 (43)		1338 (48)		
Marital Status:	Married	991 (72)		2083 (74)		.10
	Divorced/separated/widowed	257 (19)		498 (18)		
	Never married	133 (9)		220 (8)		
Predictor Variables:						
GAD		171 (12)		232 (8)		<.001
MDD		121 (9)		155 (6)		<.001

Table 4. Characteristics of those with and without hypertension

Both GAD and MDD were associated with an elevated risk of hypertension in fully-adjusted models, although the association was stronger for MDD than GAD on this occasion. Of the participants with co-morbid GAD and MDD, 72 (47%) were hypertensive. Both GAD, MDD, and comorbidity were associated with an increased risk of hypertension in age-adjusted analyses, but when adjusting for all other covariates, only comorbidity was significantly related to hypertension, although there was a trend for a relationship with GAD ($p = .06$).

Given that antihypertensive medication can be prescribed for conditions other than hypertension, hypertension was redefined based on only physician diagnosis and measured blood pressure. This reduced the sample to 4180 and the numbers classified as hypertensive as 1329 (32%). In the separate fully adjusted models, both GAD and MDD were positively associated with hypertension defined in this alternative fashion.

However, in the fully adjusted comorbidity competitive analysis, no statistically significant relationships emerged. The only association to approach significance was between co-morbidity and hypertension.

Over 30% of the sample met the main criteria for hypertension. This proportion is somewhat higher than that reported from studies with participants of a similar mean age (e.g., Patten, et al., 2009). However, in part this could reflect different definitions of hypertension; relying solely on reported diagnostic and medication status, and not including measured blood pressure, will almost certainly lead to an underestimate of prevalence. In addition, the present sample was clustered at the low end of the socio-economic spectrum. This might also help explain their relatively high prevalence of hypertension. Other analyses indicate an inverse gradient between socio-economic status and measured blood pressure, although a less consistent association between socio-economic position and hypertension treatment rates (Colhoun, Hemingway, & Poulter, 1998). In the present sample, however, household income in midlife was associated with hypertension.

Both GAD and MDD were positively associated with hypertension. The latter result is consistent with the cross-sectional and prospective outcomes from the Canadian National Population Health Survey (Patten et al., 2005; Patten, et al., 2009). We know of no previous studies that have examined the relationship between GAD and hypertension. However, a positive association between symptoms of anxiety and hypertension has been reported from NHANES and the Framingham study (Jonas, et al., 1997; Markovitz, et al., 1993), although no such relationship emerged from analysis of data from the CARDIA study (Yan, et al., 2003). In fully adjusted competitive analysis, we found that only the co-morbidity of GAD and MDD was significantly associated with an increased risk of hypertension. It is possible that co-morbidity signals more severe psychiatric dysfunction and that it is the severity of dysfunction that is associated with physical health outcomes, similar to the findings for mortality above. However, it is also possible that comorbidity reflects a greater negative disposition, and it is this which is associated with hypertension (Suls & Bunde, 2005). Whatever the case, given the high comorbidity of GAD and MDD, it is perhaps regrettable that studies of psychiatric disorders and physical health have focused almost exclusively on single disorders.

4.2 Limitations and mechanisms

Although we are not able to determine causality from the present cross-sectional associations, the prospective associations between MDD and hypertension (Patten et al., 2009) and symptoms of anxiety and hypertension studies (Jonas et al., 1997; Markovitz et al., 1993), cited above, make it unlikely that GAD or MDD are a psychological response to hypertension diagnosis. There are several putative pathways through which disorders such as GAD and MDD might contribute to development of hypertension. In addition, in the majority of instances in the present study, hypertension was apparently undiagnosed. Further, many of the sample had served in Vietnam. As a life event, a diagnosis of hypertension is likely to pale by comparison. The two most cited are unhealthy behaviours and physiological dysregulation. In the present analyses, the associations were still evident following adjustment for two of the most prominent unhealthy behaviours, smoking and high levels of alcohol consumption. That smokers have lower blood pressure and that alcohol consumption is positively related to hypertension are common observations (Beilin, 1987; Green, Jucha, & Luz, 1986). Although we have no data directly pertaining to the second route, others have observed altered activity of the hypothalamic-pituitary-adrenal axis in approximately 50% of depressed patients (Brown, Varghese, & McEwen, 2004), which, in turn, may increase the risk of hypertension (Torpy, Mullen, Ilias, & Nieman, 2002).

Other limitations of this analysis are that, as discussed above, the present study's participants were all men and so there is the issue of generalisation. Indeed, in the Framingham study, symptoms of anxiety predicted hypertension in middle-aged men but not middle-aged women (Markovitz et al., 1993). Accordingly, the associations reported here may pertain only for men. In addition, the present participants were largely from the lower end of the socio-economic spectrum and thus our findings may not generalise to the population as a whole. However, these analyses again indicate the importance of GAD, as well as MDD in terms of health outcomes, and particular their comorbidity.

5. Conclusion

In conclusion, the analyses discussed above indicated that both GAD and MDD were individually positively related to all-cause mortality and to hypertension in male Vietnam-era veterans. However, the strongest association with both mortality and hypertension was observed for co-morbid GAD and MDD. Further, when considering another major health outcome, the metabolic syndrome, GAD but not MDD was associated with an increased prevalence of this constellation of symptoms. Depression has been the main focus for studies of psychiatric disorders and physical health outcomes. The current data suggest that future research should perhaps pay equal attention to GAD and, for some outcomes, it seems that it is particularly its co-morbidity with MDD and/or other mental disorders which might predict poorer health. Future research remains to determine the mechanisms underlying these associations with health outcomes, through prospective assessment and a thorough inclusion of both biological and behavioural covariates.

6. Acknowledgment

Mortality surveillance of the cohort in the post-service VES was funded by the National Center for Environmental Health, Atlanta, US. The Medical Research Council (MRC) Social and Public Health Services Unit receives funding from the MRC and the Chief Scientist Office at the Scottish Government Health Directorates. The author would also like to acknowledge the involvement of Professor Douglas Carroll, Dr Catharine Gale, and Dr G. David Batty in the analyses reported

7. References

Ahern, D. K., Gorkin, L., Anderson, J. L., Tierney, C., Hallstrom, A., Ewart, C., et al. (1990). Biobehavioral variables and mortality or cardiac arrest in the Cardiac Arrhythmia Pilot Study (CAPS). *American Journal of Cardiology*, Vol.66, pp.59-62.

American Psychiatric Association, (1980). *Diagnostic and statistical manual of mental disorders* (3rd. edition). American Psychiatric Association, Washington DC.

Batty, G. D., Shipley, M. J., Mortensen, L., Boyle, S. H., Barefoot J, Grønbaek, M., et al. (2008). IQ in late adolescence/early adulthood, risk factors in middle-age, and later all-cause mortality in men: the Vietnam Experience Study. *Journal of Epidemiology and Community Health*, Vol.62, pp.522-531.

Beilin, L. J. (1987). Epidemiology of alcohol and hypertension. Adv Alcohol Subst Abuse, Vol.6, 69-87.

Boscarino, J. A. (1997). Diseases among men 20 years after exposure to severe stress: implications for clinical research and medical care. *Psychosomatic Medicine*, Vol.59, pp.605-614.

Boscarino, J. A. (2004). Posttraumatic stress disorder and physical illness: results from clinical and epidemiologic studies. *Annals of the New York Academy of Sciences*, Vol.1032, pp.141-153.

Boscarino, J. A. (2006a). External-cause mortality after psychologic trauma: the effects of stress exposure and predisposition. *Comparative Psychiatry*, Vol.47, pp.503-514.

Boscarino, J. A. (2006b). Posttraumatic stress disorder and mortality among U.S. Army veterans 30 years after military service. *Annals of Epidemiology*, Vol.16, pp.248-256.

Boscarino, J. A., & Chang, J. (1999). Higher abnormal leukocyte and lymphocyte counts 20 years after exposure to severe stress: research and clinical implications. *Psychosomatic Medicine*, Vol.61, pp.378-386.

Brown, E. S., Varghese, F. P., & McEwen, B. S. (2004). Association of depression with medical illness: does cortisol play a role? *Biological Psychiatry*, Vol.55, pp.1-9.

Chiong, J.R. (2008). Controlling hypertension from a public health perspective. *International Journal of Cardiology*, Vol. 127, pp.151-156.

Colhoun, H. M., Hemingway, H., & Poulter, N. R. (1998). Socio-economic status and blood pressure: an overview analysis. *Journal of Human Hypertension*, Vol.12, pp.91-110.

Denollet, J., & Brutsaert, D. L. (1998). Personality, disease severity, and the risk of long-term cardiac events in patients with a decreased ejection fraction after myocardial infarction. *Circulation*, Vol.97, pp.167-173.

Dohrenwend, B.P., Turner, J.B., Turse, N.A., Adams, B.G., Koenen, K.C., & Marshall, R. (2006). The psychological risks of Vietnam for U.S. veterans: a revisit with new data and methods. *Science*,Vol.313, pp.979-82.

Dohrenwend, B.P., Turner, J.B., Turse, N.A., Adams, B.G., Koenen, K.C., & Marshall, R. (2007). Continuing controversy over the psychological risks of Vietnam for U.S. veterans. *Journal of Trauma and Stress*, Vol.20, pp.449-65.

Dunbar, J. A., Reddy, P., Davis-Lameloise, N., Philpot, B., Laatikainen, T., Kilkkinen, A., et al. (2008). Depression: an important co morbidity with metabolic syndrome in a general population. *Diabetes Care*, Vol.31, pp.2368-2373.

Eaker, E. D., Sullivan, L. M., Kelly-Hayes, M., D'Agostino, R. B., Sr., & Benjamin, E. J. (2005). Tension and anxiety and the prediction of the 10-year incidence of coronary heart disease, atrial fibrillation, and total mortality: the Framingham Offspring Study. *Psychosomatic Medicine*, Vol.67, pp.692-696.

Frasure-Smith, N., & Lesperance, F. (2003). Depression and other psychological risks following myocardial infarction. *Archives of General Psychiatry*, Vol.60, 627-636.

Frasure-Smith, N., Lesperance, F., & Talajic, M. (1995). The impact of negative emotions on prognosis following myocardial infarction: is it more than depression? *Health Psychology*, Vol.14, 388-398.

Gaylord, K. M. (2006). The psychosocial effects of combat: the frequently unseen injury. *Critical Care Nursing Clinician North America*, Vol.18, pp.349-357.

Goldbacher, E. M., & Matthews, K. A. (2007). Are psychological characteristics related to risk of the metabolic syndrome? A review of the literature. *Annals of Behavioral Medicine*, Vol.34, 240-252.

Green, M. S., Jucha, E., & Luz, Y. (1986). Blood pressure in smokers and nonsmokers: epidemiologic findings. *American Heart Journal*, Vol.111, pp.932-940.

Haines, A. P., Imeson, J. D., & Meade, T. W. (1987). Phobic anxiety and ischaemic heart disease. *BMJ*, Vol.295, pp.297-299.

Hallstrom, T., Lapidus, L., Bengtsson, C., & Edstrom, K. (1986). Psychosocial factors and risk of ischaemic heart disease and death in women: a twelve-year follow-up of participants in the population study of women in Gothenburg, Sweden. *Journal of Psychosomatic Research*, Vol.30, pp.451-459.

Hankin, C. S., Spiro, A., 3rd, Miller, D. R., & Kazis, L. (1999). Mental disorders and mental health treatment among U.S. Department of Veterans Affairs outpatients: the Veterans Health Study. *American Journal of Psychiatry*, Vol.156, pp.1924-1930.

Heiskanen, T. H., Niskanen, L. K., Hintikka, J. J., Koivumaa-Honkanen, H. T., Honkalampi, K. M., Haatainen, K. M., et al. (2006). Metabolic syndrome and depression: a cross-sectional analysis. *Journal of Clinical Psychiatry*, 67, pp.1422-1427.

Herrmann, C., Brand-Driehorst, S., Kaminsky, B., Leibing, E., Staats, H., & Ruger, U. (1998). Diagnostic groups and depressed mood as predictors of 22-month mortality in medical inpatients. *Psychosomatic Medicine*, Vol.60, pp.570-577.

Herva, A., Rasanen, P., Miettunen, J., Timonen, M., Laksy, K., Veijola, J., et al. (2006). Co-occurrence of metabolic syndrome with depression and anxiety in young adults: the Northern Finland 1966 Birth Cohort Study. *Psychosomatic Medicine*, Vol.68, pp.213-216.

Hoge, C. W., Auchterlonie, J. L., & Milliken, C. S. (2006). Mental health problems, use of mental health services, and attrition from military service after returning from deployment to Iraq or Afghanistan. *Journal of the American Medical Association*, Vol.295, pp.1023-1032.

Hoge, C. W., Castro, C. A., Messer, S. C., McGurk, D., Cotting, D. I., & Koffman, R. L. (2004). Combat duty in Iraq and Afghanistan, mental health problems, and barriers to care. *New England Journal of Medicine*, Vol.351, pp.13-22.

Holwerda, T. J., Schoevers, R. A., Dekker, J., Deeg, D. J., Jonker, C., & Beekman, A. T. (2007). The relationship between generalized anxiety disorder, depression and mortality in old age. *International Journal of Geriatric Psychiatry*, Vol.22, pp.241-249.

Isomaa, B., Almgren, P., Tuomi, T., Forsen, B., Lahti, K., Nissen, M., et al. (2001). Cardiovascular morbidity and mortality associated with the metabolic syndrome. *Diabetes Care*, Vol.24, pp.683-689.

Jennings, J.R., Muldoon, M.F., Hall, M., Buysse, D.J., & Manuck, S.B. (2007). Self-reported sleep quality is associated with the metabolic syndrome. *Sleep*, Vol.30, pp.219-223.

Jonas, B. S., Franks, P., & Ingram, D. D. (1997). Are symptoms of anxiety and depression risk factors for hypertension? Longitudinal evidence from the National Health and Nutrition Examination Survey I Epidemiologic Follow-up Study. *Archives of Family Medicine*, Vol.6, pp.43-49.

Kessler, R. C., Berglund, P., Demler, O., Jin, R., Merikangas, K. R., & Walters, E. E. (2005). Lifetime prevalence and age-of-onset distributions of DSM-IV disorders in the

National Comorbidity Survey Replication. *Archives of General Psychiatry,* Vol.62, pp.593-602.

Kessler, R. C., Chiu, W. T., Demler, O., Merikangas, K. R., & Walters, E. E. (2005). Prevalence, severity, and comorbidity of 12-month DSM-IV disorders in the National Comorbidity Survey Replication. *Archives of General Psychiatry,,* Vol.62, pp.617-627.

Kessler, R. C., DuPont, R. L., Berglund, P., & Wittchen, H. U. (1999). Impairment in pure and comorbid generalized anxiety disorder and major depression at 12 months in two national surveys. *American Journal of Psychiatry,* Vol.156, pp.1915-1923.

Kinder, L. S., Bradley, K. A., Katon, W. J., Ludman, E., McDonell, M. B., & Bryson, C. L. (2008). Depression, posttraumatic stress disorder, and mortality. *Psychosomatic Medicine,* Vol.70, 20-26.

Kinder, L. S., Carnethon, M. R., Palaniappan, L. P., King, A. C., & Fortmann, S. P. (2004). Depression and the metabolic syndrome in young adults: findings from the Third National Health and Nutrition Examination Survey. *Psychosomatic Medicine,* Vol.66, pp.316-322.

Koponen, H., Jokelainen, J., Keinanen-Kiukaanniemi, S., Kumpusalo, E., & Vanhala, M. (2008). Metabolic syndrome predisposes to depressive symptoms: a population-based 7-year follow-up study. *Journal of Clinical Psychiatry,* Vol.69, pp.178-182.

Lakka, H. M., Laaksonen, D. E., Lakka, T. A., Niskanen, L. K., Kumpusalo, E., Tuomilehto, J., et al. (2002). The metabolic syndrome and total and cardiovascular disease mortality in middle-aged men. *Journal of the American Medical Association,* Vol.288, pp.2709-2716.

Lane, D., Carroll, D., Ring, C., Beevers, D. G., & Lip, G. Y. (2001). Mortality and quality of life 12 months after myocardial infarction: effects of depression and anxiety. *Psychosomatic Medicine,* Vol.63, pp.221-230.

Markovitz, J. H., Matthews, K. A., Kannel, W. B., Cobb, J. L., & D'Agostino, R. B. (1993). Psychological predictors of hypertension in the Framingham Study. Is there tension in hypertension? *Journal of the American Medical Association,* Vol.270, pp.2439-2443.

McCaffery, J. M., Niaura, R., Todaro, J. F., Swan, G. E., & Carmelli, D. (2003). Depressive symptoms and metabolic risk in adult male twins enrolled in the National Heart, Lung, and Blood Institute twin study. *Psychosomatic Medicine,* Vol.65, pp.490-497.

Murphy, J. M., Monson, R. R., Olivier, D. C., Sobol, A. M., & Leighton, A. H. (1987). Affective disorders and mortality. A general population study. *Archives of General Psychiatry,* Vol.44, pp.473-480.

Musselman, D. L., Evans, D. L., & Nemeroff, C. B. (1998). The relationship of depression to cardiovascular disease: epidemiology, biology, and treatment. *Archives of General Psychiatry,* Vol.55, pp.580-592.

O'Leary, D. A., & Lee, A. S. (1996). Seven year prognosis in depression. Mortality and readmission risk in the Nottingham ECT cohort. *British Journal of Psychiatry,* Vol.169, pp.423-429.

Osby, U., Brandt, L., Correia, N., Ekbom, A., & Sparen, P. (2001). Excess mortality in bipolar and unipolar disorder in Sweden. *Archives of General Psychiatry,* Vol.58, pp.844-850.

Patten, S. B., Beck, C. A., Kassam, A., Williams, J. V., Barbui, C., & Metz, L. M. (2005). Long-term medical conditions and major depression: strength of association for specific conditions in the general population. *Canadian Journal of Psychiatry,* Vol.50, pp.195-202.

Patten, S. B., Williams, J. V., Lavorato, D. H., Campbell, N. R., Eliasziw, M., & Campbell, T. S. (2009). Major depression as a risk factor for high blood pressure: epidemiologic evidence from a national longitudinal study. *Psychosomatic Medicine,* Vol.71, pp.273-279.

Pelle, A. J., Gidron, Y. Y., Szabo, B. M., & Denollet, J. (2008). Psychological predictors of prognosis in chronic heart failure. *Journal of Cardiac Failure,* Vol.14, pp.341-350.

Prince, M., Patel, V., Saxena, S., Maj, M., Maselko, J., Phillips, M. R., et al. (2007). No health without mental health. *The Lancet,* Vol.370, pp.859-877.

Raikkonen, K., Matthews, K. A., & Kuller, L. H. (2002). The relationship between psychological risk attributes and the metabolic syndrome in healthy women: antecedent or consequence? *Metabolism,* Vol.51, pp.1573-1577.

Raikkonen, K., Matthews, K. A., & Kuller, L. H. (2007). Depressive symptoms and stressful life events predict metabolic syndrome among middle-aged women: a comparison of World Health Organization, Adult Treatment Panel III, and International Diabetes Foundation definitions. *Diabetes Care,* Vol.30, pp.872-877.

Reeves, R. R., Parker, J. D., & Konkle-Parker, D. J. (2005). War-related mental health problems of today's veterans: new clinical awareness. *Journal of Psychosocial Nursing and Mental Health Services,* Vol.43, pp.18-28.

Riskind, J.H., Beck, A.T., Berchick, R.J., Brown, G., & Steer, R.A. (1987). Reliability of DSM-III diagnoses for major depression and generalized anxiety disorder using the structured clinical interview for DSM-III. *Archives of General Psychiatry,* Vol.44, pp.817-20.

Robins, L., Helzer, J., & Cottler, L. (1987). *Diagnostic Interview Schedule (version III-A) Training Manual.* Veterans Administration, St Louis.

Rugulies, R. (2002). Depression as a predictor for coronary heart disease. a review and meta-analysis. *American Journal of Preventative Medicin*e, Vol.23, pp.51-61.

Sareen, J., Cox, B. J., Afifi, T. O., Stein, M. B., Belik, S. L., Meadows, G., et al. (2007). Combat and peacekeeping operations in relation to prevalence of mental disorders and perceived need for mental health care: findings from a large representative sample of military personnel. *Archives of General Psychiatry,* Vol.64, pp.843-852.

Sevincok, L., Buyukozturk, A., & Dereboy, F. (2001). Serum lipid concentrations in patients with comorbid generalized anxiety disorder and major depressive disorder. *Canadian Journal of Psychiatry,* Vol.46, pp.68-71.

Skilton, M. R., Moulin, P., Terra, J. L., & Bonnet, F. (2007). Associations between anxiety, depression, and the metabolic syndrome. *Biological Psychiatry,* Vol.62, pp.1251-1257.

Spruill, T. M., Pickering, T. G., Schwartz, J. E., Mostofsky, E., Ogedegbe, G., Clemow, L., et al. (2007). The impact of perceived hypertension status on anxiety and the white coat effect. *Annals of Behavioral Medicine,* Vol.34, pp.1-9.

Strine, T. W., Mokdad, A. H., Dube, S. R., Balluz, L. S., Gonzalez, O., Berry, J. T., et al. (2008). The association of depression and anxiety with obesity and unhealthy behaviors among community-dwelling US adults. *General Hospital Psychiatry,* Vol.30, pp.127-137.

Suls, J., & Bunde, J. (2005). Anger, anxiety, and depression as risk factors for cardiovascular disease: the problems and implications of overlapping affective dispositions. *Psychological Bulletin*, Vol.131, pp.260-300.

Surtees, P. G., & Barkley, C. (1994). Future imperfect: the long-term outcome of depression. *British Journal of Psychiatry*, Vol.164, pp.327-341.

The Centers for Disease Control Vietnam Experience Study, (1987). Postservice mortality among Vietnam veterans. *Journal of the American Medical Association*, Vol.257, pp.790-795.

The Centers for Disease Control Vietnam Experience Study, (1988a). Health status of Vietnam veterans. I. Psychosocial characteristics. *Journal of the American Medical Association*, Vol.259, pp.2701-2707.

The Centers for Disease Control Vietnam Experience Study, (1988b). Health status of Vietnam veterans. II. Physical Health. *Journal of the American Medical Association*, Vol.259, pp.2708-2714.

Therrien, F., Drapeau, V., Lupien, S. J., Beaulieu, S., Dore, J., Tremblay, A., et al. (2008). Awakening cortisol response in relation to psychosocial profiles and eating behaviors. *Physiology of Behavior*, Vol.93, pp.282-288.

Thomas, G. N., Schooling, C. M., McGhee, S. M., Ho, S. Y., Cheung, B. M., Wat, N. M., et al. (2007). Metabolic syndrome increases all-cause and vascular mortality: the Hong Kong Cardiovascular Risk Factor Study. *Clinical Endocrinology*, Vol.66, pp.666-671.

Torpy, D. J., Mullen, N., Ilias, I., & Nieman, L. K. (2002). Association of hypertension and hypokalemia with Cushing's syndrome caused by ectopic ACTH secretion: a series of 58 cases. *Annals of the New York Academy of Science*, Vol.970, pp.134-144.

Trevisan, M., Liu, J., Bahsas, F. B., & Menotti, A. (1998). Syndrome X and mortality: a population-based study. Risk Factor and Life Expectancy Research Group. *American Journal of Epidemiology*, Vol.148, 958-966.

Tyrer, P., & Baldwin, D. (2006): Generalised anxiety disorder. *The Lancet*, Vol.368, pp.2156-2166.

Vaccarino, V., McClure, C., Johnson, B. D., Sheps, D. S., Bittner, V., Rutledge, T., et al. (2008). Depression, the metabolic syndrome and cardiovascular risk. *Psychosomatic Medicine*, Vol.70, pp.40-48.

van Hout, H. P., Beekman, A. T., de Beurs, E., Comijs, H., van Marwijk, H., de Haan, M., et al. (2004). Anxiety and the risk of death in older men and women. *British Journal of Psychiatry*, Vol.185, pp.399-404.

Vogt, T., Pope, C., Mullooly, J., & Hollis, J. (1994). Mental health status as a predictor of morbidity and mortality: a 15-year follow-up of members of a health maintenance organization. *American Journal of Public Health*, Vol.84, pp.227-231.

Weissman, M. M., Markowitz, J. S., Ouellette, R., Greenwald, S., & Kahn, J. P. (1990). Panic disorder and cardiovascular/cerebrovascular problems: results from a community survey. *American Journal of Psychiatry*, Vol.147, pp.1504-1508.

World Health Organisation, (1992). International Statistical Classification of Diseases and related health problems. WHO, Geneva.

Whooley, M.A., Caska, C.M., Hendrickson, B.E., Rourke, M.A., Ho, J., & Ali, S. (2007). Depression and inflammation in patients with coronary heart disease: findings from the Heart and Soul Study. *Biological Psychiatry*, Vol.62, pp.314-20.

Wulsin, L. R., Vaillant, G. E., & Wells, V. E. (1999). A systematic review of the mortality of depression. *Psychosomatic Medicine*, Vol.61, pp.6-17.

Yan, L. L., Liu, K., Matthews, K. A., Daviglus, M. L., Ferguson, T. F., & Kiefe, C. I. (2003). Psychosocial factors and risk of hypertension: the Coronary Artery Risk Development in Young Adults (CARDIA) study. *Journal of the American Medical Association*, Vol.290, pp.2138-2148.

8

Cardiac Diseases and Anxiety Disorders

Cicek Hocaoglu, Cagdas H.Yeloglu and Selim Polat
Rize University
Turkey

1. Introduction

Anxiety disorders are amongst the most common psychiatric disorders in all over the world. Its an emotion that prepares the individual to the environmental changes or helps to create a response to those changes. Also there are psychological symptoms such as distress, excitement and a precognition and fear of suddenly something bad going to happen. Anxiety is a symptom that could be seen in many organic disorder and can accompany almost any psychiatric disorder. The relationship between anxiety and cardiovascular system (CVS), is known since the first studies on individuals the 1870's so-called irritable cardiac diseases. With tachycardia and palpitations as a result of severe fear and anxiety related issues, has become a focus of interest in studies that examine the activity of CVS. Nowadays, the relationship between psychological factors and cardiac disease have been discussed. Because creation potential of the sudden death due to cardiac diseases are more sensitive to the psychiatric disorders and development of any cardiac disease might start serious mental issues. These situations are the main subjects of psychocardiology. In addition, mental disorders which has similar symptoms of cardiac diseases (panic disorder (PD), generalized anxiety disorder (GAD), post-traumatic stress disorder (PTSD), etc.) is another problem area. Anxious thoughts causes reduced autonomic variability condition which is a result of decrease in vagal tone. The first reaction to stress is muscle weakness and a feeling of heart stopping due to parasympathetic activation. A short time later, the sympathetic system is activated, sweating, palpitation, tremors, rapid and deep breathing begin. When they do challenging activities or concerned there will be cardiovascular variability and falls occur phasic parasympathetic tone. Studies on this subject emphasize cardiac sensitization caused by sympathetic activity. According to this stimulation of central and peripheral adrenergic structures, catecholamine infusion and behavioral stress can cause cardiac sensitivity in both healthy and ischemic heart. Cardiac diseases within the psychiatric views (whether or syndromal levels of disorder matter), surely, should be recognized and addressed. Patients who work under heavy stressful conditions suffers from continuous excreting of catecholamine with the further aggravated cardiac disease. At the same time, anxiety is caused by a decrease in vagal control also increases the susceptibility to coronary cardiac disease. On most cardiac diseases cases, an intense anger and hostile attitude follows the anxiety. Anxiety came out tops as a leading emotional problem for cardiac patients when it unites with other negative emotions. As a result, the importance of early diagnosis and treatment is obvious due to the reason that occurring simultaneously psychiatric views which emerges with cardiac diseases to cause the illness to worsen. Myocardial infarction, hypertension, congestive heart failure, pacemaker application in patients often accompanied by psychiatric symptoms. In this chapter the relation between cardiac diseases and the anxiety disorder will be discussed.

2. Cardiac diseases

Cardiac disease refers to any condition affecting the ability of the heart and blood vessels to function properly. There are many different kinds of cardiac disease, but they all threaten the circulatory system in one way or another (Baruah, 2010). This is what makes cardiac disease so deadly; a disruption of the blood supply to any part of the body can lead to tissue damage or death, often within a matter of minutes. Some of the major types of cardiac disease include: Coronary heart disease, hypertensive heart disease, myocardial infarction.

Nowadays, cardiac disease has emerged as the leading cause of death worldwide, particularly in developed countries. The World Health Organization (WHO) reported that 16.7 million deaths in 2003 were caused by some form of cardiovascular disease (Ahrens et al. 2010). Though the rate of cardiac disease is highest in developed countries, developing countries are seeing an increase in the occurrence of cardiac disease (Dakheel et al. 2011). The World Health Organization estimates that by 2010, cardiac disease will surpass AIDS as the leading cause of death in developing countries (WHO 2006).

2.1 Coronary heart disease (CHD)

CHD is the condition that results from the buildup of plaques within the walls of arteries that supply the heart muscle with oxygen and nutrients. CHD can lead to *heart attacks*, which occur when the buildup suddenly interrupts the heart's supply of blood, leading to the damage or death of heart tissue. This is the single largest cause of death in the world. (Furuya et al. 2001, Ko et al.2006, Ingelsson et al. 2007, Baruah, 2010).

2.2 Hypertensive heart disease (HHD)

Hypertension, also known as high blood pressure, can increase the risk for a number of other heart-related conditions, including heart attack, stroke, cardiac arrest, and congestive heart failure (Franklin et al.2011, Simões et al. 2011). In other words, hypertensive heart disease is the target organ response to arterial hypertension. Left ventricular hypertrophy represents an important predictor for cardiovascular events. Myocardial fibrosis, a common end point in hypertensive heart disease, has been linked to the development of left ventricular hypertrophy and diastolic dysfunction (Janardhanan & Kramer, 2011).

2.3 Myocardial infarction (MI)

The damage or death of an area of the heart muscle (myocardium) resulting from a blocked blood supply to the area. The affected tissue dies, injuring the heart. Symptoms include prolonged, intensive chest pain and a decrease in blood pressure that often causes shock (Gul et al.2011). About one quarter of people having an acute myocardial infarction (MI) in the USA will die of it, half of them within 1 hour of the onset of symptoms. Cardiogenic shock develops in over 5% of people surviving the first hour after an acute MI, with a mortality of 50% to 80% in the first 48 hours (Wakai 2011).

3. What is psychogenic cardiac disease?

The pathway toward the current recognition that mental stress and psychiatric illness is a cause of cardiovascular disease has been long. The adverse cardiovascular consequences of panic disorder and chronic mental stress are probable but do remain contentious. A common theme of this field is the importance of neural mechanisms, particularly those involving the sympathetic nervous system, in the origins of cardiovascular disease attributable to stress and psychiatric illness. Evidence exists affirming the mechanistic importance of extreme sympathetic nervous system activation in stress (takotsubo) cardiomyopathy of acute activation of the cardiac sympathetic outflow (Esler 2010) Takotsubo cardiomyopathy (TC) is a neurocardiological disorder presumed to be triggered by stress, which may cause reversible heart failure, usually in postmenopausal women. TC, more recently called transient left ventricular apical ballooning syndrome, is a recently described acute cardiac syndrome. The syndrome is characterised by a sudden onset of transient extensive akinesia of the left ventricle, often involving all three major coronary artery territories, in the absence of significant coronary artery stenosis. The syndrome is accompanied by angina-like chest pain, electrocardiographic changes and minimal release of cardiac enzymes and biomarker levels, mimicking an acute myocardial infarction and is often preceded by an episode of emotional or physical stress, which may play a key role in the pathogenesis of the disorder. The ECG changes are suggestive of an acute coronary syndrome with T-wave inversion with/without ST elevation, most often in the precordial leads. However, the exact mechanism still remains unknown (Sansen &, Holvoet 2007). Characteristically, there is only a limited release of cardiac enzymes disproportionate to the extent of regional wall motion abnormality. Transient right ventricular dysfunction may occur and is associated with more complications, longer hospitalisation and worse left ventricular systolic dysfunction. Serial echocardiography is useful to document improvement in cardiac function. Transient mid-cavity obstruction has been invoked with subsequent myocardial stunning in the akinetic segments. Most clinicians are unfamiliar with this disorder. Therefore, some TCs are misdiagnosed as acute myocardial infarction. The modified Mayo Clinic criteria usually confirm a diagnosis, although the diagnostic criteria for TC remain controversial. Enhanced awareness by clinicians is important when encountering patients with chest pain and elevated cardiac enzymes. Treatment is supportive. The most effective long-term management remains to be defined. Although the prognosis is good with recovery of ventricular function at about three weeks, some patients have died (Middlemost & Mabin 2008, Nussinovitch et al.2011). Complete recovery usually occurs after dramatic presentation, frequently complicated with acute heart failure. Therapy is empiric and directed towards supportive measures against cardiogenic shock, acute heart failure, dysrhythmias. In-hospital mortality rate is less than 1%, but long-term prognosis is still unknown (Putniković et al. 2010). Delineating these biological mediators of heart risk in acute mental stress has provided a potential target for pharmaceutical prevention, to inhibit platelet activation and block adrenergic cardiovascular stimulation. Agreement has been reached that the triggering of myocardial infarction and sudden death by acute mental stress is no longer a hypothetical construct only. It is now proven, is a matter of relevance to the health of the general community, and has led to preventive medical advice being incorporated into national health advisory documents (Esler 2010).

4. Anxiety disorders

Anxiety disorders are a universal phenomenon: exaggerations of evolutionarily hard- wired reactions to dangers to the body or to the psyche. Physicians in earlier times focused on the somatic manifestations of anxiety, such as palpitation, shortness of breath, and the like. Even as recently as the late nineteenth century, the various disorders subsume under the heading of anxiety were described and considered as separate entities, not yet unified as elements of particular class of disorders (Stone 2010). Today, anxiety disorders are classified by DSM-IV-R into four major categories: panic disorder with and without agoraphobia, social phobia and other phobias (eg, simple phobia and agoraphobia without a history of panic attacks), generalized anxiety disorder, posttraumatic stress disorder and obsessive compulsive disorder (Brown & Leyfer 2010).

5. Cardiac diseases and anxiety disorders

A substantial literature supports clinically important associations between psychiatric illness and chronic medical conditions. Patients with severe mental disorders have about twice the prevalence of the classic risk factors for coronary heart disease (CHD) (Birkenaes et al. 2006). Evidence from methodologically rigorous studies of a strong association between CHD and depressive disorders is especially compelling (Shapiro 2005). The prevalence of major depression in patients with CHD is much higher, especially after myocardial infarction, than in the general population. Various psychiatric symptoms are observed on the patients who had myocardial infarction (MI) on their pre, during and after treatment time periods. Also on the treatment period, anxiety, depression, hostile behaviours, aggression, denial, hardships on following medical suggestions, refusing, and as the most severe result, delirium can be observed. Anxiety, is a clinical appearance which is observed on the MI patients during the first 24 hours. With the patient's acceptance to coroner intensive care unit, the patients can show anxious suspense and with this perspective it is possible for patients to see this sickness and it's conditions as a disaster or a treat for themselves. Uncertainty cause anxiety on all patients. Sudden fear of death, the lack of autonomy, deficiency on sexuality, the change of roles on family relationships or losing their status, the fear of having a new infarction risk can cause anxiety on patients. The depression is the most frequently observed symptoms on the patients after their discharge from hospital. Depression also causes delay on the patient's psychosocial recovery. On the other hand, anxiety is frequently observed on patients after their discharge from hospital. This situation prevents the the patients to gain their functionality again on lots of their roles, mainly their sexual life (Hackett et al.1998). Most research focuses on depression, finding that depression can adversely affect self-care and increase the risk of incident cardiac diseases, complications and mortality. Anxiety is also extremely common in patients with CHD. Anxiety disorders are less well studied, but robust epidemiological and clinical evidence shows that anxiety disorders play an equally important role. Biological theories of the interactions between anxiety and cardiac diseases and chronic pain are presented. Available data suggest that anxiety disorders in medically ill patients should not be ignored and could be considered conjointly with depression when developing strategies for screening and intervention, particularly in primary care. Emerging data offer a strong argument for the role of anxiety in medical illness and suggest that anxiety disorders rival depression in terms of risk, comorbidity and outcome (Roy-Byrne et al. 2008). Several studies have suggested an increased risk of fatal CHD among patients with panic disorder, phobic anxiety and other anxiety disorders. The postulated mechanisms through which anxiety may increase the risk of fatal CHD include hyperventilation during an acute attack, which could in turn induce coronary spasm, or an acute attack of anxiety triggering an episode of fatal ventricular arrhythmias. Nonetheless, it is possible that some unmeasured confounding factors, such as diet or physical exercise, could explain the observed association. On the other hand, the specificity of the association between anxiety and sudden death makes confounding an unlikely explanation for the observed effect. If confounding by diet or exercise could explain the association, one would have expected a positive relationship of anxiety to nonfatal myocardial infarction, as well as to fatal CHD (Kawachi et al.1994). In patients with congestive heart failure, tissue nutrition disrupts due to inadequate pumping ability of heart and in this context some changes might occur in the brain. Symptoms similar to generalised anxiety disorder can be seen, such as breathing difficulties, fatigue, attention and memory deficits as well as expectation anxiety. Anxiety increases the heart rate and blood pressure which results exacerbation in myocard ischemia and worsens the heart failure. And if severity of heart failure increases anxiety increases too (Majani et al.1999, Grubb et al.2000, Aydemir 2006). In patients with chronic stress, constant catecholamine decharge worsens heart diseases even more. Also anxiety causes reduction in vagal tone and that leads to a predispozition at coroner heart diseases. Usually, in patients with heart failure, rage and hostility accompanies with anxiety. Anxiety is one of the leading emotional problems that needs to be dealt with especially if it is together with the other negative emotions. Particularly, anxiety that follows myocard infarction results as more complications and worsens the prognosis (Watkins et al., Moser & Dracup, Aydemir 2006). There are significant associations between anxiety and CHD risk, with a potential biologic link between anxiety and elevations in a biomarker with powerful prognostic factor, namely C-reactive protein (CRP). Previous studies underlined an association between CRP and depression in otherwise healthy adults as well as in CHD patients, potentially indicating a biological link between depression and cardiovascular morbidity and mortality. However, previous research seemed to mainly focus on depression and biomarkers in patients with and without CHD, not taking into account anxiety and specific anxiety disorders. It is not clear whether this association is directly causal or relates to other medical processes among patients with heightened anxiety. Several, mostly epidemiological studies underlined the impact of anxiety on CHD incidence and re-occurrence. In particular, generalized anxiety, generalized anxiety disorder (GAD), and phobic anxiety showed significant associations with CHD (Bankier et al.2008, Bankier et al.2009). Among women with suspected myocardial ischemia, the value of depression symptoms for predicting CHD events varied by the severity of comorbid anxiety. These results suggest that the clinical utility of depression measures may be improved by using them in combination with measures of anxiety (Rutledge et al.2009). Anxiety seemed to be an independent risk factor for incident CHD and cardiac mortality (Roest et al.2010). In men, aged 18 to 20 years, anxiety as diagnosed by experts according to ICD-8 criteria independently predicted subsequent CHD events (Janszky et al.2010). Anxiety is associated with elevated serotonin-mediated platelet reactivity in stable CHD patients and symptoms of anxiety show strong, independent correlations with platelet function (Zafar et al.2010). An initial clinical observation that patients with externally located cardiac pacemakers are more distressed and depressed than those with internally sited pacemakers has been confirmed. In Crisp & Stonehill's study a group of patients with cardiac pacemakers scores more highly on anxiety, phobic and depressive scales of a standardized psychoneurotic diagnostic questionnaire than do 'normal' populations (Crisp & Stonehill 1969). Patients with cardiac diseases undergoing electrophysiological studies, pacemaker implantation, and myocardial revascularization have different levels and prevalence of anxiety, but they do not show differences in the level and prevalence of depression (Carneiro et al.2009).

5.1 Cardiac diseases and panic disorder

From their symptoms, panic disorder, which gets it's name from the mythological God Pan, and consists of unexpected panic attack, can be confused with myocardial infarction. In other words, panic disorder and myocardial infarction can have the same symptom patterns. Regarding to cardiac diseases, panic disorder is the most mentioned anxiety disorder. On major numbers of patients whom suspected to have coroner artery disease, were diagnosed panic disorder with further inspections. On the case of young age group patients complaining especially about chest pain, it is essential to think this as a significant symptom of panic disorder (Halperin 1996). Panic disorder is associated prospectively with coronary artery disease, but the risk of acute myocardial infarction associated with panic disorder has not been specifically investigated. Panic disorder which characterized with the increased oscillation on sympathatic nervous system, increase the risk of cardiac disease due to noradrenergic system disregulation on locus cereleus. It was identified as an independent risk factor for subsequent acute myocardial infarction. Comprehensive multidisciplinary approaches are needed to optimize primary and secondary prevention of acute myocardial infarction among patients with panic disorder (Chen et al. 2009). A possible association between the level of anxiety illness severity and sympathovagal balance, which may imply greater cardiac risk. Panic disorder (PD) patients have a heightened or deregulated autonomic nervous system at rest and during autonomic challenge compared with healthy controls (HC) (Martinez et al.2010). Multifiber sympathetic nerve recording has documented massive stimulation of the sympathetic nervous system during panic attacks, accompanied by a surge of epinephrine secretion from the adrenal medulla. Sympathetic nervous tone at rest is normal, but the sympathetic nerves of panic disorder sufferers have been demonstrated to release epinephrine as a cotransmitter. This epinephrine in sympathetic nerves of panic disorder sufferers is presumably taken up from plasma during panic attacks or synthesized in situ by the epinephrine-synthesizing enzyme phenylethanolamine methyltransferase, which has been shown in experimental animals to be induced by chronic mental stress and is present in the sympathetic nerves of patients with panic disorder. This sympathetic nerve epinephrine cotransmission is potentially a cause of cardiac arrhythmias (Esler 2010). Panic disorder has been associated with both an increased risk of coronary events. Hemoconcentration, with both a decrease in plasma volume and an increase in plasma viscosity, is a possible contributor to the risk of acute ischemic events. The acute hemoconcentration observed in relation to pentagastrin-induced panic symptoms may be relevant to the increased risk of stroke and acute coronary events found in patients with panic disorder (Le Melledo et al.2011). In patients with complicated hypertension, panic atack and anxiety has been seen more frequently (Aydemir 2006). Frequency of panic disorders in hypertension patients was reported as 13% (Davies et al.1999).

5.2 Cardiac diseases and post-traumatic stress disorder (PTSD)

PTSD occurcs after traumatic life events, appears under circumstances reminds situations like facing death or death related events and charecterized by couple of symptoms such as avoiding behaviour,living the event in an unpealsant way over and over again during a dream or in memory and accompanied with severe anxiety. Especially in patients who recognizes MI as a trauma, often PTSD can be observed. Whenever patient perceives a heart related stimulant he goes back to the beginning and live the event all over again (Aydemir 2006). PTSD makes MI hard to be dealt with for the patient and physiologically it might delay trombolysis (Alonzo 1999).

6. Treatment

Psychiatric disorders are common feature of heart disease patients and possibly stem from their common biochemical background. Depression, anxiety and heart failure co-morbidity has several clinical implications on the prognosis of these patients. Furthermore antidepressant drugs have known cardiovascular side effects, while their safety and efficacy in heart failure has not been fully elucidated yet. The right choice of antidepressant treatment in cardiac diseases an issue of high importance as it can affect the clinical outcome of these patients. Even though certain conclusions cannot be drawn yet, evidence suggests that the use of selective serotonin reuptake inhibitors may have a beneficial effect on clinical outcome of heart failure patients (Tousoulis et al.2010). Tricyclic antidepressants and SSRIs may be associated with increased risk of mortality, and SSRIs with increased risk of hemorrhagic and fatal stroke, although absolute event risks are low (Smoller et al.2009). The quinidine-like effects of some antidepressant drugs (particularly tricyclic antidepressants) and depression in patients with major mental illness. The tricyclic antidepressants (TCAs) have various effects on the cardiovascular system, including Type IA antiarrhythmic activity that has been associated with an increased risk of mortality in post-myocardial infarction patients. This is especially true among elderly patients with existing risk factors for corrected QT (QTc) interval prolongation. Vieweg et al. (2009) used PubMed, previously reported review articles and the extensive personal files of the authors to identify cases of subjects aged>or=60 years who developed QTc interval prolongation, polymorphic ventricular tachycardia (PVT)/torsade de pointes (TdP) and/or sudden cardiac death while taking antipsychotic or antidepressant drugs or a combination of these medications. They identified 37 patients who had taken, in total, 46 antipsychotic or antidepressant drugs. Their most striking finding was that almost four-fifths of their cases involved women. When the 14 critically ill subjects receiving haloperidol intravenously were excluded, 91.3% of their subjects were women. Almost three-quarters of their study subjects had cardiovascular disease. Specifically, such clinicians treating elderly patients with antipsychotic and antidepressant drugs that may prolong the QTc interval should aggressively obtain a baseline ECG for elderly female patients with additional risk factors such as personal or family history of pre-syncope or syncope, electrolyte disturbances or cardiovascular disease. Elderly male patients are also subject to QTc interval prolongation when such risk factors are present. It is important that the clinicians themselves inspect ECGs. If the QT interval is more than half the RR interval, QTc interval prolongation is likely to be present (Vieweg et al. 2009). Some antidepressant agents can cause electrophysiological changes of cardiac function leading to ventricular arrhythmias and sudden death. However, antidepressants have also protective effects on the heart through their capacity to modulate cardiac autonomic-mediated physiological responses. Heart rate variability and QTc length are two strictly linked parameters that allow us to appreciate the effects of different drugs on cardiac physiology. Heart rate variability reflects functioning of the autonomic nervous system and possibly also regulation by the limbic system. Autonomic regulation of cardiac activity influences also cardiac repolarization and QT length, both directly and via its effects on heart rate (Sala et al. 2009). There is a significant body of evidence suggesting that the presence of depression is independently associated with a decline in health status and an increase in the risk of hospitalization and death for patients with coronary artery disease or congestive heart failure. Novel treatment modalities such as selective serotonin re-uptake inhibitors (SSRIs) may improve depressive symptoms, anxiety symptoms and prognosis of post-myocardial infarction and heart failure patients interacting with the common pathophysiologic mechanisms of depression and cardiovascular disease (Paraskevaidis et al. 2006). SSRIs are established agents for the treatment of depression and are well tolerated in patients with cardiac disease. SSRIs are a heterogeneous group of antidepressants, which apart from their common mechanism of action, differ substantially in their chemical structure, metabolism and pharmacokinetics. Intervention with sertraline has the potential to provide depressed patients with cardiac disease relief from their depressive symptoms, improvement in quality of life and a potential benefit in their cardiovascular risk profile (Parissis et al.2007). But, escitalopram overdose leading to prolongation of the QTc interval has only twice been previously described in the literature. In the event of an overdose, QT prolongation can occur and ECG monitoring should take place for at least 2 days after ingestion in order to prevent life-threatening arrhythmias such as torsades de pointes (tdp). Other factors and drugs that could contribute to prolongation of the QT interval should be taken into account when determining the time period needed for ECG monitoring in the individual patient (Mohammed et al. 2010). Tianeptine therapy for affective disorders concurrent with MI causes an evident reduction in psychopathological symptomatology and a statistically significant decrease in Hamilton Depression Rating Scale and Hamilton Anxiety Rating Scale scores (Vasiuk et al.2010). There is some evidence for the safe and at least modestly effective use of psychotherapy and antidepressants to treat depression and anxiety disorder in heart failure patients. Cognitive behavioral psychotherapy and selective serotonin reuptake inhibitors are first line treatments. The efficacy of depression treatment in altering cardiac outcomes in heart failure patients has yet to be established (Shapiro 2009). The SSRI paroxetine was compared with a therapeutic level of the TCA nortriptyline in a randomized, controlled study and demonstrated a benign cardiovascular profile, while the TCA induced a significantly higher rate of serious adverse cardiovascular events. On the basis of this favorable cardiovascular profile, the SSRIs should therefore be the preferred choice for the treatment of most patients with comorbid depression and cardiovascular disease. Investigation of putative pathophysiologic mechanisms linking depression and cardiovascular mortality, such as the role of platelet activation, will form the basis for further investigation of antidepressant treatments in order to establish if the antidepressants have a beneficial effect on the prognosis of cardiovascular diseases (Roose 2001).

7. Conclusion

Anxiety disorders those occur along with a cardiac disease must be recognesed in early stages and must be treated with care. The effects of the drugs over heart and drug-drug interactions must taken into account of medical treatment. İf we apply all these principles, the results would be pleasing. During the treatment clinicians must be sensitive about their patient's psychiatric symptoms and disorders.

8. Acknowledgment

We offer thanks to our team for suggesting that we write a book about.

9. References

Ahrens, I.; Lip, G.Y.H. & Peter, K. (2010). New oral anticoagulant drugs in cardiovascular Disease.*Thrombosis and Haemostasis*. Vol.104, No.1,(July 2010), pp. 49-60, ISSN: 0340-6245

Alonzo, A.A. (1999). Acute myocardial infarction and posttraumatic stres disorder: The consequences of cumulative adversity. *Journal Cardiovascular Nursing*,Vol. 13, pp. :33-45.

Aydemir, O. (2006). Psychocardiology. *Turkiye Clinics Journal of International Medicine Sciences*, Vol. 47, No.2, pp.57-63.

Bankier, B.; Barajas, J. & Martinez-Rumayor, A. (2009). Association Between Anxiety and C-Reactive Protein Levels in Stable Coronary Heart Disease Patients. *Psychosomatics*, Vol. 50, No. 4, (July 2009), pp. 347 - 353.

Bankier, B.; Barajas J. & Martinez-Rumayor. (2008). Association between C-reactive protein and generalized anxiety disorder in stable coronary heart disease patients. *European Heart Journal*, Vol. 29, No. 18, (September 2008), pp. 2212 - 2217.

Baruah, D.K. (2010) What is the cardiac diseas.http://www.dkbaruah-cardiology.com/

Birkenaes, A.B.;, Søgaard, A.J.& Engh, J.A.(2006). Sociodemographic characteristics and cardiovascular risk factors in patients with severe mental disorders compared with the general population. *Journal Clinical Psychiatry*, Vol.67, No.3, (March 2006), pp.425-433.

Brown, A.T & Leyfer, O. Classification of Anxiety Disorders, In: *Textbook of Anxiety Disorders*, D. Stein, E. Hollander & B. Rothbaum (Eds),pp.(17-35), American Psychiatric Publishing, ISBN 978-1-58562-254-2, Arlington, VA.

Carneiro, A.F.; Mathias, L.A. & Rassi, J.A. (2009). Evaluation of preoperative anxiety and depression in patients undergoing invasive cardiac procedures.*Revista Brasileira Anestesiologia* , Vol. 59, No. 4, (Jul-Aug; 2009), pp.431-438.

Chen, Y.H.; Tsai, S.Y & Lee, H.C. (2009). Increased Risk of Acute Myocardial Infarction for Patients With Panic Disorder: A Nationwide Population-Based Study. *Psychosomotic Medicine*, Vol.71, No. 7, (September 2009), pp. 798 - 804.

Crisp, A.H. & Stonehill, E. (1969). Aspects of the psychological status of patients treated with cardiac pacemakers. *Postgradute Medical Journal*, Vol. 45, No. 525, (July 1969), pp. 423-427.

Dakheel, F.I.; Smko, R. & Negrat, K. (2011). Using Data Mining Techniques for Finding Cardiac Outlier Patients. *Engineering and Technology, Vol.* 73, pp. 442-447.

Davies, S.J.; Ghahramani, P. & Jackson, P.R.(1999). Association of panic disorder and panic attacks with hypertension. *American Journal Medicine*, Vol. 107, pp.310-316.

Esler, M. (2010). The 2009 Carl Ludwig Lecture: pathophysiology of the human sympathetic nervous system in cardiovascular diseases: the transition from mechanisms to medical management. *Journal of Applied Physiology*, Vol.108, No.2, (February 2010), pp. 227 - 237.

Franklin, S.S.; Chow, V.H. & Mori, A.D. (2011). Wong ND. The significance of low DBP in US adults with isolated systolic hypertension. *Journal of Hypertension,* 2011 Apr 8.

Furuya, H.; Nagaoka, T.& Mizushima, S. (2001). Coronary risk appraisal for primary prevention of coronary heart disease in a community. *Nippon Koshu Eisei Zasshi ,* Vol. 48, No.4, (April 2001), pp.276-288.

Gul, E.E.; Nikus, K.C. & Sonmez, O.(2011). Dilemma in predicting the infarct-related artery in acute inferior myocardial infarction: A case report and review of the literature. *Cardiology Journal,* Vol.18, No. 2, pp. 204-216.

Grubb, N.R.; Simpson, C.& Fox, K.A. (2000) Memory function in patients with stable, moderate to severe cardiac failure. American Heart Journal, Vol.140, pp.1-5.

Hackett, T.P.; Rosenbaum, J.F.& Tesar, G.(1998). Emotion, Psychiatric Disorders, and the Heart, In: *Textbook of Cardiovascular Medicine,* Braunwald E (ed), 3rd ed., WB Saunders Company, p.1883-1899, Philadelphia.

Halperin, P. (1996). Heart Disease, In: *Textbook of Consultation-Liaison Psychiatry,* Rundell JR., Wise MG (Eds), pp.(550-560), 1st ed, The American Psychiatric Press,Washington.

Ingelsson, E.; Schaefer, E.J.&, Contois, J.H. (2007). Clinical utility of different lipid measures for prediction of coronary heart disease in men and women. *JAMA.* Vol. 298, No.7, (August 2007), pp.776-785.

Janardhanan, R. & Kramer, C.M. (2011). Imaging in hypertensive heart disease. *Expert Review Cardiovascular Therapy,* Vol.9, No.2, (February 2011), pp. 199-209.

Janszky, I.; Ahnve, S. & Lundberg, I. (2010). Early-Onset Depression, Anxiety, and Risk of Subsequent Coronary Heart Disease 37-Year Follow-Up of 49,321 Young Swedish Men. *Journal of the American College Cardiology,* Vol.56, No.1,(June 29), pp. 31 - 37.

Kawachi, I.; Sparrow, D. & Vokonas, P.S. (1994). Symptoms of anxiety and risk of coronary heart disease. *Circulation,* Vol. 90, pp. 2225-2229, ISSN: 1524-4539

Ko, M.; Kim, M.T. &, Nam, J.J. (2006). Assessing risk factors of coronary heart disease and its risk prediction among Korean adults: the 2001 Korea National Health and Nutrition Examination Survey. *International Journal of Cardiology,* Vol.110, No. 2, (June 2006), pp.184-190.

Le Melledo, J.M.; Perez-Parada, J. & Morrow, J. (2011). Pentagastrin-induced hemoconcentration in healthy volunteers and patients with panic disorder: effect of pretreatment with ethinyl estradiol.*Journal of Psychopharmacology,* Vol. 25, No.1, (January), pp. 71 - 77.

Majani, G.; Pierobon, A. & Giardini, A. (1999). Relationship between psychological profile and cardiological variables in chronic heart failure. The role of patient subjectivity. *Eurepoan Heart Journal,* Vol. 20,pp. 1579-86.

Martinez, J.M.; A. Garakani, A. & Kaufmann, H. (2010). Heart Rate and Blood Pressure Changes During Autonomic Nervous System Challenge in Panic Disorder Patients. *Psychosomotic Medicine,* Vol. 72, No. 5, (June 1), pp. 442 - 449.

Middlemost, S. & Mabin, T. (2008). Takotsubo cardiomyopathy: an acute and reversible cardiomyopathy mimicking acute myocardial infarction. *Cardiovascular Journal of Africa.* Vol. 19, No.1, (Jan-Feb 2008), pp.33-38.

Mohammed, R.; Norton, J.& Geraci, S.A.(2010), Prolonged QTc interval due to escitalopram overdose. *Journal Mississipi State Medical Association,* Vol. 51, No.12, (December 2010), pp.350-353.

Moser, D.K.& Dracup, K.(1996). Is anxiety early after myocardial infarction associated with subsequent ischemic and arrhythmic events?. *Psychosomotic Medicine,* Vol.58, pp.395-401.

Nussinovitch, U.; Goitein, O. & Nussinovitch, N. (2011). Distinguishing a Heart Attack From the "Broken Heart Syndrome" (Takotsubo Cardiomyopathy). *Journal of Cardiovascular Nursing.* 2011 Mar 2. Pubmed ID 21372731

Paraskevaidis, I.; Parissis, J.T.& Fountoulaki, K. (2006). Selective serotonin re-uptake inhibitors for the treatment of depression in coronary artery disease and chronic heart failure: evidence for pleiotropic effects. *Cardiovascular Hematological Agents Medicinal Chemistry,* Vol.4, No.4,(October 2006), pp.361-367.

Parissis, J.; Fountoulaki, K.& Paraskevaidis, I. (2007). Sertraline for the treatment of depression in coronary artery disease and heart failure. *Expert Opinion Pharmacotherapy,* Vol. 8, No. 10, (July 2007), pp.1529-1537.

Putniković, B.; Cvorović, V. & Panić, M. (2010). Takotsubo cardiomyopathy: report of the first case series in Serbia and review of the literature. *Medicinski Pregled.* Vol. 63, No. 1-2, (Jan-Feb 2010), pp.75-81.

Roest, A.M.; Martens, E.J. & Jonge, P.(2010).Anxiety and Risk of Incident Coronary Heart Disease A Meta-Analysis. *Journal of the American College Cardiology,* Vol. 56,pp:38-46.

Roose, S.P.(2001). Depression, anxiety, and the cardiovascular system: the psychiatrist's perspective.*Journal Clinical Psychiatry,* Vol. 8, pp.19-22.

Roy-Byrne, P.P.; Davidson, K.W. & Kessler, R.C. (2008). Anxiety Disorders and Comorbid Medical Illness. *Focus,* Vol. 6, No. 4, (October 2008), pp. 467 - 485.

Rutledge, T.; Linke, S.E. & Krantz, D.S. (2009). Comorbid Depression and Anxiety Symptoms as Predictors of Cardiovascular Events: Results From the NHLBI-Sponsored Women's Ischemia Syndrome Evaluation (WISE) Study. *Psychosomotic Medicine,* Vol. 71, No. 9, (November 2009) pp. 958 - 964.

Tousoulis, D.; Antonopoulos, A.S.& Antoniades, C.(2010).Role of depression in heart failure--choosing the right antidepressive treatment. *International Journal Cardiology,* Vol.140, No.1, (April 2010), pp. 12-8.

Sala, M.; Lazzaretti, M. & Vidovich, G. (2009). Electrophysiological changes of cardiac function during antidepressant treatment. *Therapeutic Advances in Cardiovascular Disease,* Vol. 3, No. 1, (February 2009),pp. 29 - 43.

Sansen, V.& Holvoet, G. (2007). Takotsubo cardiomyopathy presenting as multivessel coronary spasm syndrome: case report and review of the literature. *Acta Cardiology.* Vol. 62, No. 5, (October 2007), pp. 507-511.

Shapiro, P.A.(2009).Treatment of depression in patients with congestive heart failure. *Heart Failure Reviews,* Vol.14, No.1, (March 2009), pp. 7-12.

Simões, M.R.; Ribeiro, J. R.F. & Vescovi, M.V. (2011). Acute Lead Exposure Increases Arterial Pressure: Role of the Renin-Angiotensin System. *PLoS One,* Vol. 6, No.4, (April 2011), pp. e18730.

Stone, M.H. (2010). History of Anxiety Disorders, In: *Textbook of Anxiety Disorders,* D. Stein, E. Hollander & B. Rothbaum (Eds),pp.(3-17), American Psychiatric Publishing, ISBN 978-1-58562-254-2, Arlington, VA.

Smoller, J.W.; Allison, M.& Cochrane, B.B.(2009). Antidepressant use and risk of incident cardiovascular morbidity and mortality among postmenopausal women in the Women's Health Initiative study. *Archives Internal Medicine*, Vol.169, No.22, (December 2009), pp.2128-2139.

Vasiuklu, A.; Lebedev, A.V.& Dovzhenko, T.V.(2010).Affective disorders in acute myocardial infarction and possibilities of their correction with tianeptin.*Terapevticheskil Arkhiv*, Vol.82, No.10, pp.28-33.

Vieweg, W.V.; Wood, M.A.& Fernandez, A. (2009). Proarrhythmic risk with antipsychotic and antidepressant drugs: implications in the elderly. *Drugs Aging*, Vol. 26, No. 12, pp. 997-1012.

Wakai, A.P. (2011). Myocardial infarction (ST-elevation). *Clinical Evidence (Online),* (January 2011), pii: 0202.

Watkins, L.L.; Blumenthal, J.A.& Carney, R.M.(2002). Association of anxiety with reduced baroreflex cardiac control in patients after acute myocardial infarction. American Heart Journal, Vol. 143, pp.460-466.

World Health Organization, "*The World Health Report 2006 – working together for health*", http://www.who.int/whr/2006/en/index.html. 2006.

Zafar, M.U; Paz-Yepes, M.N & Shimbo, D. (2010). Anxiety is a better predictor of platelet reactivity in coronary artery disease patients than depression. *European Heart Journal.* Vol. 31, No. 13, pp. 1573-1582.

9

The Transformation of Post-Traumatic Stress Disorder: From Neurosis to Neurobiology

Tanja C. Mletzko and Boadie W. Dunlop
Department of Psychiatry and Behavioral Sciences
Emory University School of Medicine, Atlanta, Georgia
USA

1. Introduction

Lives can be severely disrupted after a momentous negative experience. Particularly potent are unexpected negative events, or "traumas," such as a near death experience, a severe injury, or being exposed to intense interpersonal violence or a natural disaster. Although most people recover from these traumatic events, many do not, and experience persistent fear, anxiety and/or depression following the event. In the past, these maladaptations after trauma were considered to be a reflection of personal weaknesses and were stigmatized. Now, after 30 years of research, the physiological responses to severe stress and trauma are being increasingly understood, as are the risk factors for a pathological response to trauma. These gains from the study of memory and neurohormonal reactivity and control systems hold forth the promise of improved, biologically-informed, psychotherapeutic and pharmacologic interventions for the prevention and treatment of post-traumatic stress disorder (PTSD) in the future.

2. History and development

2.1 Origins of PTSD

That the severe stress of military combat exposure could cause disabling psychiatric symptoms among soldiers had long been recognized, and was identified by a variety of names across wars, such as *shell shock*, *battle fatigue*, and *traumatic war neurosis*. These reactions are characterized by a period of emotional numbness, depersonalization or derealization in the days after the trauma, followed by a longer period of anxiety, insomnia, nightmares, painful memories and phobic avoidance. However, these symptoms were considered to be time-limited responses to combat or other sudden, unexpected trauma, much as grief was a time-limited reaction to personal loss (McHugh & Treisman, 2007). In 1952, with the creation of the first edition of the DSM (DSM-I), the American Psychiatric Association included the diagnosis of '*gross stress reaction*' in its nosologic classification system and defined it as a response to an extreme physical or mental stressor by an otherwise normal person. By definition, the response needed to be short-lived in nature, and if persistent, required the diagnosis of another, more enduring diagnosis unrelated to trauma (Andreasen, 2010). PTSD became a formal psychiatric diagnosis with its inclusion in the 3rd edition of the Diagnostic and Statistical Manual of Mental Disorders, DSM-III

(American Psychiatric Association [APA], 1980). The diagnosis emerged from the work of American psychiatrists opposed to the Vietnam War, who documented symptoms of severe stress among war veterans that continued for years after having returned home (Scott, 1990).The emergence of PTSD in DSM-III, involved two key changes to the classic stress reaction construct: 1) eliminating the time frame as a temporary reaction; and 2) eliminating the requirement that the individual experiencing symptoms after a traumatic event had to be 'otherwise normal.'

The DSM-III defined a traumatic event as a catastrophic stressor experienced by an individual that was outside the realm of normal human experience, be it natural, such as hurricanes or floods, or man-made, such as war, torture, rape or plane crashes. By design, commonly occurring stressful experiences for individuals, such as divorce, loss of employment and illnesses were excluded as traumatic events due to the assumption that these experiences were relatively common and ordinary stressors (APA, 1980). Initially, motor vehicle accidents as well as traumatic experiences in childhood, such as sexual or physical abuse, were not thought to elicit a traumatic stress response of an intensity warranting the diagnosis. This distinction was altered in the fourth version of the DSM (DSM-IV). The traumatic stressor required for a diagnosis of PTSD in the DSM-IV is defined in the "A"-criterion: the experience of an event that involves an actual or threatened death or serious injury, or threat to the physical integrity of oneself or another person, or learning about the unexpected or violent death, serious harm or threat of death or injury to somebody close to oneself (Criterion A1). In addition, the individual response must involve fear, helplessness or horror (Criterion A2) (APA, 1994).

Although the concept of PTSD has received broad acceptance in psychiatry, there continues to be ongoing controversy about the diagnosis, particularly regarding the breadth of experiences and phenomenology it encompasses (McHugh & Treisman, 2007; McNally 2003). The expansion of the events considered as 'stressors' for the "A1" criterion from the DSM-III to DSM-IV has been criticized for weakening the criterion from traumatic exposure to oneself (e.g. rape) to simply hearing about something traumatic happening to another person. No longer does the stressor need to be "outside the range of normal human experience." By grouping such distinct types of events under one "trauma" rubric, the potential to identify biological substrates of PTSD may be weakened, and the potential for misuse of the diagnosis for political or personal benefit is increased.

In the National Comorbidity Survey-Revised (NCS-R), a community survey of American adults, 60% of men and 51% of women had experienced at least one traumatic event in their lives; other surveys have found higher rates (Kessler et al., 2005; Breslau et al., 2009). The types of trauma experienced varies between genders, with men being exposed to more life-threatening accidents or events involving weapons, while women more frequently experience events involving sexual exploitation, such as rape or sexual assault (Kessler et al., 1995). Furthermore, the risk for PTSD varies across types of trauma. For example, development of PTSD after a natural disaster (men 3.7%, women 5.4%) is typically much less common than after rape (men 65%, women 46%) (Kessler, 2000).

2.2 Social repercussions resulting from the formal introduction of PTSD

The inclusion of PTSD as a formal psychiatric diagnosis has had substantial social impact. It has provided psychiatrically distressed patients a means for naming and conceptualizing how their lives have been altered by traumatic life events, thereby providing reassurance they are not "going crazy". However, the impact of PTSD on the larger culture is continuing to evolve. Because the symptoms of PTSD are purely subjective, can overlap with other illnesses and are easily faked, malingering to obtain the diagnosis for secondary gains is a concern. For example, several investigators have identified over-reporting of symptoms or dishonesty among substantial numbers of Vietnam veterans, who can receive disability payments if diagnosed with life-impairments stemming from PTSD (Burkett & Whitley 1998; Frueh et al., 2000; Frueh et al., 2005). Similar concerns have arisen in the civilian arena, where diagnoses of PTSD have been increasingly used in litigation against employers (Guriel & Fremouw, 2003). Furthermore,, the potential loss of disability payments that would occur if a patient with PTSD recovers or improves function may act to perpetuate symptoms and maintain the disabled state. Another social consequence has been the widespread adoption of the practice of bringing counselors to sites of disasters or other traumas, with the aim of preventing the development of PTSD in those exposed to the event, although evidence of the benefit of these programs is scarce.

3. Diagnosis

Being exposed to a traumatic event does not inevitably lead to PTSD. Most people exposed to traumatic events experience a few psychiatric symptoms, such as insomnia or anxiety, but then re-adjust to their pre-trauma life as symptoms subside over a few weeks. Moreover, ongoing psychiatric symptoms following a trauma in some patients may be better characterized as major depressive disorder (MDD) or another anxiety disorder rather than PTSD. Maladaptation after the traumatic exposure with consistent re-experiencing and phobic avoidance symptoms which persist one month after the trauma justify consideration of a diagnosis of PTSD over other diagnoses. A comparison of diagnostic criteria for other potential post-trauma diagnoses is presented in **Table 1**.

3.1 Acute stress disorder, adjustment disorder and PTSD

3.1.1 Acute stress disorder

Re-experiencing of symptoms, avoidance and hyper-arousal are common and expected following a traumatic situation, and thus PTSD cannot be formally diagnosed until one month after the traumatic event. For the first month following a trauma, symptomatic patients may meet criteria for Acute Stress Disorder (ASD). The diagnosis of ASD requires the experience of three or more dissociative symptoms within 4 weeks of the traumatic event, together with re-experiencing parts of the trauma, avoidance of memories, increased arousal, and significant impairment in occupational and social functioning. These symptoms must not be better accounted for by another mental disorder (such as brief psychotic disorder). Important associated symptoms of hopelessness and despair are also often present. A co-morbid diagnosis of Major Depressive Disorder may be warranted (APA, 1994).

The diagnosis of ASD may change to PTSD if the symptoms do not resolve within 4 weeks and the criteria for PTSD are met. ASD was introduced into DSM-IV with the aims of improving prediction of PTSD and developing interventions to prevent the development of PTSD. Roughly 10-25% of people exposed to an interpersonal trauma or motor vehicle accident will develop ASD (Elklit, 2002; Harvey & Bryant, 1998). Of those who develop ASD and are not treated, roughly 80% will go on to meet criteria for PTSD. (Harvey & Bryant, 1998). However, many victims of trauma will later meet criteria for PTSD despite not meeting criteria for ASD. These patients often do not experience sufficient dissociative

	Posttraumatic Stress Disorder Symptoms	Acute Stress Disorder	Adjustment Disorder
Trauma exposure	**Cluster A (exposure): the individual has been exposed to a traumatic event and both of the following 2 conditions were present:** (A1): person experienced, witnessed or was confronted with 1 or more event(s) involving the actual or threatened death or serious injury or a threat to the physical integrity of self or others.	Identical to Posttraumatic Stress Disorder	The onset of the behavioral or emotional problems lay within 3 months of the onset of the stressor, irrespective of (A1) and (A2).
	(A2): The person's response involved intense fear, helplessness and horror	Identical to Posttraumatic Stress Disorder	Marked distress, in excess of what would be expected given the stressor
Cluster B Re-experiencing	**One** (or more) of the following experiences: (B1) recurrent and intrusive distressing recollections of the event, including images, thoughts or perceptions (B2) recurrent distressing dreams of the event (B3) acting or feeling as if the traumatic event was happening again, including flashbacks, reliving the experience, illusions or hallucinations (B4) intense psychological distress at exposure to internal of external reminders that symbolize or resemble an aspect of the traumatic event (B5) physiological reactivity on exposure to internal or external cues that symbolize or resemble	**One** (or more) of the following experiences: (B1) numbing (B2) reduction of awareness (B3) derealization (B4) depersonalization (B5) inability to recall important aspects of the trauma	Not applicable
Cluster C Avoidance	**Three** (or more) of the following experiences (C1) avoidance of thoughts, feelings or conversations associated with the trauma (C2) efforts to avoid activities, places, or people that trigger memories of the trauma. (C3) inability to recall an important aspect of the trauma (C4) marked reduced interest in previously important activities (C5) feeling of detachment of estrangement from others (C6) restricted range of affect (no loving feelings) (C7) sense of a foreshortened future (does not expect to have a career, marriage, family, or normal life span)	Marked avoidance of reminders of the traumatic event (number of experiences not specified)	Not applicable
Cluster D Arousal	**Two** (or more) of the following experiences: (D1) difficulty falling or staying asleep (D2) irritability or outbursts of anger (D3) difficulty concentrating (D4) hypervigilance (D5) exaggerated startle	Marked symptoms of anxiety and arousal (number of experiences not specified)	Not applicable
Criterion D	Duration of disturbance (Cluster B, C and D) is more than one month	Duration of disturbance is more the 2 days but less than 28 and occurs within 4 weeks of the traumatic event	Duration of disturbance does not exceed 6 months after the stressor has been removed/ended
Criterion F	The disturbances cause clinically significant distress or impairment in social, occupational or other important areas of functioning	The disturbance causes significant distress in social, occupational or other important areas of functioning	Significant impairment in social or occupational functioning

Table 1. Differential features of post-trauma diagnoses

symptoms after the trauma to warrant an ASD diagnosis, but do experience other ASD symptoms that put them at risk for PTSD. Thus, when present, ASD indicates a need for treatment intervention, but the absence of ASD does not eliminate the need for ongoing follow-up to monitor for the emergence of PTSD symptoms.

3.1.2 PTSD, current definition

As shown in **Table 1,** the diagnosis of PTSD requires multiple criteria. The two A-criteria that are required are: (A1) witnessing, experiencing or being confronted with the actual or threatened death of serious injury or violation of physical integrity to oneself or others, and (A2) the response consisted of intense fear, helplessness or horror.

The "B" symptom cluster involves the re-experiencing of the traumatic event identified by criterion A in at least one way. These include recurrent, intrusive memories of the trauma [including images, thoughts or perceptions that cause considerable distress, and/or recurrent distressing dreams of the event and/or reliving of the experience through illusions, hallucinations or flashbacks (including upon awakening and while intoxicated)], as well as experiencing psychological distress or physical reactions upon exposure to internal or external reminders of the trauma. The "C" symptom cluster incorporates avoidance symptoms, such as thoughts and feelings about the trauma, and places, people and situations that are associated with the trauma. A numbing of experienced emotions, a reduced interest in activities, and feelings of detachment and estrangement from others are also considered to be avoidance symptoms. Finally, the "D" symptom cluster incorporates symptoms of hyperarousal, such as insomnia, irritability and anger, concentration problems, hypervigilance, and increased startle responsiveness. The condition must be present at least one month after the occurrence of the criterion "A" event, and, as with all major disorders in the DSM, the illness must cause clinically significant distress or functional impairment.

Full PTSD symptom criteria lasting for less than 3 months is considered "Acute" PTSD, while "Chronic" PTSD refers to duration of PTSD symptoms for more than 3 months. It is important to note that the onset of PTSD may not start immediately after the traumatic experience and thus the sub-classification 'with delayed onset' is given if symptoms started 6 months or longer after the event occurred. A several-year delay of symptom-onset is possible in some cases.

A potential subtype that is not part of DSM-IV, but is worthy of clinical consideration is "PTSD with psychotic symptoms." Some severely ill patients with PTSD experience frank hallucinations, despite never having had psychotic symptoms prior to their trauma. Just as MDD can become sufficiently severe to develop psychotic symptoms, a similar process may occur in PTSD patients. Under current DSM-IV criteria, PTSD patients experiencing psychotic symptoms after a traumatic event would be diagnosed with PTSD and co-morbid "Psychotic Disorder, not otherwise specified."

3.1.3 Adjustment disorder

Adjustment Disorder is a diagnosis designed to capture the presence of clinically significant psychiatric symptoms that fall short of a more definitive diagnosis, such as MDD or PTSD. Adjustment disorders occur following a stressful life event, cause significant impairment or distress, and may require treatment. Unlike ASD and PTSD, the stressful events qualifying for an adjustment disorder need not be traumatic; for example, events such as divorce, sudden unemployment or involuntarily dropping out of college are considered non-traumatic stressors. Per definition, an Adjustment Disorder is a temporary impairment that must resolve within 6 months of the stressor onset, unless the stressor persists (e.g. an ongoing severe medical condition).

3.1.4 Anxiety disorder not otherwise specified (NOS)

Patients who, after the resolution of a traumatic event, still experience ongoing clinically significant anxiety symptoms falling short of ASD or PTSD criteria per the DSM-IV definitions should be diagnosed with Anxiety Disorder NOS. Such "sub-syndromal" PTSD patients may still be substantially impaired and/or distressed by their symptoms and usually require a treatment intervention. Furthermore, subsyndromal ASD increases the risk of later developing PTSD.

3.2 Complex PTSD

Although not part of DSM-IV, "Complex PTSD" (also referred to as Disorders of Extreme Stress Not Otherwise Specified, or DESNOS) has increasingly become a focus of research (Herman, 1997; Ford, 1999). The concept of Complex PTSD reflects the variety of psychological consequences of being emotionally or physically controlled by others, under the belief that such long-term captivity (literal or figurative) changes the person's sense of self and reactions to stress. Examples of such situations include prisoner of war camps, a prostitution brothel, or situations of long-term child abuse or domestic violence. In addition to classic PTSD symptoms of avoidance, re-experiencing and hyper-arousal, Complex PTSD is proposed to include distorted perceptions of both the self and the perpetrator, and a tendency to pursue a pattern of chronic victimization. Greater than 90% of people who meet criteria for Complex PTSD also meet criteria for DSM-IV-defined PTSD, which led to its exclusion from the DSM-IV. However, the concept has clinical utility in differentiating between PTSD patients who may need broader or more intense forms of treatment.

3.3 Differential diagnosis of PTSD symptoms, and the problem of comorbidity

Symptoms resembling PTSD can be attributed to other psychopathologies as well. Of crucial importance in differential diagnosis is clarifying which, if any, symptoms preceded rather than followed the traumatic event. For instance, recurrent intrusive thoughts can occur in Obsessive-Compulsive Disorder (OCD). The differentiating characteristic of intrusive thoughts in PTSD is that these thoughts and memories relate to the traumatic event, whereas in OCD the intrusive thoughts are unrelated to a traumatic event and the patient at some point in their life should have recognized the thoughts as being inappropriate. Flashbacks (i.e., highly vivid sensory experiences of the trauma occurring while awake) reflect re-experiencing the traumatic event, and differ from sensory hallucinations of non-existent stimuli, such as occur in substance-abuse or psychotic disorders. Also, PTSD Cluster C symptoms, such as loss of interest in activities, can also occur in Major Depressive Disorder as well as other anxiety disorders. The overlap of PTSD symptoms with MDD, bipolar disorder or other anxiety disorders is especially problematic for the Cluster D symptoms (particularly sleep disturbances, irritability, and concentration difficulties). It is important to note that the DSM permits the simultaneous diagnosis of PTSD with MDD, OCD, or other mood, anxiety or psychotic disorders if they also meet criteria for those disorders.

The co-occurrence of 2 or more psychiatric conditions is referred to as comorbidity. When PTSD is comorbid, it may precede or follow the development of other psychiatric conditions. On the one hand, pre-existing diagnoses, such as bipolar disorder and substance dependence, may increase the probability of traumatic exposure, thus increasing the risk for PTSD (Rakofsky et al., 2011). Conversely, data from the National Comorbidity Study (NCS) demonstrated that individuals with PTSD have an increased risk for developing substance use disorders, as well as mood and other anxiety disorders post trauma, compared to individuals with no PTSD diagnosis (Kessler et al., 2000).

3.3.1 Substance abuse

Patients with PTSD have a 3-4 fold increased risk of an alcohol or drug use disorder (Read et al., 2003). Most studies find that PTSD precedes the development of a substance abuse problem, and that experienced distress seems to serve as a key long-term risk factor for developing abuse (Read et al., 2004). Abuse of alcohol and other sedatives (e.g. benzodiazepines) may arise from an attempt to suppress the intrusion of distressing memories, so called "self-medication." Substantial research has identified connections between early-life traumatic experiences, such as childhood physical or sexual abuse, the development of PTSD, and subsequent drug abuse in adolescents (Kilpatrick et al., 2003). In one study of urban primary care patients, the number of traumatic events and a history of cocaine dependence both predicted current PTSD symptomatology, and this effect was independent of exposure to trauma during adulthood (Khoury et al., 2010). Comorbid PTSD has also been found to predict poorer outcomes of treatment for substance abuse (Ouimette et al., 1997). The clear implications for clinical practice are that all patients with a substance use disorder should be evaluated for PTSD, and vice versa.

3.3.2 Suicidality

Individuals with PTSD have a six-fold increased risk of attempted suicide (Kessler, 2000). The increased risk of both suicide ideation and attempts in patients with PTSD is present in both developed and developing countries (Nock et al., 2009). A well-designed prospective study examining suicidal ideation in women either with or without MDD and PTSD found that, after controlling for trauma history, MDD and PTSD independently predicted suicidal ideation, as did a history of interpersonal violence victimization. Women with PTSD alone reported more suicide attempts than women with MDD only. Among women with comorbid PTSD and MDD, 63% had experienced suicidal ideation and 14.4% had attempted suicide (Cougle, et al., 2009). Notably, thoughts of death or suicide are not a diagnostic criterion for PTSD, unlike for MDD. Nevertheless, inquiry and monitoring about suicidal thoughts is clearly of importance in the assessment and treatment of patients with PTSD.

4. Epidemiology

Lifetime exposure to traumatic events is estimated to range from 50-90% of the general population (Kessler et al., 1995; Darves-Bornoz et al., 2008; Breslau et al., 1998). There is substantial variability between countries, and even between cultures within countries, in terms of exposure to trauma and prevalence of PTSD. Chronic traumatic experiences, such as prolonged ethnic violence or civil wars increase the conditional risks of developing PTSD; thus, in less developed countries where these circumstances occur, rates of PTSD are higher. However, the likelihood of developing PTSD after specific types of traumatic exposure is relatively similar across countries (Wittchen et al., 2009). For example, professional Firefighters in the United States, Canada and Germany exhibit comparable conditional risks for PTSD after traumatic experiences (Wagner et al, 1998; Corneil et al, 1999). Even after the most distressing events, the probability of developing PTSD is less than 50%, and for most traumas the risk is much lower (Wittchen et al., 2009; Breslau, 2009). Nevertheless, many victims of trauma who do not meet criteria for PTSD may still notice psychological changes after the trauma. For example, among survivors who were in the Twin Towers during the September 11, 2001 terrorist attacks, 15% had probable PTSD 2-3 years later, but 96% reported at least one post-trauma symptom, the most common being hypervigilance and increased startle reactivity (DiGrande et al., 2011).

The first National Comorbidity Survey, which conducted interviews of a nationally representative sample of about 8,000 American adults in the 1990's found the lifetime prevalence of PTSD to be 7.8%. The prevalence among women (10.4%) was twice that of men (5%) (Kessler et al., 1995). These estimates were confirmed in the US National Comorbidity Survey - Replication (NCS-R), conducted about 10 years later, in which the lifetime prevalence of PTSD was 6.8%, with 9.7% of women and 3.6% of men affected. (Kessler et al., 2005).

Important unresolved issues in the epidemiology of PTSD are the rates of recovery and recurrence of the disorder. As occurs in MDD and several anxiety disorders, such as GAD and panic disorder, symptoms of the illness typically wax and wane over time. They tend to worsen at times of stress, particularly with the occurrence of a new traumatic event. For example, among patients who experienced active PTSD symptoms over many years, the majority experienced extended periods of times with only limited symptom severity or impairment (Breslau et al., 1998). Thus, it appears that patients with chronic PTSD often do not meet full criteria for the illness continually, but rather enter periods of remission or partial remission from their symptoms, even without treatment.

4.1 Risk factors for the development of PTSD

A broad range of factors have been identified to predict greater risk of PTSD, though there is great variability between studies regarding the relative importance of these factors. Although earlier work suggested that mere exposure to prior trauma was a risk factor for developing PTSD, longitudinal data indicate that only prior traumas that result in PTSD increase the risk of PTSD from subsequent traumatic events (Breslau et al., 2008). Pre-existing (i.e. pre-trauma) risk factors include female gender, pre-existing psychiatric disorders, substance use disorders, low socioeconomic status, lower intelligence, and adverse early life experiences. Risk factors associated with the traumatic event itself and its associated context are probably more significant predictors for PTSD than pre-trauma factors, and include the severity of the trauma, social support post-trauma, physical injuries, and the development of ASD (Berwin et al., 2000). Additionally, psychological factors such as humiliation, guilt and self-blame for actions taken during the event may arise in the aftermath of trauma, and may increase risk for developing PTSD (Yehuda, 2002).

A "dose-response" model postulates that PTSD symptoms increase with the severity of the stressor (March, 1993). This model is supported by some studies (e.g. greater proximity to the epicenter of an earthquake increases risk for PTSD symptoms) but not others (e.g. greater severity of motor vehicle accidents do not increase PTSD, (Pynoos et al., 1993; Schnyder et al., 2001). In accordance with the dose-response theory, the risk of a comorbid psychiatric disorder does appear to increase with the intensity and severity of the PTSD symptomatology. A non-linear dose model posits that the most significant risk for developing PTSD occurs once a certain threshold of trauma severity occurs, but greater trauma severity beyond that threshold adds little to increased risk (Harvey & Yehuda, 1999).

4.2 Recent disasters and PTSD

Improvements in survey methodology have allowed for initial evaluation and follow-up for PTSD surveillance among survivors exposed to traumas in recent years. **Table 2** presents findings from some more notable recent disasters. The consistent finding is that symptoms of PTSD are common in the days to weeks after an event, but for the majority of those exposed, return to normal functioning occurs. Notable in Table 2 is that mass disasters appear to induce higher rates of PTSD (25-50%) than smaller scale natural disasters that were previously found to carry PTSD rates of about 5% (Kessler, et al., 1995). Although most people are resilient to trauma, particularly for non-interpersonal events, when the scale of destruction is immense, and produces social breakdown and mass casualties, greater rates of PTSD can be expected. One shortcoming to these data is the limited amount of detailed surveillance data from disasters occurring in poorer nations.

The World Trade Center terrorist attacks on September 11, 2001 have been the focus of several investigations into the psychiatric effects of mass trauma. Consistent with the dose-response model, likelihood of having PTSD 2-3 years after the attacks was directly correlated with the number of types of trauma experienced by the victims during the attacks, and with presence on a higher floor of the buildings at the time of the attacks (DiGrande et al., 2011). Nearly 6 out of 10 people living in lower Manhattan at the time of the attacks experienced at least one PTSD symptom, most commonly insomnia and intrusive memories (Galea et al., 2002). One unique feature of this event was the massive and detailed media coverage, as extensive video footage of the disaster was replayed extensively in the weeks afterwards. The effects of media coverage appeared to be deleterious, as a phone survey performed the weekend after the attack found 44% of adults and 35% of children were experiencing at least one symptom of substantial stress, with higher rates associated with greater extent of television viewing of the disaster (Schuster et al., 2001). Restricting children's exposure to televised traumatic events is recommended by several professional organizations.

4.3 Gender differences in prevalence

Men experience more traumatic events over their lifetime than women, with only rape and childhood sexual abuse traumata occurring more commonly in females (Kessler et al., 1995). Despite their greater exposure to trauma, men have consistently lower rates of lifetime PTSD across studies than women. This pattern is consistent with all anxiety disorders, except OCD, which is equally common between genders. Of particular relevance to PTSD risk, women have greater risk for repeated, uncontrollable interpersonal trauma, such as childhood sexual abuse. Furthermore, traumas like these which violate the physical and emotional integrity of the victim may contribute to greater severity of subsequent symptoms (Pratchett et al., 2010). The loss of personal control over one's physical integrity as well as the extreme helplessness experienced may contribute to the high rate of PTSD following rape for both genders: 65% in men and 46% in women (Kessler, 2000). Furthermore, compared to men, women with PTSD are nearly twice as likely to have comorbidity with another anxiety disorder or depression (Breslau et al., 1997). These differences in types of trauma and rates of comorbidity may explain the higher rates of PTSD among women, though a gender-related biological vulnerability, perhaps related to sex steroid function and stress reactivity, must also be considered (J.B. Becker et al., 2007).

Region/ Year	Disaster type	General Disaster Impact	Sample size	Time point of sampling	% PTSD Diagnosis	Other Diagnoses	Reference
Italy 2009	Earthquake	309 deaths, 1,600 injuries 65,000 displacements	512 students	10 months after disaster	37.5% PTSD, 29.9% partial PTSD		Dell'Osso et al. (2011)
China 2008	Earthquake	69,227 deaths, 374,176 injuries 4.8million displacements	2250 students 446 adults (aged 15 or older)	6 months post disaster 2.5months post disaster	15.8% PTSD 45.5% PTSD	40.5% Anxiety, Overall 48.6% of students had 1 or more diagnosis, 24.5% MDD,	Fan et al. (2011) and Kun et al. (2009)
Peru 2007	Earthquake	596 deaths,	298 adults	5 months post disaster	25.2 % PTSD		Cairo et al. (2010)
Armenia 1988	Earthquake	25.000 deaths 700,000 displacements	1785 adults	12-24 months post disaster	49.6% PTSD	82% fulfilling at least one comorbid psychiatric disorder	Armenian et al. (2000)
Turkey 1999	Earthquake	18,243 deaths, 250,000 displacements	774 adults	40 months post disaster	37.2% PTSD	67.5% comorbid PTSD/MDD, 25.2% Depression	Salcioglu et al. (2007)
USA 2005	Hurricane Katrina	1,800 deaths, 500,000 displacements	101 adults	12 months	50% above PTSD cut-off score		LaJoie et al. (2010)
Indian Ocean 2004	Earthquake Tsunami	230,210 deaths, 125,000 injuries, 1.69 million displacements	1505 vacationing Swedish adults	14 months post disaster	13-56% above PTSD cut-off score depending on trauma exposure		Wahlstroem et al. (2008)

Table 2. Recent large disasters and incidence of PTSD

4.4 PTSD among children and adolescents

The National Survey of Adolescents interviewed over 4000 American adolescents and found that 25% of the 12-17-year olds had experienced a sexual (8.1%) or physical (17.4%) assault (Kilpatrick et al., 2003). In this study, significant PTSD symptomatology was identified in 30% of girls with a sexual abuse history, and one third of the sexually assaulted girls reported substance abuse in their lifetime compared to 5% of non-sexually assaulted girls. Other studies indicate that natural disasters are equally as traumatizing for children and adolescents as they are for adults. Recent data from earthquakes in Italy and China (Dell'Osso et al., 2011; Fan et al., 2011) show PTSD rates between 15 and 37% in children, with almost half of the children displaying more than one psychiatric disorder. Although considerable research has been done on the commission of harm (such as sexual or physical abuse), the omission of care (e.g. loss of a parent, physical or emotional neglect) may also produce traumatic responses in children. The implications of childhood trauma for the person's life trajectory are profound, and are an urgent area for further research.

4.5 Civilian trauma vs. combat trauma

Although there is substantial resilience among soldiers in the face of trauma, an estimated 10-20% of currently deployed soldiers in the ongoing wars in the Middle East will develop PTSD (Hoge et al., 2004). The development of PTSD in soldiers often occurs in conjunction with depression, aggression, substance abuse and increased rates of suicide. One compelling difference between retired soldiers with PTSD and civilians with PTSD is the decreased threshold for intimate partner violence in veterans; rates of domestic violence in veterans with PTSD is 3 times higher than in veterans without PTSD or civilians (Jordan et al., 1992). Differences in civilian versus combat PTSD are also seen in responses to treatment. Many, but not all, studies of medications to treat PTSD have found poorer responses among patients with PTSD related to combat than other traumas (Benedek et al., 2009; Martenyi & Soldatenkova, 2006).

4.6 Traumatic brain injury and PTSD

Traumatic brain injuries (TBI) can be a result of concussions, originate from vehicle or fire-arm accidents, or open head injuries such as being shot during combat. Distinguishing PTSD and TBI is complicated due to the overlapping symptoms of both illnesses. Both conditions include fatigue, anxiety, insomnia, poor memory and concentration as well as irritability, anger and depression (Institute of Medicine, 2008). TBI may contribute to the development of PTSD, and they increase the morbidity of soldiers returning from deployment. In fact, rates of PTSD among US soldiers with a TBI incurred during the Iraq War, have been reported as high as 43% (Hoge et al., 2008). TBI-PTSD patients may have greater difficulty benefiting from psychotherapy interventions, due to reduced concentration and other cognitive impairments.

4.7 PTSD and medical conditions

Chronic stress has long been thought to contribute to physical disease, with particular concern about cardiovascular consequences. Persistent re-experiencing of a traumatic event as occurs in PTSD may be considered a form of chronic stress. Recent prospective cohort studies of male Vietnam veterans have identified PTSD symptom level as an independent risk factor for nonfatal and fatal cardiovascular disease (CVD), even after controlling for several other risk factors for CVD, including smoking status, family history of CVD and education level (Kubzansky et al., 2007; Boscarino, 2008). This finding was replicated in a study of PTSD patients who had been deported to Siberia during childhood. These patients also showed an increased prevalence of cardiovascular disease, as well as diabetes, and hearing difficulties compared to age-matched controls (Walczewska et al., 2011). One theorized mechanism for this association with heart disease is that high levels of catecholamines present in PTSD (see below) could lead to damage of the intimal endothelium of coronary vessels, enhancing the progression of atherosclerosis.

5. Biology

Our current understanding of the biology of PTSD has derived primarily from animal models of fear learning and extinction in animals, and through cross-sectional comparison of a variety of biological markers and genes in PTSD patients versus unafflicted healthy controls. The most extensively studied biological alterations in patients with PTSD are disturbances in functioning of the hypothalamic-pituitary-adrenal (HPA) axis and the sympathetic nervous system (SNS), which are key drivers of the "fight or flight" response to fear. Encoding (i.e. storing into memory) of fearful events through activity in the amygdala and hippocampus is thought to depend on the function of the HPA axis and SNS systems (Cahill et al., 1994). Pathologic fear memory formation, and the failure to learn or access safety memories (extinction), are thought to be fundamental to the development of PTSD. The two systems interact, with glucocorticoids produced through activation of the HPA axis having inhibitory effects on the SNS system (Tsigos & Chrousos, 2002).

5.1 Sympathetic nervous system

SNS activation involves increased signaling by the catecholamines norepinephrine (NE, also known as noradrenaline) and epinephrine. Activation of the adrenal medulla produces NE and epinephrine for the body periphery, whereas the locus ceruleus (LC) is the primary source of NE in the central nervous system (CNS). Inputs from the amygdala and hypothalamus, both key fear processing brain regions, drive LC activation. In turn, the LC projects to a variety of stress-responsive brain regions, including the amygdala, hippocampus, hypothalamus, thalamus, prefrontal cortex and periaqueductal gray area. The post-synaptic alpha-1, beta-1 and beta-2 receptors in the CNS mediate the NE signal, and pre-synaptic alpha-2 receptors serve as a negative feedback signal to reduce NE signaling. Greater NE activity in the CNS found in PTSD patients may serve a key role in the pathogenesis of core PTSD symptoms, particularly fear learning, hyperarousal and heightened startle response.

Greater SNS activity in PTSD patients is reflected in higher greater heart rate, blood pressure and skin conductance, than healthy controls, particularly in response to reminders of a traumatic event. Moreover, elevated heart rate and epinephrine levels immediately following trauma may predict later development of PTSD (Delahanty & Nugent, 2006). Yohimbine, an alpha-2 receptor antagonist, which acts by blocking the negative feedback effects mediated by this receptor and thus increases NE signaling, can induce flashbacks and SNS activation in PTSD patients (Southwick et al.,1999). Traumatic reminders also induce greater cerbrospinal fluid concentrations of NE in PTSD patients than controls (Geracioti et al., 2008).

Serotonin is another neurotransmitter that has been studied in PTSD, in part because medications that affect serotonin transmission have some efficacy in treating the disorder (see below). Moreover, abnormalities in serotonin signaling have been associated with greater rates of hostility, impulsivity and suicide, which are often present in PTSD (Dunlop et al., 2009). However, to date, evidence linking serotonin system dysfunction to PTSD is not compelling.

5.2 Hypothalamic-pituitary-adrenal axis

The HPA axis is a hormonal circuit that controls the stress response. Corticotropin releasing hormone (CRH, also referred to as corticotropin releasing factor), is released from the hypothalamus along with arginine vasopressin (AVP). In concert with AVP, CRH then acts on the anterior pituitary gland, where it binds to CRH receptors to trigger the release of adrenocorticotropin (ACTH) and endorphins (endogenous opioids). ACTH released from the pituitary into the systemic circulation then acts on the adrenal cortex, inducing the release of cortisol. Cortisol is the main effector hormone of the stress response. In addition it exerts negative feedback effects on the HPA circuit by binding to glucocorticoid and mineralocorticoid receptors in the hypothalamus, pituitary and hippocampus. These signaling cascades act relatively quickly, and apparently have evolved to provide the organism with a rapid, short-lived response to acutely threatening situations. However, exposure to high levels of cortisol over time leads to a loss of dendritic branching in the hippocampus, potentially reducing hippocampal volume (Sapolsky et al., 1990).

Cortisol's effect on the body's organ systems are mediated via two types of corticosteroid receptors. When cortisol concentrations are low, the type I (mineralocorticoid, or MR) is thought to mediate cortisol's effects. The type II (glucocorticoid, or GR) becomes relevant as cortisol levels increase, as happens as part of the circadian rhythm or in the face of stress. Under these conditions the MRs saturate, and cortisol signaling occurs through GRs, inducing the negative feedback signal. After binding cortisol, both MRs and GRs translocate to the nucleus, where they interact with DNA to induce changes in gene expression (Raison & Miller, 2003).

Cortisol plays a significant role in memory consolidation, and also limits memory retrieval in emotionally-charged situations (for a review see, de Quervain et al., 2009). Most individuals lose retrieval of the specific emotional memory over time, but this is not the case in patients suffering from PTSD, for whom the traumatic memory is easily and vividly accessed and thus relived unexpectedly, or reactivated due to an external event or situation that triggers the memory. Reduced cortisol concentrations immediately following trauma may allow sustained activity of the SNS and CRF systems, thus prolonging fear processing and thereby laying the groundwork for traumatic memory formation and PTSD (Pacak et al., 1995). Indeed, low cortisol concentrations measured shortly after trauma predicts development of PTSD, as do heightened levels of SNS activity after trauma (Yehuda et al., 1998). Whether these findings reflects a low basal level of cortisol or impaired HPA axis activation in the face of trauma is uncertain. Also problematic is that activity of the HPA axis post-trauma may vary considerably by the time of measurement (i.e. circadian rhythm factors) and duration in days since trauma, indicating the need for tight control over these variables in assessing hormonal states after trauma (McFarlane et al., 2010).

Studies comparing basal cortisol levels in PTSD patients versus controls have had inconsistent findings (depending on control groups and populations studied), though reduced cortisol levels in PTSD patients is suggested by several studies (Meewisse et al., 2007). Inconsistent findings have also emerged from studies of HPA axis function in PTSD patients undergoing psychological stressors, such as exposure to reminders of trauma or cognitive stress tests (Miller et al., 2007). Patients with PTSD do show greater suppression of HPA axis function when administered a low dose of dexamethasone as part of the dexamethasone suppression test than do healthy controls (deKloet et al., 2006). In addition, CSF concentrations of CRH have been found to be elevated in PTSD (Baker et al., 1999), and CRH stimulation in PTSD patients produces less ACTH response than in healthy controls, both of which suggest that CRH receptors in the pituitary are down-regulated (Yehuda, 2006). Taken together, these data suggest that the PTSD is associated with a dysregulated HPA axis, though whether this disruption reflects a risk factor for, or consequence of, PTSD is uncertain.

5.3 Other signaling systems

Limited data support the potential involvement of other systems in the biology of PTSD. Reduced benzodiazepine receptor expression in the frontal cortex, thalamus and hippocampus has been identified in combat-PTSD patients, suggesting diminished inhibitory capacity in PTSD, as in other anxiety disorders (Bremner et al., 2000a; Geuze et al., 2008a). Brain derived neurotrophic factor (BDNF) is a protein involved in neurogenesis and the maturation, differentiation, migration and survival of neurons, and is particularly concentrated in brain regions involved in learning and memory, including hippocampus, amygdala, cerebral cortex and cerebellum. Studies of peripheral and CSF concentrations of

BDNF have found diverging results (Rakofsky et al., n.d.). However, in a small study, lower serum BDNF concentrations in patients with chronic PTSD predicted greater responses to 12-weeks of treatment with the antidepressant escitalopram (Berger et al., 2010). Neuropeptide Y (NPY) is an anxiolytic CNS protein which may serve as a protective factor against PTSD. NPY appears to diminish sensitivity to stress, perhaps through its ability to inhibit activity in CRH and NE circuits. In a small study, soldiers exposed to combat who had not developed PTSD had greater NPY plasma concentrations than veterans with PTSD (Yehuda et al., 2006). Finally, expression of a protein important for the transport of neurotransmitters and for cell cycle progression, p11 (also known as S100-A10), may serve as a biomarker to distinguish PTSD from mood disorders. In peripheral blood mononuclear cells, p11 was downregulated in PTSD patients, whereas patients with MDD or bipolar disorder had increased levels of p11 versus controls (Ursano et al., 2010).

Pituitary adenylate cyclase-activating polypeptide (PACAP) performs a variety of functions in the body relating to stress reactivity, including regulating CRH release and SNS function. In an urban primary-care population at high risk for PTSD, peripheral blood levels of PACAP directly correlated with posttraumatic stress symptoms in women, but not in men. Moreover, the gene for the PAC1 receptor (ADCYAP1R1), which binds PACAP, has a functional single nucleotide polymorphism (SNP) in an estrogen-response binding element. A SNP in this region of the PAC1 gene in women predicted PTSD diagnosis and symptom burden in the same study (Ressler et al., 2011).

5.4 Structural and functional neuroimaging

To date, the primary brain regions implicated as being altered in PTSD include the amygdala, hippocampus, anterior cingulate cortex (ACC) and the orbitofrontal cortex (OFC). The medial component of the OFC, the rostral and ventral components of the ACC, and the medial PFC are included in the brain region referred to by some authors as the ventromedial prefrontal cortex (vmPFC). Current models of the development of PTSD propose that exaggerated amygdala response to fearful stimuli lead to powerful encoding of fear memories and expression of fear reactions. The hippocampus is heavily interconnected with the amygdala, is thought to provide contextual information regarding danger, and also has crucial roles in forming explicit (i.e. conscious) memories, and in cortisol-mediated feedback after HPA-axis activation. Impaired hippocampal function in PTSD may contribute to failure to appreciate safe versus dangerous contexts following trauma. Reduced ACC and OFC function impair extinction of fear responding, and alter attention and response to fear-related stimuli (Rauch et al., 2006). Greater resting state activity of the dorsal ACC and mid-cingulate cortex may represent a risk factor for developing PTSD after trauma exposure (Shin et al., 2009).

5.4.1 Hippocampus

The hippocampus is considered particularly vulnerable to disruption in PTSD, based on the neurotoxicity hypothesis, which posits that chronic increased levels of corticosteroids resulting from stress cause atrophy and reduced dendritic branching of hippocampal neurons (Sapolsky et al., 1990). A reduced hippocampal volume may potentially limit the neuroendocrine response of the HPA axis, as shown in monkeys, who, when stressed, show increased cortisol production (Lyons et al., 2001).

Reduced hippocampal volumes are present in patients with chronic PTSD (Bremner et al., 2000b). However, it remains unclear whether smaller hippocampal volumes are present prior to the trauma (i.e. represent a risk factor for PTSD), are a consequence of developing PTSD, or are combination of both mechanisms. (Gilbertson et al., 2002; Felmingham et al., 2009). Impairment of hippocampal function is also suggested from functional magnetic resonance imaging (fMRI) studies, in which the activity of brain regions is extrapolated from blood flow changes over time. For example, when engaged in verbal learning tasks PTSD patients demonstrate lower levels of hippocampal activation than matched non-PTSD control subjects (Bremner et al., 2003; Shin et al., 2004). Sustained treatment of PTSD for several months with the antidepressant paroxetine produced increases in hippocampal volume and cognitive function (Vermetten et al., 2003).

5.4.2 Amygdala and vmPFC

The amygdala is a crucial component of the neural circuitry controlling fear, and is the primary site involved in associating stimuli with danger. Localized lesions in the amygdala result in docile and unfearful animals (Weiskrantz, 1956). Amygdala volumes have not been shown to differ between PTSD and healthy control subjects. However, abnormalities of amygdala function in PTSD have been identified using challenge (i.e. symptom provocation) studies, in which patients are exposed to reminders of their trauma, such as words or pictures. Using these paradigms, several researchers have identified a consistent pattern of hyperactive amygdala and hypoactive vmPFC function, though some discrepant findings have been reported (reviewed in Rauch et al., 2006). Moreover, greater amygdala activity in response to subliminally presented fearful or angry faces occurs in PTSD patients, reflecting greater threat-related reactivity (Rauch et al., 2000; Armony et al., 2005).

In structural imaging studies, patients with PTSD demonstrate reduced overall prefrontal cortex volume compared to healthy controls, as well as specific reductions in anterior ACC and vmPFC volumes (Geuze et al., 2008b). Women with sexual abuse-related PTSD demonstrate hypoactivation of the OFC and medial PFC during fear extinction learning compared to healthy control women (Bremner et al., 2005). These findings are of significance because the quality of memory extinction in humans is correlated with vmPFC thickness (Milad et al., 2005), and recall of extinguished memories is associated with activation of the vmPFC in healthy controls (Milad et al., 2007).

A meta-analysis of emotion processing studies found that PTSD patients, compared to healthy control subjects, demonstrate greater activity in the amygdala, parahippocampal gyrus, insula, mid-cingulate cortex and precuneus during emotion processing tasks (Etkin & Wagner, 2007). Amygdala and insula hyperactivation also occur in other phobic disorders, such as specific and social phobias. However, reduced activation in certain brain regions versus healthy controls was found only in PTSD patients. The regions of hypoactivation in PTSD patients include the vmPFC, rostral ACC, dorsal ACC and anterior hippocampus (Etkin & Wagner 2007). Lower levels of medial prefrontal cortex activation has been associated with greater PTSD symptom severity. Hypoactivations in the ACC occur in conjunction with hyperactivation of the amygdala and insula, indicating diminished frontal control over emotion-generating limbic regions. These findings are consistent with reports of diminished ACC grey matter volume and integrity of white matter tracts connecting limbic regions with the ACC in patients with PTSD (Kasai et al., 2008; Schuff et al., 2011).

In summary, the neural network model of PTSD proposes that the illness arises from an overly powerful fear-learning process, mediated primarily by the amygdala, which occurs in conjunction with deficient control over fear and stress responses and memories due to inadequate vmPFC and hippocampal activity and/or connectivity.

5.5 Startle

The startle reflex is the involuntary response to an intense unexpected stimulus, and involves flexing of the body and forward thrusting of the head. Startle is believed to indicate autonomic excitability, which can be measured by heart rate, blood pressure and skin conductance (Grossman et al., 2002). The intensity of the startle reflex can be assessed through auditory startle testing, in which the subject hears a loud unexpected noise, and the subsequent amplitude and latency of eyeblinking is measured. "Fear-potentiated startle" refers to the greater startle responding that occurs by cueing the subject that an aversive stimulus is coming so that their level of fear is heightened (Grillon, 2002). A simple 3-neuron subcortical circuit mediates the startle response but, importantly, it is modulated by inputs from the amygdala and other limbic structures (M. Davis, 1992). Startle responding patterns have been used to distinguish PTSD and non-PTSD subjects, and to differentiate between patients with PTSD versus MDD. Enhanced startle responding was found only in PTSD patients, with MDD patients not differing from controls, which suggests that startle responding may serve as a biomarker for PTSD (Jovanovic et al., 2009; Jovanovic et al., 2010a). Fear-potentiated startle assessed among healthy police academy cadets predicted development of PTSD symptom severity after one year of police work (Pole et al., 2009). This finding suggests that greater sensitivity to contextual and explicit threats and slower habituation to repeated aversive stimuli may represent risk factors for PTSD symptoms after trauma. Recent work in highly traumatized patients found greater concentrations of baseline and post-dexamethasone plasma ACTH to be correlated with greater fear-potentiated startle, thus linking abnormal HPA axis feedback with this innovative biomarker (Jovanovic et al., 2010b).

5.6 Genetics

As is the case for all psychiatric disorders, identifying specific genetic associations with PTSD is challenging due to the need for large numbers of subjects to detect small gene effects, and the variability introduced by imperfect phenotype definitions. The importance, of gene-environment interactions in PTSD is gaining increased attention, though definitive identification of PTSD risk alleles awaits further research (Mehta & Binder, 2011). The insertion-deletion functional polymorphism of the promoter region of the serotonin transporter gene (SLC6A4) in some studies modified the effects of environmental risks (e.g. trauma load or post-trauma social support) for PTSD (Koenen et al., 2009; Xie et al., 2009). Even stronger evidence is emerging for the role of FKBP5 (also known as the FK506 binding protein 51), an important intracellular regulator of the glucocortiocoid receptor complex. Functional polymorphisms of the FKBP5 gene are associated with glucocorticoid receptor resistance and consequently impaired negative HPA axis feedback after stress (Binder et al., 2008). Alleles that induce high expression of FKBP5 may serve to increase the risk of PTSD or MDD after early trauma.

6. Prevention

Some traumatic experiences cannot be avoided and are a part of our human existence (i.e., natural disasters or accidents), yet, not every individual with trauma exposure goes on to develop ASD or PTSD. Three levels of prevention to reduce the risk of mental disorders have been proposed by Mrazek & Haggerty (1994): universal, selected and indicated preventions. With regard to PTSD, universal or primary prevention encompasses general prevention of traumatic experiences; examples include sexual assault or child maltreatment awareness programs. Individuals with identified risk factors for developing PTSD are targeted in selected prevention programs, e.g. soldiers prior to deployment or first-response disaster relief workers. These individuals have had previous exposure to potentially traumatizing situations and are offered brief psychotherapy by mental health counselors. The third and last level of prevention targets individuals who exhibit subsyndromal symptoms (e.g., irritability, dissociation, sleep disturbances) of PTSD but do not meet full criteria yet. Patients with Acute Stress Disorder or Adjustment Disorder would benefit from an indicated prevention in order to prevent chronicity and/or worsening of impairments.

6.1 Treating the acutely traumatized individual

6.1.1 Psychological first aid

In the immediate aftermath of a traumatic event, basic steps can be taken to diminish the psychological devastation felt by victims. Such "psychological first aid" has the goals of creating an environment that: 1) provides safety; 2) is calming; 3) allows connectedness to others; 4) enhances self-efficacy, and; 5) instills hope. **Table 3** provides some guidance for people assisting in the aftermath of a trauma.

DO	DON'T
Help meet basic needs (food, shelter, medical care)	React negatively to traumatized people who are upset and being difficult
Listen to people who want to talk about their trauma experience	Force people to share their experiences with you
Provide accurate information about the trauma that has occurred	Make promises that cannot be kept
Help people contact relatives and friends	Criticize existing relief activities in front of people experiencing the trauma
Provide suggestions for people to help themselves	Tell people how they should be thinking, feeling or acting after the trauma
Remind people more help is on the way (if this is indeed the case)	Give simple reassurance such as "Everything will be OK"
Establish routines, particularly for sleep/wake cycles	Limit exposure of people to information about the trauma (such as repeated news reports or video)

Table 3. Do's and don'ts of psychological first aid

The principles of psychological first aid in the prevention of PTSD and adverse psychiatric sequelae after trauma were applied in the case of 33 Chilean miners who were trapped deep in a mine after a structural collapse in August 2010. Their plight underground captured worldwide attention until they were rescued after 69 days. Their situation was certainly considered a traumatic event - a sudden experience of being trapped underground, and for the first several weeks they did not know if people on the surface knew they were alive.

By all accounts, the men coped remarkably well in their dire situation. A number of psychological first aid measures likely contributed to the good outcomes. First, by having a group of 33 trapped together, feelings of isolation were reduced, and a sense of camaraderie could be built. Importantly, a senior miner exercised judicious leadership of the men, maintaining order and social structure. He divided them into teams and assigned duties to maximize their survival and comfort. Later, rescuers provided tasks for the men to do to aid in the rescue efforts, which reduced helplessness and provided a sense of control.

When rescuers successfully established contact with the miners through a small drilled hole, it provided reassurance that help was coming, and provided a means by which the men could be informed of the rescue efforts and receive notes from loved ones. The miners maintained a 24 hour light-dark schedule using truck batteries to ensure adequate rest. Initial food and water supplies were carefully apportioned, and later supplemented by supplies from rescuers. Fortunately, none sustained significant injuries from the accident, which would have increased the psychological stress of the situation. Thus, by attending to physical needs, maintaining daily routines, establishing basis for hope and contact with loved ones, and by giving the miners a role in their own rescue, the risks for severe psychological breakdown were minimized.

Websites with information regarding trauma and PTSD that victims and families may find useful are listed in **Table 4**.

ORGANIZATION	INTERNET ADDRESS
American Psychological Association	http://www.apa.org/topics/ptsd/index.aspx
Anxiety Disorders Association of America	http://www.adaa.org/understanding-anxiety/posttraumatic-stress-disorder-ptsd
United States Department of Veterans Affairs/ The National Center for PTSD	http://www.ptsd.va.gov/
PTSD-help network (veteran-to-veteran network)	http://www.ptsdhelp.net/
Deployment Health Clinical Center	http://www.pdhealth.mil/clinicians/ptsd.asp
The PTSD Alliance	http://www.ptsdalliance.org/
National Institute of Mental Health	http://www.nimh.nih.gov/health/topics/post-traumatic-stress-disorder-ptsd/index.shtml
Victim Assistance Online	http://www.vaonline.org/trauma.html
The European Society for Traumatic Stress Studies	https://www.estss.org/learn-about-trauma/
The National Crime Victims Research and Treatment Center	http://colleges.musc.edu/ncvc/
National Child Traumatic Stress Network	http://www.nctsn.org/

Table 4. Internet resources for PTSD

6.1.2 Psychological debriefing

Psychological Debriefing refers to psychological interventions initiated within days after a traumatic event that aim to prevent maladaptive responses to trauma. Psychoeducation about expected reactions to trauma exposure is a component of all debriefing techniques. Perhaps the most widely used form of acute post-trauma intervention is Critical Incident Stress Debriefing (CISD). Originally developed for occupations frequently exposed to potentially traumatizing situations, such as emergency medical personnel, firefighters or police officers, CISD has been increasingly applied to the direct victims of trauma (Mitchell & Everly, 2001). CISD typically is performed in the course of a single, several-hour group session and involves several phases. Besides psychoeducation, other key components of CISD are the elicitation of thoughts and feelings experienced during the trauma, recounting the worst part of the incident, and identification of stress reactions and how to manage them. Although CISD has been employed in a wide range of group-trauma situations, there is now substantial doubt about the intervention's effectiveness. Meta-analyses of clinical trials have not shown CISD to prevent the development of PTSD (van Emmerik et al., 2002); in fact some studies suggest CISD may produce an increase in psychopathology over untreated controls. (Bledsoe, 2003; Mayou et al., 2000). Adverse outcomes may be due in part to the group setting in which everybody is invited to share their experiences, irrespective of the extent of their traumatization, which may add to the sense of carnage and danger. Additionally, sharing personal reactions to a traumatic situation with strangers may heighten anxiety in vulnerable individuals.

6.1.3 Early pharmacological interventions

Given that resilience is the typical response to trauma, the use of *a priori* medication approaches as a selected preventive treatment immediately after trauma may reflect a therapeutic over-reach, particularly given our limited understanding of the biology of PTSD (Sones et al., 2011). Nevertheless, the inroads made in understanding PTSD pathophysiology have led to the exploration of several pharmacological approaches to prevent PTSD development, with particular focus on the noradrenergic and HPA axis systems. To inhibit the effects of greater SNS activation and NE signaling among people who will eventually develop PTSD after a trauma, the beta-adrenergic receptor antagonist ("beta-blocker") propranolol has been studied as a prospective treatment for emergency room trauma and surgical trauma patients. Despite early data suggesting benefit in reducing traumatic memory consolidation (Brunet et al., 2008), subsequent studies have not found propranolol effective at preventing PTSD in these settings (Hoge et al., 2011; M.B. Stein et al., 2007). Clonidine, an alpha-2 receptor antagonist that acts to reduce norepinephrine release, has also been proposed as a preventative treatment for PTSD, though there are no controlled studies of this intervention. Finally, based on the finding of low cortisol concentrations post-trauma in patients who later develop PTSD, administration of hydrocortisone (a glucocorticoid) soon after trauma was found to prevent the development of PTSD in small studies, a finding worthy of further pursuit (De Quervain & Margraf, 2008).

Two recent naturalistic studies of physically injured patients suggest that administration of an opiate medication, morphine, immediately after trauma may lessen later PTSD severity (Bryant et al., 2009; Holbrook et al., 2010). Opioids reduce norepinephrine transmission, though wheher any preventive effects derive from that mechanism, which would imply benefit in non-injured patients, or simply through the benefits of pain control are unknown.

7. Treatment

7.1 Treatment of acute stress disorder

Cognitive behavioural therapy (CBT) approaches incorporating a combination of prolonged exposure and cognitive restructuring have been the most extensively studied treatments for ASD. Several studies have demonstrated that a short course (approximately 5 sessions) of CBT is effective in preventing the progression of ASD to PTSD, and that the gains can be maintained for years following treatment (Bryant et al., 2003). There is growing evidence that the prolonged exposure component, rather than cognitive restructuring, is the more potent part of the therapy (Bryant et al., 2008), which is consistent with the growing focus on prolonged exposure for the treatment of PTSD. An Israeli study that compared cognitive therapy, prolonged exposure therapy, escitalopram 10-20 mg/d or placebo found substantial superiority in preventing PTSD for both psychotherapies over the antidepressant, which did not separate from either placebo or an untreated control group (Shalev, 2007).

7.2 Treatment of PTSD

All the leading guidelines and evidence-based reviews of treatments for PTSD recommend some form of psychotherapy as the preferred first line treatment for PTSD. However, controversy arises regarding the stage at which pharmacotherapy should be considered. The Institute of Medicine (2008) report goes so far as to assert there is insufficient evidence for the efficacy of pharmacotherapy, though it should be noted that this report did not definitively conclude that medications were ineffective for PTSD. Some national guidelines recommend SSRI medication or psychotherapy as first line treatments (Baldwin et al., 2005; Swinson et al., 2006; Ursano et al., 2004; Benedek et al., 2009) whereas others recommend relegating medications to second line treatments to be used only if psychotherapy fails or is unavailable (Forbes et al., 2007; National Collaborating Centre for Mental Health, 2005). Actual treatment choices in clinical practice are influenced by other factors, including treatment availability, patient preference, and the presence of significant comorbid disorders, such as depression, bipolar disorder, or other anxiety disorders (Rakofsky & Dunlop, 2011).

7.2.1 Psychotherapies

CBT refers to a variety of psychological interventions that address the dysfunctional thoughts and maladaptive behaviors that serve to maintain a state of mental illness. For PTSD, the behavioral intervention of exposure is a key component of CBT treatment, and includes the confrontation of the traumatic memory in a safe, therapeutic setting. Once the trauma memory is activated, the patient processes the information and the emotion repeatedly ("habituation"), ultimately forming new, non-fear inducing memories of the traumatic event ("extinction"). CBT also commonly includes cognitive restructuring of maladaptive beliefs, such as guilt and overly pessimistic views about the world and self, by identifying and replacing excessively negative perceptions and interpretations with more realistic appraisals (Bryant et al, 2008).

7.2.1.1 Prolonged exposure

A specific form of CBT often used for PTSD, called Prolonged Exposure, is delivered over the course of 9-12 ninety minute sessions (Foa et al., 1999). Initial sessions involve education about common reactions to trauma and breathing control for relaxation. Subsequently, prolonged and repeated recounting of the memory is performed (called "imaginal exposure"), during which the patient is encouraged to include as much sensory and emotional detail of their traumatic experience as possible. Between sessions, patients are assigned homework, which includes listening once or twice daily to an audiotape of their imaginal exposure created in session with the therapist. Later in therapy in vivo exposure is introduced, in which patients confront places and objects in the real world they have avoided due to their association with the traumatic event, but when in fact they are objectively safe. Throughout the treatment, the therapist discusses with the patient their thoughts and feelings related to the exposure experiences. All these components are intended to directly challenge the fear associated with the trauma.

Prolonged exposure is the only treatment with sufficient scientific support to be recommended by the Institute of Medicine (2008) for the treatment of PTSD. Unlike other psychotherapies that have demonstrated benefit only in relation to a no-treatment wait-list control condition (which fail to control for the non-specific effects of therapy), prolonged exposure has demonstrated benefit in reducing PTSD symptoms beyond other non-trauma-related treatment, such as present-centered therapy (Schnurr et al., 2007) and narrative therapy (Bichescu et al., 2007). Exposure therapy has demonstrated maintenance of treatment gains for up to 5 years post-treatment (for further review, see Ponniah & Hollon, 2009). The primary drawback from prolonged exposure treatment is patient drop-out, presumably due to distress induced by the procedure. Moreover, it may be difficult to get patients with high levels of avoidance to agree to this form of treatment. Unfortunately, prolonged exposure therapy is not yet routinely used in clinical practice, due to inadequate training of therapists, as well as excessive concerns about re-traumatization or decompensation of the patient.

7.2.1.2 Eye movement desensitization and reprocessing (EMDR)

EMDR uses two simultaneous attention tasks to enable the patient to process the traumatic event. The patient is asked to focus on the negative, fear-inducing emotions and thoughts (a form of exposure) while simultaneously engaging in a repetitive task, such as hand tapping, eye-movements, tactile stimulation or sounds. These are done together until the initially felt distress wanes and can be replaced by positive or neutral trauma-related thoughts (Shapiro, 1989). Benefits of EMDR have been demonstrated in various patient populations, such as rape victims (Rothbaum, 1997), combat veterans (Carlson et al., 1998) or interpersonal violence victims (van der Kolk et al., 2007). The concept of EMDR is not without criticism, especially the eye-movement component (Institute of Medicine, 2008). Critics note that treatment success may be obtained solely through the cognitive and emotional processing of the traumatic memory as well as the learning of coping skills, rather than from the eye-movement technique itself.

7.2.1.3 Cognitive processing therapy (CPT)

CPT is a form of CBT often used in the treatment of PTSD (Resick & Schnicke, 1993). CPT conceptualizes PTSD as a *disorder of non-recovery* in which maladaptive beliefs surrounding the traumatic event cause strong negative emotions that prevent the natural cognitive processing of the situation. The goal is for the patient to understand the pattern of trauma memory avoidance and associated belief systems. Problematic belief systems, such as survivor guilt, are identified as 'stuck points' that interfere with resolving the traumatic event. Traditionally, patients are asked to write a detailed emotional account of their traumatic experiences and read them out loud to the therapist, thus breaking the pattern of avoidance. Utilizing Socratic dialogue (i.e., asking questions to enable the patient's own insights instead of providing advice), as well as teaching the patient cognitive skills to identify and modify affected belief systems (such as safety, trust and control) are effective ways to teach the patients to cope with the traumatic event. CPT has demonstrated superiority over wait-list control groups for veterans with PTSD (Monson et al., 2006), and has been found to be equally effective as prolonged exposure among female rape victims (Resick et al., 2002).

7.2.1.4 Stress inoculation training

SIT, also referred to as Stress-Management training, is not trauma-specific and includes relaxation techniques as well as stress-inoculation training. The patient learns skills such as abdominal breathing, progressive muscle relaxation, positive statements, distraction, and assertiveness. The primary focus of SIT is to help the patient increase confidence in his or her ability to cope with the fear and anxiety that arise from reminders of their trauma. SIT is sometimes used as an active control comparison condition in psychotherapy studies of anxiety disorders, but it has also been found to be as effective as PE in some studies (Foa, et al., 1999).

7.2.2 Pharmacotherapies

7.2.2.1 Monotherapy

Selective serotonin reuptake inhibitors (SSRIs) are the preferred initial medication treatment for PTSD. Two SSRIs, paroxetine and sertraline, have received regulatory approval for the treatment of PTSD in the United States and Europe. A recent Cochrane Collaboration meta-analysis found that among medication treatments for PTSD, SSRIs had the most convincing effect, and that the included trials were of relatively high quality (D.J. Stein et al., 2006). Several other agents also have data suggesting efficacy, including venlafaxine, mirtazapine, some tricyclic antidepressants (TCAs, amitriptyline, imipramine) and the monoamine oxidase inhibitor (MAOI) phenelzine. Mirtazapine positively affects sleep, and is recommended as a second line agent by many guidelines. The clinical trials supporting the use of TCAs and MAOIs for PTSD had methodological limitations, but these medications can be effective for some patients. An exception is the reversible MAOI brofaromine, which showed no benefit in two large placebo-controlled trials (Baker et al., 1995). TCAs and MAOIs are usually prescribed only after failure with SSRIs, SNRIs or mirtazapine, due to their potential for serious cardiovascular events and drug interactions.

An additional agent used for the treatment of PTSD is nefazodone. This 5HT2a receptor antagonist and weak serotonin reuptake inhibitor has support of efficacy from a placebo-controlled trial, and has been widely employed in the treatment of combat veterans (L.L. Davis et al., 2004). Use in recent years has declined due to its association with a low-risk of hepatotoxicity (the estimated rates of liver failure are 1 case per 30,000 - 250,000 patient-years of exposure), relegating its use to patients unresponsive to other treatments.

Dose ranges for medications used to treat PTSD are similar to those required to treat MDD, and should be up-titrated at 4 week intervals until remission is obtained or intolerance occurs. Response to medication may take 1-3 months. More sustained treatment can provide further gains and reduced likelihood of relapse (Davidson et al., 2002). Should the first SSRI treatment prove ineffective or intolerable, a second SSRI or venlafaxine should be tried (Davidson et al., 2006).

7.2.2.2 Augmentation

Pharmacological treatment decisions become more challenging when medication provides a clear benefit, but the patient continues to have some significant ongoing symptoms. In these cases, it is probably better to add a second medication ("augmentation") rather than switch to another monotherapy. There is some evidence that the atypical antipsychotics olanzapine and risperidone can augment SSRI response in patients with PTSD (M.B. Stein et al., 2003; Bartozkis et al., 2005). Open-label data suggest that quetiapine may also have value in the treatment of PTSD, particularly for sleep-related symptoms (Robert et al., 2005). However, the side effect risks with these medications, including significant risk for weight gain and metabolic disturbances, argue that they should be reserved for the most treatment-resistant cases. The choice of augmenting medication may be guided in part by the types of persisting symptoms.

Prazosin, at a dose of 2-15 mg/day, has demonstrated specific effects on sleep quality and nightmares in patients who were also receiving other medications for PTSD (Raskind et al., 2003; Raskind et al., 2007; Taylor et al., 2008). Other adrenergic agents sometimes used adjunctively in combat veterans are guanfacine and clonidine. In contrast to prazosin, which is an alpha-1 receptor antagonist, these alpha-2 receptor agonists, which act to reduce noradrenergic signaling via inhibitory feedback, did not prove superior to placebo (Neylan et al., 2006). The efficacy of beta-blockers in chronic PTSD have not been studied in controlled trials.

Another medication with positive sleep effects is mirtazapine, which is recommended as a second line agent by many guidelines. The anti-epileptic agent and GABA modulator valproic acid was not found to be effective as a monotherapy in an 8-week placebo-controlled trial in veterans with PTSD (L.L. Davis et al., 2008). Nevertheless, valproic acid is sometimes used as an adjunctive agent, particularly among combat veterans with prominent hyperarousal symptoms (Fesler, 1991; Clark et al., 1999).

Other anti-epileptic agents have been studied for use in chronic PTSD. The most promising is topiramate, an agent thought to act by blocking voltage-gated sodium channels, which significantly reduced re-experiencing symptoms and improved remission rates in a 12-week placebo-controlled study (Tucker et al., 2007). A very small randomized trial suggested efficacy for lamotrigine, another voltage-gated sodium channel antagonist (Hertzberg et al., 1999). In contrast, tiagabine, a GABA reuptake inhibitor, proved ineffective compared to placebo in a large 12-week trial (Davidson et al., 2007). In addition, small open label studies suggest potential benefits for phenytoin, levetiracetam, and carbamazepine (reviewed in Berger et al., 2009).

Benzodiazepines are commonly used to treat anxiety, but there is little support for their use in PTSD. A specific concern about benzodiazepines is their impairing effect on learning. Recovery from PTSD is thought to require new learning about the meaning of stimuli and contexts associated with the trauma, and benzodiazepines may diminish that ability. It is important to note that very little research on the use of benzodiazepines to treat PTSD has been performed, so a definitive statement about inefficacy cannot be made (Braun et al., 1990). Nevertheless, they should not be considered as monotherapy agents for patients with PTSD, and generally should not be used to treat anxiety in the acute aftermath of a traumatic event (Gelpin et al., 1996; Mellman et al., 2002).

A consistent finding across nearly all medication trials for PTSD is that patients with civilian trauma demonstrate more benefit from active medication than patients with combat-related trauma. It is important to note that no guidelines recommend the use of bupropion as a standard agent for the treatment of PTSD, and a large placebo-controlled trial showed no benefit for this medication in treating PTSD (M.E. Becker et al., 2007). Unfortunately, no large trials have compared different pharmacotherapies, so support for the relative efficacy of one class of medications over another does not exist, and there are no predictors for which medication is best suited for a particular individual. Rather, issues of cost, availability, potential side effects and other comorbid illnesses often guide treatment selection.

Other problems that complicate treatment choices for PTSD are the relative paucity of studies of long-term outcomes, and minimal study among patients with prominent comorbid conditions (e.g. substance abuse), or treated in primary care settings. Thus, the generalizability of findings from clinical trials remains uncertain. In general, comorbid substance abuse should be treated before or simultaneously with treatment for PTSD. Also, in patients with comorbid bipolar disorder, optimization of mood stabilization treatment should usually be the initial focus of treatment (Rakofsky & Dunlop, 2011).

DRUG	MECHANISM	CLINCIALTRIALS.GOV IDENTIFIER(S)
Aprepitant	Antagonist of neurokinin type 1 receptors, thereby blocking effect of Substance P. May reduce alcohol cravings in PTSD patients with alcohol dependence	NCT00896038
Carvedilol	Beta receptor blocker; blocks the effect of norepinephrine at these receptors. Being studied in low dose form.	NCT01221792
D-Cycloserine	Glutamate receptor modulator. May improve extinction learning in PE	NCT00356278; NCT00875342
Ganaxolone	Synthetic neurosteroid; modulates GABA-A receptors.	NCT01339689
GSK561679	CRH type 1 receptor antagonist.	NCT01018992
Hydrocortisone	Synthetic glucocorticoid; acts like cortisol. Being studied as monotherapy and adjunctively to improve extinction learning in PE.	NCT00706173; NCT01090518; NCT00751855
Ketamine	NMDA glutamate receptor antagonist	NCT00749203
Methylene Blue	Metabolic enhancer; increases brain utilization of oxygen. May improve extinction learning in PE	NCT01188694
Nepicastat	Inhibits enzyme dopamine beta hydroxylase, thereby reduces norepinephrine production	NCT00659230

(GABA: Gamma-aminobutyric acid; NMDA: N-methyl D-aspartic acid; PE: prolonged exposure therapy)

Table 5. Exploratory pharmacologic interventions for PTSD

7.2.3 Sleep therapies

Sleep disturbances in PTSD are extremely common and often become a focus of treatment. Specific sleep problems in PTSD include insomnia and recurrent nightmares. It is unclear whether nightmares occur during rapid-eye-movement (REM) sleep or non-REM sleep, or both. Nightmares can contribute to sleep-related anxiety, such as fear of going to sleep, fear of going back to sleep after awakening, and fear of the dark. Sleep-related anxieties may be particularly evident among PTSD patients whose trauma is associated with nighttime or beds, such as rape victims. Often, to combat insomnia and nightmares, patients will use alcohol to induce sleep and suppress dreams. Although alcohol may provide these short-term benefits, there are long-term consequences from sustained alcohol use including sleep fragmentation, rebound REM sleep from alcohol withdrawal, and risk of abuse and dependence (Lamarche & De Koninck, 2007).

Despite the high frequency of subjective complaints about sleep disruption, objective assessments of sleep in patients with PTSD have been very inconsistent, with no clear abnormalities identified. One large community-based polysomnography study found only that PTSD patients had more frequent brief arousals after REM sleep than control patients; (Breslau et al., 2004). This study suggests that some PTSD sleep complaints may be stem from greater subjective perceptions of brief awakenings, though whether this effect represents a vulnerability for PTSD or a consequence of the illness is unknown. In general, patients with PTSD should be screened for the presence of any other sleep disorders that may aggravate insomnia, such as obstructive sleep apnea and restless legs syndrome;

treatment of these comorbid conditions may improve PTSD treatment outcome (Lamarche & DeKoninck, 2007).

Sleep problems that persist despite psychological or pharmacological interventions for PTSD can be addressed through insomnia-specific treatments. CBT packages developed specifically to treat insomnia, which include strategies like sleep restriction, stimulus control, education, and alteration of beliefs about insomnia, have been successfully applied in patients with PTSD (Ulmer et al., 2011). To target nightmares specifically, imagery rehearsal therapy (IRT) has demonstrated benefit among civilian PTSD patients. In IRT, patients write down the recurring dream(s), then re-write it into a non-threatening form, and finally use imagery to rehearse the revised dream as practice during the day (Krakow et al., 2001).

In addition to the use of prazosin for nightmares, and mirtazapine for insomnia, additional medications are often used for sleep complaints in PTSD patients. Trazodone (dosed at 50-200 mg at bedtime) and the non-benzodiazepine sedatives, such as zolpidem, are among the most commonly employed, although there are no placebo-controlled studies of these medications for PTSD-specific insomnia. Low dose quetiapine (25-200 mg at bedtime) is also used for severe sleep complaints, but this medication requires ongoing monitoring for metabolic and movement disorder risks.

8. Future of PTSD

Our understanding of PTSD continues to evolve. Significant advances in the coming years are likely in the areas of the characterization of the illness, approaches to treatment, and our understanding of decision-making in PTSD patients.

8.1 Diagnostic criteria

A new edition of the DSM, DSM-V, is expected to be published in the near future (http://www.dsm5.org/ProposedRevisions/Pages/proposedrevision.aspx?rid=165). Major proposed revisions to the DSM-IV criteria for PTSD include:

1. Dropping the A2 criterion, due to a lack of evidence that experiencing a sense of horror, terror or helplessness at the time of the trauma has any diagnostic utility.
2. A revised definition of "trauma" that better specifies what experiences are considered to cross the "traumatic threshold."
3. Separating the current "C"-criteria into two categories: one specifically for avoidance of reminders of the trauma, and the second focusing on overall negative emotional experiences, chosen from factor analyses of symptoms.
4. Eliminating the distinction between Acute and Chronic PTSD due to lack of evidence supporting this distinction.

8.2 New treatments

A key component of prolonged exposure therapy is the reactivation of the traumatic memory as intensely and thoroughly as possible. To enhance this process, computers can be used to augment the sensory experiences associated with the memory. Virtual reality is a computer-based form of prolonged exposure therapy in which the patient actively participates in a three-dimensional virtual world by means of head-mounted displays. The virtual reality device incorporates display screens for eyes, as well as earphones and head-tracking devices. If desired, vibration platforms and olfactory stimuli can be integrated, creating a maximally real sensory experience. Immersion in this virtual world enhances the emotional engagement with the traumatic memory, as well as controlling all stimuli relevant to the individual trauma (Rothbaum et al., 2010). In this therapeutic model, patients are gradually exposed to their traumatic event and the therapist adjusts the multimodal stimuli to elicit the appropriate anxiety response. Pilot studies suggest benefit of the use of virtual reality in exposure therapies, and large trials of this treatment modality are underway.

New medications currently in clinical trials for PTSD are listed in Table 5 Most new treatment approaches to PTSD look to build on our increasingly sophisticated understanding of memory formation and extinction (e.g. Ressler et al., 2004). Several medications are being explored as means to augment the extinction learning that occurs in prolonged exposure therapy. The most advanced of these medications is D-Cycloserine (DCS), a drug previously used to treat tuberculosis, which acts as a partial NMDA (N-methyl-D-aspartate)-glutamatergic receptor agonist and thereby enhances synaptic formation during learning. Indeed, DCS has been found to enhance memory in humans (Tsai et al., 1999). Multiple trials have also demonstrated benefit of DCS over placebo in enhancing exposure-based treatments for phobic disorders (for review, see M. Davis et al., 2006). In these studies, DCS is dosed approximately one hour prior to each exposure therapy session (usually about 5 total sessions); the medication is not taken on a daily basis between therapy visits. Current studies combining DCS with exposure therapy, including virtual reality prolonged exposure for war veterans with PTSD, will soon determine whether the benefits of DCS enhancement of psychotherapy observed in other anxiety disorders can be extended to PTSD.

Memory erasure represents the ultimate manipulation of memory processes. Although in its infancy, this approach proposes to eliminate the powerful emotions developed in connection to the memory a traumatic event, rather than simply reduce their impact, as occurs through extinction learning in current PE treatment. Recent work in mice identified that fear reactions associated with a newly-learned memory can be erased through subsequent behavioral experience by removing certain calcium-permeable alpha-amino-3-hydroxyl-5-methyl-4-isoxazole-propionate (AMPA) receptors from the synapses in the lateral amygdala during a short time window after fear learning has occurred (Clem & Huganir, 2010). Manipulating this process in humans may allow for complete erasure of a traumatic memory, though the ethical implications of memory erasure shall need consideration as this research goes forward.

More traditional medication-based symptom-suppression approaches are also being explored. Theories postulating dysfunction in the HPA axis in PTSD (and MDD) have spawned a significant effort to discover agents that can modify this system (Holsboer & Ising 2008). Several CRH type 1 receptor antagonists have been developed, but none have yet proven superior to placebo in the treatment of MDD. Whether these agents may be of benefit in PTSD will be determined from an ongoing trial.

8.3 Decision making

Imaging research to date has focused primarily on the fear, anxiety and impaired cognition of patients with PTSD. However, a diagnostic criterion present in most patients with PTSD is a markedly diminished interest or participation in activities. This hedonic item reflects a change in risk-reward experience in PTSD. As discussed by Stein & Paulus (2009), this change represents a manifestation of a new homeostatic steady state between approach and avoidance. Emerging work employing neuroeconomic approaches to analyze decision-making in patients with many psychiatric disorders, including PTSD, may greatly inform the underlying biological disruptions in these conditions, and identify targeted approaches for psychotherapeutic and pharmacologic treatments (Elman et al., 2009).

9. Conclusion

PTSD is now firmly established as a characteristic psychological reaction to a sudden, unexpected terrible event. Although much more work is required to further delineate the biology of this disorder, the ability to model fear responding in animals gives hope that this disorder will be one of the more tractable psychiatric illnesses in the years ahead. If applied with rigor and concerned caring, cognitive behavioral forms of psychotherapy can be tremendously helpful to many patients with PTSD. Much remains to be done to improve pharmacotherapy approaches for PTSD, for which new neurobiological discoveries are necessary to guide innovation. Perhaps most promising is the potential to combine psychotherapy with medication, such as with D-cycloserine, to enhance outcomes combined with prolonged exposure therapy. Though the illness of PTSD is daunting for patients and clinicians alike, there is a justifiable basis for optimism about future treatment of this condition.

10. References

American Psychiatric Association Committee on Nomenclature and Statistics. (1952). *Diagnostic and Statistical Manual of Mental Disorders*. American Psychiatric Association, Washington, D.C.

American Psychiatric Association Committee on Nomenclature and Statistics. (1980). *Diagnostic and Statistical Manual of Mental Disorders* (3rd edition), American Psychiatric Association, Washington, D.C.

American Psychiatric Association Committee on Nomenclature and Statistics. (1994). *Diagnostic and Statistical Manual of Mental Disorders* (4th edition), American Psychiatric Association, Washington, D.C.

Andreasen, N.C. (2010).Posttraumatic stress disorder: a history and a critique. *Annals of the New York Academy of Sciences*, Vol. 1208, pp. 67-71.

Armenian, H.K., Morikawa W., Melkonian, A.K., Hovanesian, A.P., Haroutunian, N., Saigh, P.A. et al. (2000). Loss as a determinant of PTSD in a cohort of adult survivors of the 1988 earthquake in Armenia: implications for policy. *Acta Psychiatrica Scandinavica,* Vol. 102, pp. 58-64.

Armony, J.L, Corbo, V., Clement, M.H. & Brunet, A. (2005). Amygdala response in patients with acute PTSD to masked and unmasked emotional facial expressions. *American Journal of Psychiatry*, Vol. 162, pp. 1961–1963.

Baker, D.G., Diamond, B.I., Gillette, G. , Hamner, M., Katzelnick, D., Keller, et al. (1995). A double-blind, randomized, placebo-controlled, multi-center study of brofaromine in the treatment of post-traumatic stress disorder. *Psychopharmacology,* Vol. 122, pp. 386–389.

Baker, D.G., West, S.A., Nicholson, W.E., Ekhator, N.N., Kasckow, J.W., Hill, et al. (1999). Serial CSF corticotropin-releasing hormone levels and adrenocortical activity in combat veterans with posttrauamatic stress disorder. *American Journal of Psychiatry*, Vol. 156, pp. 585-588.

Baldwin, D.S., Anderson, I.M., Nutt, D.J., Badndelow, B., Bond, A, Davidson, J.R.T., et al. (2005). Evidence-based guidelines for the pharmacological treatment of anxiety disorders: recommendations from the British Association for Psychopharmacology. *Journal of Psychopharmacology,* Vol. 19, pp. 567-596.

Bartzokis, G., Lu, P.H., Turner, J., Mintz, J. & Saunders, C.S. (2005). Adjunctive risperidone in the treatment of chronic combat-related posttraumatic stress disorder. *Biological Psychiatry*. Vol. 57, pp. 474-479.

Becker, J.B., Monteggia, L.M., Perrot-Sinal, T.S., Romeo, R.D., Taylor, J.R., Yehuda, R., et al. (2007). Stress and disease: is being female a predisposing factor? *Journal of Neuroscience,* Vol. 27, pp. 11851-11855.

Becker, M.E., Hertzberg, M.A., Moore, S.D., Dennis, M.F., Bukenya, D.S. & Beckham, J.C. (2007). A placebo-controlled trial of bupropion SR in the treatment of chronic posttraumatic stress disorder. *Journal of Clinical Psychopharmacology,* Vol. 27, pp. 193-197.

Benedek, D.M., Friedman, M.J., Zatzick, D., Ursano, R.J. (2009). Guideline Watch (March 2009). *Practice Guideline for the Treatment of Patients with Acute Stress Disorder and Posttraumatic Stress Disorder*. American Psychiatric Association, Washington, D.C.

Berger, W., Mendlowicz, M.V., Marques-Portella, C., Kinrys, G., Fontenelle, L.F., Marmar, C.R., et al. (2009). Pharmacologic alternatives to antidepressants in posttraumatic stress disorder: A systematic review. *Progress in Neuro-psychopharmacology and Biological Psychiatry,* Vol. 33, pp. 169-180.

Berger, W., Mehra, A., Lenoci, M., Metzler, T.J., Otte, C., Tarasovsky, G., et al. (2010) Serum brain-derived neurotrophic factor predicts responses to escitalopram in chronic posttraumatic stress disorder. *Progress in Neuropsychopharmacology and Biological Psychiatry,* Vol. 34, pp. 1279-1284.

Berwin, C.R., Andrews, B. & Valentine, J.D. (2000). Meta-analysis of risk factors for posttraumatic stress disorder in trauma-exposed adults. *Journal of Consulting and Clinical Psychology,* Vol. 68, pp. 748-766.

Bichescu, D., Neuner, F., Schauer, M. & Elbert, T. (2007). Narrative exposure therapy for political imprisonment-related chronic posttraumatic stress disorder and depression, *Behaviour Research and Therapy,* Vol. 45, pp. 2212–2220.

Binder, E.B., Bradley, R.G., Liu, W., Epstein, M.P., Deveau, T.C., Mercer, K.B., et al. (2008). Association of FKBP5 polymorphisms and childhood abuse with risk of posttraumatic stress disorder symptoms in adults. *Journal of the American Medical Association*, Vol. 299, pp. 1291-1305.

Bledsoe, B.E. (2003). Critical Incident Stress Management (CISM): Benefit or risk for emergency services? *Prehospital Emergency Care;* Vol. 7, pp. 272-279.

Boscarino, J.A. (2008). A prospective study of PTSD and early-age heart disease mortality among Vietnam veterans: Implications for surveillance and prevention. *Psychosomatic Medicine,* Vol. 70, pp. 668-676.

Braun, P., Greenberg, D., Dasberg, H. & Lerer, B. (1990). Core symptoms of posttraumatic stress disorder unimproved by alprazolam treatment. *Journal of Clinical Psychiatry,* Vol. 51, pp. 236–238.

Bremner, J.D., Innis, R.B., Southwick, S.M., Staib, L., Zoghbi, S. & Charney, D.S. (2000a). Decreased benzodiazepine receptor binding in prefrontal cortex in combat-related posttraumatic stress disorder. *American Journal of Psychiatry,* Vol. 157, pp. 1120-1126.

Bremner, J.D., Narayan, M., Anderson, E.R., Staib, L.H., Miller, H.L. & Charney, D.S. (2000b). Hippocampal volume reduction in major depression. *American Journal of Psychiatry,* Vol. 157, pp. 115-127.

Bremner, J.D., Vythilingam, M., Vermetten, E., Southwick, S.M., McGlashan, T., Staib, L.H., et al. (2003). Neural correlates of declarative memory for emotionally valenced words in women with posttraumatic stress disorder related to early childhood sexual abuse. *Biological Psychiatry* Vol. 53, pp. 879–889.

Bremner, J.D., Vermetten, E., Schmahl, C., Vaccarino, V., Vythilingam, M., Afzal, N., et al. (2005). Positron emission tomographic imaging of neural correlates of a fear acquisition and extinction paradigm in women with childhood sexual-abuse-related post-traumatic stress disorder. *Psychological Medicine,* Vol. 35, pp. 791-806.

Breslau, N., Davis, G.C., Andreski, P., Peterson, E.L. & Schultz, L.R. (1997). Sex differences in posttraumatic stress disorder. *Archives of General Psychiatry,* Vol. 54, pp. 1044-1048.

Breslau, N., Kessler, R.C., Chilcoat, H.D., Schultz, L.R., Davis, G.C. & Andreski, P. (1998). Trauma and posttraumatic stress disorder in the community: The 1996 Detroit area survey of trauma. *Archives of General Psychiatry,* Vol. 55, pp. 626-632.

Breslau, N., Roth, T., Burduvali, E., Kapke, A., Schultz, L. & Roehrs, T. (2004). Sleep in lifetime posttraumatic stress disorder. *Archives of General Psychiatry,* Vol. 61, pp. 508-516.

Breslau, N., Peterson, E. L., & Schultz, L. R. (2008). A second look at prior trauma and the posttraumatic stress disorder effects of subsequent trauma: A prospective epidemiologic study. *Archives of General Psychiatry,* Vol. 65, pp. 431-437.

Breslau, N. (2009). The epidemiology of trauma, PTSD, and other posttrauma disorders. *Trauma, Violence, and Abuse,* Vol. 10, pp. 198-210.

Brunet, A., Orr, S.P., Tremblay, J., Robertson, K., Nader ,K. & Pitman, R.K.(2008). Effect of post-retrieval propranolol on psychophysiologic responding during subsequent script-driven traumatic imagery in post-traumatic stress disorder. *Journal of Psychiatric Research,* Vol. 42, pp. 503-506.

Bryant, R.A, Moulds, M.L. & Nixon, R.V. (2003). Cognitive behaviour therapy of acute stress disorder: a four-year follow-up. *Behavioral Research and Therapy,* Vol. 41, pp. 489-494.

Bryant, R.A., Mastrodomenico, J., Felmingham, K.L., Hopwood, S., Kenny, L., Kandris, E., et al. (2008). Treatment of acute stress disorder: a randomized controlled trial. *Archives of General Psychiatry,* Vol. 65, pp. 659-667.

Bryant, R.A., Creamer, M.C., O'Donnell, M.L., Silove, D., & McFarlane, A.C. (2009). A Study of the protective function of acute morphine administration on subsequent posttraumatic stress disorder. *Biological Psychiatry,* Vol. 65, pp. 438-440.

Burkett BG, Whitley G. (1998). *Stolen Valor: How the Vietnam Generation Was Robbed of its Heroes and History.* Verity, Dallas, TX.

Cahill, L., Prins, B., Weber, M. & McGaugh, J.L. (1994). Beta-adrenergic activation and memory for emotional events. *Nature,* Vol. 371, pp. 702-704.

Cairo, J.B., Dutta, S., Nawaz, H., Hashmi, S., Kasl, S. & Bellido, E. (2010). The prevalence of Posttraumatic Stress Disorder among adult earthquake survivors in Peru. *Disaster Medicine and Public Health Awareness,* Vol. 4, pp. 39-46.

Carlson, J., Chemtob, C.M., Rusnak, K., Hedlun, N.L. & Muraoka, M.Y. (1998). Eye movement desensitization and reprocessing (EMDR): Treatment for combat-related post-traumatic stress disorder. *Journal of Traumatic Stress,* Vol. 11, pp. 3-24.

Clark, R.D., Canive, J.M., Calais, L.A., Qualls, C.R. & Tuason, V.B. (1999). Divalproex in posttraumatic stress disorder: An open-label clinical trial. *Journal of Traumatic Stress,* Vol. 12, pp. 395–401.

Clem, R.L. & Huganir, R.L. (2010). Calcium-permeable AMPA receptor dynamics mediate fear memory erasure. *Science,* Vol. 330, pp. 1108-1112.

Corneil, W., Beaton, R., Murphy, S., Johnson, C. & Pike, K. (1999). Exposure to traumatic incidents and prevalence of posttraumatic stress symptomatology in urban firefighters in two countries. *Journal of Occupational Health Psychology,* Vol. 4, pp. 131-141.

Cougle, J.R., Keough, M.E., Riccardi, C.J. & Sachs-Ericsson, N. (2009). Anxiety disorders and suicidality in the National Comorbidity Survey-Replication. *Journal of Psychiatric Research,* Vol. 43, pp. 825-829.

Darves-Bornoz, J.M., Alonso, J., de Girolamo, G., de Graaf, R., Haro, J.M., Kovess-Masfety, V., et al. (2008). Main traumatic events in Europe : PTSD in the ESEMeD Survey. *Journal of Traumatic Stress,* Vol. 32, pp. 455-462.

Davidson, J.R., Pearlstein, T., Londborg, P., Brady, K.T., Rothbaum, B., Bell, J. (2002). Efficacy of sertraline in preventing relapse of posttraumatic stress disorder: Results of a 28-week double-blind, placebo-controlled study. *American Journal of Psychiatry,* Vol. 158, pp. 1974-1981.

Davidson, J., Baldwin, D., Stein, D.J., Kuper, E., Benattia, I., Ahmed, S., et al. (2006). Treatment of posttraumatic stress disorder with venlafaxine extended release: A 6-month randomized controlled trial. *Archives of General Psychiatry,* Vol. 63, pp. 1158-1165.

Davidson, J.R.T., Brady, K.M., Mellman, T.M., Stein, M.B. & Pollack, M.H. (2007). The efficacy and tolerability of tiagabine in adult patients with post-traumatic stress disorder. *Journal of Clinical Psychopharmacology,* Vol. 27, pp. 85–88.

Davis, L.L., Jewel, M.E., Ambrose, S., Farley, J., English, B., Bartolucci, A., et al. (2004). A placebo-controlled study of nefazodone for the treatment of chronic posttraumatic stress disorder: a preliminary study. *Journal of Clincial Psychopharmacology,* Vol. 24, pp. 291-297.

Davis, L.L., Davidson, J.R.T., Ward, L.C., Bartolucci, A., Bowden, C.L. & Petty, F. (2008) Divalproex in the treatment of posttraumatic stress disorder: A randomized, double-blind, placebo-controlled trial in a veteran population. *Journal of Clinical Psychopharmacology,* Vol. 28, pp. 84–88.

Davis M. (1992). The role of the amygdala in fear and anxiety. *Annual Review of Neuroscience,* Vol. 15, pp. 353-375.

Davis, M., Ressler, K.J., Rothbaum, B.O. & Richardson, R. (2006). Effects of D-cycloserine on extinction: Translation from preclinical to clinical work. *Biological Psychiatry,* Vol. 60, pp. 369-375.

de Kloet, C.S., Vermetten, E., Geuze, E., Kavelaars, A., Heijnen, C.J. & Westenberg, H.G. (2006). Assessment of HPA-axis function in posttraumatic stress disorder: pharmacological and non-pharmacological challenge tests, a review. *Journal of Psychiatric Research,* Vol. 40, pp. 550-567.

De Quervain, D. & Margraf, J. (2008). Glucocorticoids for the treatment of post-traumatic stress disorder and phobias: a novel therapeutic approach. *European Journal of Pharmacology,* Vol. 583, pp. 365-371.

De Quervain, D., Aerni, A., Schelling, G & Roozendaal, B. (2009). Glucocorticoids and the regulation of memory in health and disease. *Frontiers in Neuroendocrinology,* Vol. 30, pp. 358-370.

Delahanty, D.L. & Nugent, N.R. (2006). Predicting PTSD prospectively based on prior trauma history and immediate biological responses. *Annals of the New York Academy of Sciences,* Vol. 1071, pp. 27-40 .

Dell-Osso, L., Carmassi, C., Massimetti, G., Daneluzzo, E., Di Tommaso, S. & Rossi, A. (2011). Full and partial PTSD among young adult survivors 10 months after the L'Aquila 2009 earthquake: Gender differences, *Journal of Affective Disorders,* Vol. 131, pp.79-83.

DiGrande, L., Neria, Y., Brackbill, R.M., Pullimam, P. & Galea, S. (2011). Long-term post-traumatic stress symptoms among 3,271 civilian survivors of the September 11, 2001 terrorist attacks on the World Trade Center, *American Journal of Epidemiology,* Vol. 173, pp. 271-281.

Dunlop, B.W., Garlow, S. & Nemeroff, C.B. (2009). The neurochemistry of depressive disorders: Clinical studies. *Neurobiology of Mental Illness, 3rd Ed.,* D. Charney D & E.J. Nestler, pp. (435-460), Oxford University Press, New York, NY .

Ehring, T., Ehlers, A., Clear, A. & Glucksman, E. (2008). Do acute psychological and psychobiological responses to trauma predict subsequent symptom severities and PTSD and depression? *Psychiatric Research,* Vol. 161, pp. 67-75.

Elklit, A. (2002). Acute Stress Disorder in victims of robbery and victims of assault. *Journal of Interpersonal Violence,* Vol. 17, pp. 872-887.

Elman, I., Lowen, S., Frederick, B,B., Chi, W., Becerra, L. & Pitman, R.K. (2009). Functional neuroimaging of reward circuitry responsivity to monetary gains and losses in posttraumatic stress disorder. *Biological Psychiatry,* Vol. 66, pp. 1083-1090.

Etkin, A., Wager, T.D. (2007). Functional neuroimaging of anxiety: A meta-analysis of emotional processing in PTSD, social anxiety disorder, and social phobia. *American Journal of Psychiatry,* Vol. 164, pp. 1476-1488.

Fan, F., Zhang, Y., Yang, Y., Mo, L. & Liu, X. (2011). Symptoms of posttraumatic stress disorder, depression, and anxiety among adolescents following the 2008 Wenchuan earthquake in China. *Journal of Traumatic Stress,* Vol. 24, pp. 44-53.

Felmingham, K., Williams, L.M., Whitford,T.J., Falconer, E., Kemp, A.H., Peduto, A., et al. (2009). Duration of posttraumatic stress disorder predicts hippocampal grey matter loss. *Neuroreport,* Vol.20, pp. 1402–1406.

Fesler, F.A. (1991). Valproate in combat-related posttraumatic-stress-disorder. *Journal of Clinical Psychiatry,* Vol. 52, pp. 361–364.

Foa, E.B., Dancu, C.V., Hembree, E.A., Jaycox, L.H., Meadows, E.A. & Street, G.P. (1999). A comparison of exposure therapy, stress inoculation training, and their combination for reducing posttraumatic stress disorder in female assault victims. *Journal of Consulting and Clinical Psychology,* Vol. 67, pp. 194-200.

Forbes, D., Creamer, M., Phelps, A., Bryant, R., McFarlane, A., Grant, J., et al. (2007). Australian guidelines for the treatment of adults with acute stress disorder and post-traumatic stress disorder. *Australian and New Zealand Journal of Psychiatry.* Vol. 41, pp. 637-648.

Ford, J. D. (1999). Disorders of extreme stress following war-zone military trauma: Associated features of posttraumatic stress disorder or comorbid but distinct syndromes? *Journal of Consulting and Clinical Psychology,* Vol. 67, pp. 3-12 .

Frueh, B.C., Hamner, M.B., Cahill, S.P., Gold, P.B. & Hamlin, K.L. (2000). Apparent symptom overreporting in combat veterans evaluated for PTSD. *Clinical Psychology Reviews,* Vol. 20, pp. 853-885.

Frueh, B.C., Knapp, R.G., Cusack, K.J., Grubaugh, A.L., Sauvageot, J.A., Cousins, V.C., et al. (2005). *Psychiatric Services,* Vol. 56, pp. 1123-1133.

Galea, S., Resnick, H., Ahern, J., Gold, J., Bucuvalas, M., Kilpatrick, D., et al. (2002). Posttraumatic stress disorder in Manhattan, New York City, after the September 11th terrorist attacks. *Journal of Urban Health,* Vol. 79, pp. 340-353.

Gelpin, E., Bonne, O., Peri, T., Brandes, D. & Shalev, A.Y. (1996). Treatment of recent trauma survivors with benzodiazepines: A prospective study. *Journal of Clinical Psychiatry,* Vol. 57, pp. 390–394.

Geracioti, T.D. Jr, Baker, D.G., Kasckow, J.W., Strawn, J.R., Mulchahey, J., Dashevsky, B.A., et al. (2008). Effects of trauma-related audiovisual stimulation on cerebrospinal fluid norepinephrine and corticotropin-releasing hormone concentrations in post-traumatic stress disorder. *Psychoneuroendocrinology.* Vol. 33, pp. 416-24.

Geuze, E., van Berckel, B.N.M., Lammertsma, A.A., Boellaard, R., de Kloet, C.S., Vermetten, E., et al. (2008). Reduced GABAA benzodiazepine receptor binding in veterans with post-traumatic stress disorder, *Molecular Psychiatry,* Vol. 13, pp. 74-83.

Geuze, E., Westenberg, H.G., Heinecke, A., de Kloet, C.S., Goebel, R. & Vermetten, E. (2008). Thinner prefrontal cortex in veterans with posttraumatic stress disorder. *Neuroimage,* Vol. 41, pp. 675-681.

Gilbertson, M.W., Shenton, M.E., Ciszewski, A., Kasai, K., Lasko, N.B., Orr, S.P., et al. (2002). Smaller hippocampal volume predicts pathologic vulnerability to psychological trauma. *Nature Neuroscience,* Vol. 5, pp. 1242-1247

Grillon, C. (2002). Startle reactivity and anxiety disorders: Aversive conditioning, context and neurobiology. *Biological Psychiatry,* Vol. 52, pp. 958-975.

Grossman, R., Buchsbaum, M.S. & Yehuda, R. (2002). Neuroimaging studies in post-traumatic stress disorder. *Psychiatric Clinics of North America,* Vol. 25, pp. 317-340.

Guriel, J. & Fremouw, W. (2003) Assessing malingered posttraumatic stress disorder: a critical review. *Clinical Psychology Reviews,* Vol. 23, pp. 881 –904.

Harvey, A.G. & Bryant, R.A. (1998). The relationship between Acute Stress Disorder and Posttraumatic Stress Disorder: A prospective evaluation of motor vehicle accident survivors. *Journal of Consulting and Clinical Psychology,* Vol. 66, pp. 507-512.

Harvey, A.G. & Yehuda, R. (1999). Strategies to study risk for the development of PTSD. In: *Risk Factors for Posttraumatic Stress Disorder*, R. Yehuda, pp. (1-22), American Psychiatric Press, Washington, D.C.

Herman, J. (1997). *Trauma and recovery: The aftermath of violence from domestic abuse to political terror*. New York: Basic Books

Hertzberg, M.A., Butterfield, M.I., Feldman, M.E., Beckham, J.C., Sutherland, S.M., Connor, K.M., et al. (1999). A preliminary study of lamotrigine for the treatment of posttraumatic stress disorder. *Biological Psychiatry*, Vol. 45, pp. 1226–1229.

Hoge, C.W., Castro, C.A., Messer, S.C., McGurk, D., Cotting, D.I. & Koffman, R.L. (2004). Combat duty in Iraq and Afghanistan, mental health problems, and barriers to care. *New England Journal of Medicine*, Vol. 351, pp. 13-22

Hoge, C.W., McGurk, D., Thomas, J.L., Cox, A.L., Engel, C.C. & Castro, C.A. (2008). Mild traumatic brain injury in U.S. soldiers returning from Iraq. *New England Journal of Medicine*, Vol. 358, pp. 453-463.

Hoge, E.A., Worthington, J.J., Nagurney, J.G., Chang, Y., Kay, E.B., Feterowski, C.M., et al. (2011). Effect of acute posttrauma propranolol on PTSD outcome and physiological responses during script-driven imagery. *CNS Neuroscience and Therapeutics*, epub ahead of print, January 10, 2011.

Holbrook, T.L., Galarneau, M.R., Dye, J.L., Quinn K. & Dougherty, A.L. (2010). Morphine use after combat injury in Iraq and post-traumatic stress disorder. *New England Journal of Medicine*, Vol. 362, pp. 110-117.

Holsboer, F. & Ising, M. (2008). Central CRH system in depression and anxiety - evidence from clinical studies with CRH-1 receptor antagonists. *European Journal of Pharmacology*, Vol. 583, pp. 350-357.

Institute of Medicine (2008). *Treatment of Posttraumatic Stress Disorder: An Assessment of the Evidence*, National Academy of Sciences. National Academies Press. Washington, D,C. http://books.nap.edu/catalog/11955.html

Jordan, B.K., Marmar, C.R., Fairbank, J.A., Schlenger, W.E., Kulka, R.A., Hough, R.L., et al. (1992). Problems in families of male Vietnam veterans with posttraumatic stress disorder. *Journal of Consulting and Clinical Psychology*, Vol. 60, pp. 916-926.

Jovanovic, T., Blanding, N.Q., Norrholm, S.D., Duncan, E., Bradley, B. & Ressler, K. (2009). Childhood Abuse is associated with increased startle reactivity in adulthood. *Depression and Anxiety*, Vol. 26, pp. 1018-1026.

Jovanovic, T., Norrholm, S.D., Blanding, N.Q., Davis, M., Duncan, E., Bradley, B., et al. (2010). Impaired fear inhibition is a biomarker of PTSD but not depression. *Depression and Anxiety*, Vol. 27, pp. 244-251.

Jovanovic, T., Norrholm, S.D., Blanding, N.Q., Phifer,J.E., Weiss, T., Davis, M., et al., (2010). Fear potentiation is associated with hypothalamic-pituitary-adrenal axis function in PTSD. *Psychoneuroendocrinology*, Vol. 35, pp. 846-857.

Kasai, K., Yamasue, H., Gilbertson, M.W., Shenton, M.E., Rauch, S.L. & Pitman, R.K. (2008). Evidence for acquired pregenual anterior cingulate gray matter loss from a twin study of combat-related posttraumatic stress disorder. *Biological Psychiatry*, Vol. 63, pp. 550-556.

Kessler, R.C., Sonnega, A., Bromet, E., Hughes, M. & Nelson, C.B. (1995). Posttraumatic Stress Disorder in the national comorbidity survey. *Archives of General Psychiatry*, Vol. 52, pp. 1048-1060.

Kessler, R.C. (2000). Posttraumatic Stress Disorder: The burden to the individual and to society. *Journal of Clinical Psychiatry*, Vol. 61 [suppl 5], pp. 4-12.

Kessler, R.C., Chiu, W.T., Demler, O., Merikangas, K.R. & Walters, E.E. (2005). Prevalence, severity, and comorbidity of 12-month DSM-IV disorders in the National Comorbidity Survey Replication. *Archives of General Psychiatry*, Vol. 62, pp. 617-627.

Khoury, L., Tang, Y.L., Bradley, B., Cubells, J.F. & Ressler, K.J. (2010). Substance use, childhood traumatic experience, and posttraumatic stress disorder, in an urban civilian population. *Depression and Anxiety*, Vol. 27, pp. 1077-1086.

Kilpatrick, D.G., Saunders, B.E. & Smith, D.W. (2003). *Youth Victimization: Prevalence and Implications*, U.S. Department of Justice, Office of Justice Program, National Institute of Justice, Rockville, MD. Available from: http://www.ncjrs.gov/pdffiles1/nij/94972.pdf

Koenen, K.C., Amstadter, A.B. & Nugent, N.R. (2009). Gene-environment interaction in posttraumatic stress disorder: an update. *Journal of Traumatic Stress*, Vol. 22, pp. 416-426 .

Krakow, B., Hollifield, M., Johnston, L., Koss, M., Schrader, R., Warner, T.D., et al. (2001). Imagery rehearsal for chronic nightmares in sexual assault survivors with posttraumatic stress disorder: A randomized trial. *Journal of the American Medical Association*, Vol. 286, pp. 537-545.

Kubzansky, L.D., Koenen, K.C., Spiro, A. 3rd, Vokonas, P.S. & Sparrow, D. (2007). Prospective study of posttraumatic stress disorder symptoms and coronary heart disease in the Normative Aging Study. *Archives of General Psychiatry*, Vol. 64, pp. 109-116.

Kun, P., Han, S., Chen, X. & Yao, L. (2009). Prevalence and risk factors for posttraumatic stress disorder: a cross-sectional study among survivors of the Wenchuan 2008 earthquake in China. *Depression and Anxiety*, Vol. 26, pp. 134-1140.

LaJoie, A.S., Sprang, G. & McKinney, W.P. (2010). Long-term effects of Hurricane Katrina on the psychological well-being of evacuees. *Disasters*, vol. 34 (4), pp. 1031-1044.

Lamarche, L.J. & De Koninck, J. (2007). Sleep disturbances in adults with posttraumatic stress disorder: a review. *Journal of Clinical Psychiatry*, Vol. 68, pp. 1257-1270.

Lyons, D.M., Yang, C., Sawyer-Glover, A.M., Moseley, M.E. & Schatzberg, A.F. (2001). Early life stress and inherited variation in moneky hippocampal columes. *Archives of General Psychiatry*, Vol. 58, pp. 1145-1151.

March, J. (1993). What constitutes a stressor? The "Criterion A" issue, In: *Posttraumatic Stress Disorder: DSM-IV and Beyond*, Davidson J, Foa E , pp. (37-54), American Psychiatric Press, Washington, D.C.

Martenyi, F. & Soldatenkova, V. (2006). Fluoxetine in the acute treatment and relapse prevention of combat-related post-traumatic stress disorder: analysis of the veteran group of a placebo-controlled, randomized clinical trial. *European Neuropsychopharmacology*, Vol. 16, pp. 340–349.

Mayou, R.A., Ehlers, A. & Hobbs, M. (2000). Psychological debriefing for road traffic accident victims. Three year follow-up of a randomised controlled trial. *British Journal of Psychiatry*, Vol. 176, pp. 589-593.

McFarlane, A.C., Barton, C.A., Yehuda, R. & Wittert, G. (2010). Cortisol response to acute trauma and risk of posttraumatic stress disorder. *Psychoneuroendocrinology*, Vol. 36, pp. 720-727.

McHugh, P.R. & Treisman, G. (2007). PTSD: a problematic diagnostic category. *Journal of Anxiety Disorders*, Vol. 21, pp. 211-222.

McNally, R.J. Progress and controversy in the study of posttraumatic stress disorder. (2003). *Annual Review of Psychology*, Vol. 54, pp. 229-252.

Meewisse, M.L., Reitsma, J.B., de Vries, G.J., Gersons, B.P. & Olff. M. (2007). Cortisol and post-traumatic stress disorder in adults: systematic review and meta-analysis. *British Journal of Psychiatry*, Vol. 191, pp.387-392.

Mehta, D. & Binder, E.B. (2011). Gene x environment vulnerability factors for PTSD: The HPA axis. *Neuropharmacology*, epub ahead of print, March 23, 2011.

Mellman, T.A., Bustamante, V., David, D. & Fins, A.I. (2002). Hypnotic medication in the aftermath of trauma. *Journal of Clinical Psychiatry*, Vol. 63, pp. 1183–1184.

Milad, M.R., Quinn, B.T., Pitman, R.K., Orr, S.P., Fischl, B. & Rauch, S.L. (2005). Thickness of ventromedial prefrontal cortex in humans is correlated with extinction memory. *Proceedings of the National Academy of Sciences*,Vol. 102, pp. 10706-10711.

Milad, M.R., Wright, C.I., Orr, S.P., Pitman, R.K., Quirk, G.J. & Rauch, S.L. (2007). Recall of fear extinction in humans activates the ventromedial prefrontal cortex and hippocampus in concert. *Biological Psychiatry*, Vol. 62, pp. 446-454.

Miller, G.E., Chen, E. & Zhou, E.S. (2007). If it goes up, must it come down? Chronic stress and the hypothalamic-pituitary- adrenocortical axis in humans. *Psychological Bulletin*, Vol. 133, pp. 25-45.

Mitchell, J.T. & Everly, G.S. Jr. (2001). *Critical Incident Stress Debriefing: An Operations Manual for CISD, Defusing, and Other Group Crisis Intervention Services, 3rd Ed.*, Chevron Publishing, Ellicott City, MD .

Monson, C.M., Schnurr, P.P., Resick, P.A., Friedman, M.J., Young-Xu, Y. & Stevens, S.P. (2006). Cognitive processing therapy for veterans with *Journal of Traumatic Stress*, Vol. 74, pp. 898–907.

Mrazek, P.G. & Haggerty, R.J. (1994). *Reducing Risk for Mental Disorders: Frontiers for Preventative Intervention Research*, National Academies Press, Washington, D.C.

National Collaborating Centre for Mental Health. (2005). *The Management of Post Traumatic Stress Disorder in Primary and Secondary Care*, National Institute for Clinical Excellence, London, U.K.

Neylan, T.C., Lenoci, M., Samuelson, K.W., Metzler, T.J., Henn-Haase, C., Hierholzer, R.W., et al. (2006). No improvement of posttraumatic stress disorder symptoms with guanfacine treatment. *American Journal of Psychiatry*, Vol. 163, pp. 2186–2188.

Nock, M.K., Hwang, I., Sampson, N., Kessler, R.C., Angermeyer, M., Beautrais, A., et al. (2009). Cross-national analysis of the associations among mental disorders and suicidal behavior: Findings from the WHO World Mental Health Surveys, *PLOS Medicine*, 6:e1000123.

Ouimette, P.C., Ahrens, C., Moos, R.H.& Finney, J.W. (1997). Posttraumatic stress disorder in substance abuse patients: Relationship to 1-year posttreatment outcomes. *Psychology of Addictive Behaviors*, Vol. 11, pp. 34–47.

Pacak, K., Palkovits, M., Kopin, I.J. & Goldstein, D.S. (1995). Stress-induced norepinephrine release in the hypothalamic paraventricular nucleus and pituitary-adrenocortical and sympathoadrenal activity: in vivo microdialysis studies. *Frontiers in Neuroendocrinology*, Vol. 16, pp. 89–150.

Pitman, R.K., Sanders, K.M., Zusman, R.M., Healy, A.R., Cheema, F., Lasko, N.B., et al. (2002). Pilot study of secondary prevention of posttraumatic stress disorder with propranolol. *Biological Psychiatry*, Vol. 51, pp. 189-192.

Pole, N., Neylan, T.C., Otte, C., Henn-Hasse, C., Metzler, T.J. & Marmar, C.R. (2009). Prospective prediction of posttraumatic stress disorder symptoms using fear potentiated auditory startle responses. *Biological Psychiatry*, Vol. 65, pp. 235-240.

Ponniah, K. & Hollon, S.D. (2009). Empirically supported psychological treatments for adult acute stress disorder and posttraumatic stress disorder: a review. *Depression and Anxiety*, Vol. 26, pp. 1086–1109.

Pratchett, L.C., Pelcovitz, M.R. & Yehuda, R. (2010). Trauma and Violence: Are women the weaker sex? *Psychiatric Clinics of North America*, Vol. 33, pp. 465-474.

Pynoos, R.S., Goenjian, A., Karakashian, M., Tashjian, M., Manjikian, R., Manoukian, G., et al. (1993). Posttraumatic stress reactions in children after the 1998 Armenian earthquake. *British Journal of Psychiatry*, Vol. 163, pp. 239-247.

Raison, C.L. & Miller, A.H. (2003). When not enough is too much: the role of insufficient glucocorticoid signaling in the pathophysiology of stress-related disorders. *American Journal of Psychiatry*, Vol. 160, pp. 1554-1565.

Rakofsky, J.J., Ressler, K.J., Dunlop,B.W. (n.d.) BDNF function as a potential mediator of bipolar disorder and posttraumatic stress disorder comorbidity. *Molecular Psychiatry, submitted.*

Rakofsky, J.J., Levy, S.T., Dunlop, B.W. (2011) Conceptualizing treatment nonadherence in patients with bipolar disorder and post-traumatic stress disorder. *CNS Spectrums*, Vol. 16, *ePub ahead of print*

Raskind, M.A., Peskind, E.R., Kanter, E.D., Petrie, E.C., Radant, A., Thompson, C.E., et al. (2003). Reduction of nightmares and other PTSD symptoms in combat veterans by prazosin: A placebo-controlled study. *American Journal of Psychiatry*, Vol. 160, pp. 371–373.

Raskind, M.A., Peskind, E.R., Hoff, D.J., Hart, K.L., Holmes, H.A., Warren, D., et al. (2007). A parallel group placebo controlled study of prazosin for trauma nightmares and sleep disturbance in combat veterans with posttraumatic stress disorder. *Biological Psychiatry*, Vol. 61, pp. 928–934.

Rauch, S.L., Whalen, P.J., Shin, L.M., McInerney, S.C., Macklin, M.L., Lasko, N.B., et al. (2000). Exaggerated amygdala response to masked facial stimuli in posttraumatic stress disorder: a functional MRI study. *Biological Psychiatry*, Vol. 47, pp. 769-776.

Rauch, S..L, Shin, L.M. &, Phelps, E.A. (2006). Neurocircuitry models of posttraumatic stress disorder and extinction: human neuroimaging research - past, present, and future. *Biological Psychiatry*, Vol. 60, pp. 376-382.

Read, J.P., Bollinger, A.R. & Sharkansky, E.J. (2003). Assessment and diagnosis of PTSD-Substance Abuse. In: *Trauma and Substance Abuse: Causes, Consequences, and Treatment of Comorbidity*, P.C. Ouimette and P. Brown, pp. (111-125), American Psychological Association, Washington, D.C.

Read, J.P., Brown, P. & Kahler, C.W. (2004). Substance abuse and posttraumatic stress disorders: Symptom interplay and effects on outcome. *Addictive Behaviors*, Vol. 29, pp.1665-1672.

Resick, P.A. & Schnicke, M.K. (1993). *Cognitive Processing Therapy for Rape Victims: A Treatment Manual*, Sage, Newbury Park, CA

Resick, P.A., Nishith, P., Weaver, T.L., Astin, M.C. & Feuer, C.A. (2002). A comparison of cognitive-processing therapy with prolonged exposure and a waiting condition for the treatment of chronic posttraumatic stress disorder in female rape victims, *Journal of Consulting and Clinical Psychology*, Vol. 70, pp. 867–879.

Ressler, K.J., Rothbaum, B.O., Tannenbaum, L., Anderson, P., Graap, K., Zimand, E., et al. (2004). Cognitive enhancers as adjuncts to psychotherapy: Use of D-cycloserine in phobics to facilitate extinction of fear, *Archives of General Psychiatry*, Vol. 61, pp. 1136–1144.

Ressler, K.J., Mercer, K.B., Bradley, B., Jovanovic, T., Mahan, A., Kerley, K., et al. (2011). Post-traumatic stress disorder is associated with PACAP and the PAC1 receptor. *Nature*, Vol. 470, pp. 492-497.

Robert, S., Hamner, M.B., Kose, S., Ulmer, H.G., Deitsch, S.E. & Lorberbaum, J.P. (2005). Quetiapine improves sleep disturbances in combat veterans with PTSD - Sleep data from a prospective, open-label study. *Journal of Clincial Psychopharmacology*, Vol. 25, pp. 387–388.

Rothbaum, B.O., Rizzo, A. & Difede, J. (2010). Virtual reality exposure therapy for combat-related posttraumatic stress disorder. *Annals of the New York Academy of Sciences*. Vol. 1208, pp. 126-132.

Rothbaum, B. (1997). A controlled study of eye movement desensitization and reprocessing in the treatment of post-traumatic stress disordered sexual assault victims. *Bulletin of the Menninger Clinic*, Vol. 61, pp. 317-334.

Salcioglu, E., Basoglu, M. & Livanou M. (2007). Post-traumatic stress disorder and comorbid depression among survivors of the 1999 earthquake in Turkey. *Disasters*, Vol. 31(2), pp. 115-129.

Sapolsky, R.M., Uno, H., Rebert, C.S. & Finch, C.E. (1990). Hippocampal damage associated with prolonged glucocorticoid exposure in primates. *Journal of Neuroscience*, Vol. 10, pp. 2897-2902.

Schuff, N., Zhang, Y., Zhan, W., Lenoci, M., Ching, C., Boreta, L., et al. (2011). Patterns of altered cortical perfusion and diminished subcortical integrity in posttraumatic stress disorder: an MRI study. *Neuroimage*, Vol. 54, pp. S62-S68.

Schnurr, P.P., Friedman, M.J., Engel, C.C., Foa, E.B., Shea, M.T., Chow, B.K., et al. (2007). Cognitive behavioral therapy for posttraumatic stress disorder in women. *Journal of the American Medical Association*, Vol. 297, pp. 820-830.

Schnyder, U., Moergeli, H., Klaghofer, R. & Buddeberg, C. (2001). Incidence and prediction of posttraumatic stress disorder symptoms in severely injured accident victims. *American Journal of Psychiatry*, Vol. 158, pp. 594–599.

Schuster, M.A., Stein, B.D., Jaycox, L.H., Collins, R.L., Marshall, G.N., Elliott, M.N., et al. (2001). A national survey of stress reactions after the 2001 Sep 11, Terrorist attacks. *New England Journal of Medicine*, Vol. 345, pp. 1507-1512.

Scott, W.J. (1990). PTSD in DSM-III: A case in the politics of diagnosis and disease. *Social Problems*, Vol. 3, pp. 294-310.

Shalev, A.Y., Freedman, S., Dessky, R. & Israeli-Shalev, Y. (2007). Prevention of PTSD by early treatment: A randomized controlled study. Preliminary results from the Jerusalem Trauma Outreach and Prevention Study (J-TOP). *Program Book of the*

American College of Neuropsychopharmacology 46th Annual Meeting. Boca Raton, FL., pp. 63. Available from: http://acnp.org/annualmeeting/programbooks.aspx

Shapiro, F. (1989). Efficacy of the eye movement desensitization procedure in the treatment of traumatic memories. *Journal of Traumatic Stress*, Vol. 2, pp. 199-223.

Shin, L.M., Shin, P.S., Heckers, S., Krangel, T., Macklin, M.L., Orr, S.P., et al. (2004). Explicit memory and hippocampal function in posttraumatic stress disorder. Hippocampus Vol. 14, pp. 292–300.

Shin, L.M., Lasko, N.B., Macklin, M.L., Karpf, R.D., Milad, M.R., Orr, S.P., et al. (2009). Resting metabolic activity in the cingulate cortex and vulnerability to posttraumatic stress disorder. *Archives of General Psychiatry*, Vol. 66, pp. 1099-1107.

Sones, H.M., Thorp, S.R. & Raskind, M. (2011). Prevention of posttraumatic stress disorder. *Psychiatric Clinics of North America*, Vol. 34, pp. 79-94.

Southwick, S.M., Bremner, J.D., Rasmusson, A., Morgan, C.A., Arnsten, A. & Charney, D.S. (1999). Role of norepinephrine in the pathophysiology and treatment of posttraumatic stress disorder. *Biological Psychiatry*, Vol. 46, pp. 1192-1204.

Stein, D.J., Ipser, J.C. & Seedat, S. (2006). Pharmacotherapy for post traumatic stress disorder (PTSD). *Cochrane Database of Systematic Reviews*, (1):CD002795.

Stein, M.B., Kline, N.A. & Matloff, J.A. (2003). Ajdunctive olanzapine for SSRI-resistant combat-related PTSD: A double-blind, placebo-controlled study. *American Journal of Psychiatry*, Vol. 159, pp. 1777-1779.

Stein, M.B., Kerridge, C., Dimsdale, J.E. & Hoyt, D.B. (2007). Pharmacotherapy to prevent PTSD: results from a randomized controlled poof-of-concept trial in physically injured patients. *Journal of Traumatic Stress*, Vol. 10, pp. 923-32.

Stein, M.B., Paulus, M.P. (2009). Imbalance of approach and avoidance: The yin and yang of anxiety disorders. *Biological Psychiatry*, Vol. 66, pp. 1072-1074.

Swinson, R.P., Antony, M.M., Bleau, P.B., Chokka, P., Craven, M, Fallu, A., et al. (2006). Clinical Practice Guidelines: Management of Anxiety Disorders. *Canadian Journal of Psychiatry*,51 (suppl 2):1-92.

Taylor, F.B., Martin, P., Thompson, C., Williams, J., Mellman, T.A., Gross, C., et al. (2008). Prazosin effects on objective sleep measures and clinical symptoms in civilian trauma posttraumatic stress disorder: A placebo-controlled study. *Biological Psychiatry*, Vol. 63, pp. 629–632.

Tsai, R., Falk, W., Gunther, J. & Coyle, J. (1999). Improved cognition in Alzheimer's disease with short-term D-cycloserine treatment. *American Journal of Psychiatry*, Vol. 156, pp. 467-469.

Tsigos, C., Chrousos, G.P. (2002). Hypothalamic-pituitary-adrenal axis, neuroendocrine factors and stress. Journal of Psychosomatic Research, Vol. 53, pp. 865-871.

Tucker, P., Trautman, R.P., Wyatt, D.B., Thompson, J., Wu, S.C., Capece, J.A., et al. (2007). Efficacy and safety of topiramate monotherapy in civilian posttraumatic stress disorder: a randomized, double-blind, placebo-controlled study. *Journal of Clinical Psychiatry*, Vol. 68, pp. 201–206.

Ulmer, C.S., Edinger, J.D. & Calhoun, P.S. (2010). A multi-component cognitive-behavioral intervention for sleep disturbance in veterans with PTSD: A pilot study. *Journal of Clinical Sleep Medicine*, Vol. 7, pp. 57-68.

Ursano, R.J., Bell, C., Eth, S., Friedman, M., Norwood, N., Pfefferbaum, B., et al. (2004). Practice guideline for the treatment of patients with acute stress disorder and posttraumatic stress disorder. *American Journal of Psychiatry*, Vol. 161 (suppl. 11), pp. 3-31.

Ursano, R.J., Godlenberg, M., Zhang, L., Carlton, J., Fullerton, C.S., Li, H., et al. (2010). Posttraumatic stress disorder and traumatic stress: from bench to bedside, from war to disaster. *Annals of the New York Academy of Sciences*, Vol. 1208, pp. 72-81.

Van der Kolk, B., Spinazzola, J., Blaustein, M., Hopper, J., Hopper, E., Korn, D., et al. (2007). A randomized clinical trial of EMDR, fluoxetine and pill placebo in the treatment of PTSD: Treatment effects and long-term maintenance. *Journal of Clinical Psychiatry*, Vol. 68, pp. 37-46.

van Emmerik, A.A., Kamphuis, J.H., Husbosch, A.M.& Emmelkamp, P.M. (2002). Single session debriefing after psychlogical trauma: a meta-analysis. *Lancet*, Vol. 360, pp. 766-771.

Vermetten, E., Vythilingam, M., Southwick, S.M., Charney, D.S. & Bremner, J.D. (2003). Long-term treatment with paroxetine increases verbal declarative memory and hippocampal volume in posttraumatic stress disorder. *Biological Psychiatry*, Vol. 54, pp.693-702.

Wagner, D., Heinrichs, M. & Ehlert, U. (1998). Prevalence of symptoms of posttraumatic stress disorder in German professional firefighters. *American Journal of Psychiatry*, Vol. 155, pp. 1727-1732.

Walczewska, J., Rutkowski, K., Wizner, B., Cwynar, M. & Grodzicki, T. (2011). Stiffness of large arteries and cardiovascular risk in patients with post-traumatic stress disorder. *European Heart Journal*, Vol. 32, pp. 730-736.

Wahlstroem, L., Michelsen H., Schulman, A. & Backheden M. (2008). Different types of exposure to the 2004 Tsunami are associated with different levels of psychological distress and posttraumatic stress. *Journal of Traumatic Stress*, 21(5), pp.463-470.

Weiskrantz, L. (1956). Behavioral changes associated with ablation of the amygdaloid complex in monkeys. *Journal of Comparative and Physiological Psychology*, Vol. 49, pp. 381-39.

Wittchen, H.U., Gloster, A., Beesdo, K., Schonfeld, S. & Perkonigg, A. (2009). Posttraumatic stress disorder: Diagnostic and epidemiological perspectives. *CNS Spectrums*, Vol. 14 (Suppl 1), pp. 5-12.

World Health Organization (2008). *The Global Burden of Disease: 2004 Update*, World Health Organization, Geneva, Switzerland

Xie, P., Kranzler, H.R., Poling, J., Stein, M.B., Anton, R.F., Brady, K., et al. (2009). Interactive effect of stressful life events and the serotonin transporter 5-HTTLPR genotype on posttraumatic stress disorder diagnosis in 2 independent populations. *Archives of General Psychiatry*, Vol. 66, pp.1201-1209.

Yehuda, R., McFarlane, A.C., Shalev, A.Y. (1998). Predicting the development of posttraumatic stress disorder from the acute response to a traumatic event. *Biological Psychiatry*, Vol. 44, pp. 1305-1212.

Yehuda, R. (2002). Post-traumatic stress disorder. *New England Journal of Medicine*, Vol. 346,pp. 108-114.

Yehuda, R. (2006). Advances in understanding neuroendocrine alterations in PTSD and their therapeutic implications. *Annals of the New York Academy of Sciences*, Vol. 1071, pp.137-166.

Yehuda, R., Brand, S. & Yang, R.K. (2006). Plasma neuropeptide Y concentrations in combat exposed veterans: relationship to trauma exposure, recovery from PTSD and coping. *Biological Psychiatry*, Vol. 59, pp. 660-663.

10

Anxiety in Vestibular Disorders

Ágnes Szirmai
Semmelweis University, Faculty of Medicine
Department of Oto-Rhino-Laryngology and Head and Neck surgery, Budapest
Hungary

1. Introduction

Vertigo is one of the most common symptom and complaint in the clinical practice.

A frequent question in neurootological expertise is whether the vertigo of psychiatric patients suffering from anxiety disorder is caused by vestibular dysfunction or the vertigo is originated from psychiatric disease.

Several possibilities exist in the relationships between psychiatric disorders and otoneurological diseases. When organic cochleovestibular lesion occurred in a patient with normal mental state, the neurootologist must treat patients according to the cochleovestibular examination results. When the dizzy patients have normal vestibular function, the patient must be referred to the psychiatrist. The most challenging are the cases of a combined lesion: psychiatric disorder and organic cochleovestibular disease. A very interesting question is exactly why vertigo is the main symptom in such patients, whereas panic disease or anxiety disorder in other patients can cause other severe symptoms resembling heart attack, dyspnoea, and abdominal crisis. Vestibular neuronitis, benign positional vertigo, Ménière's disease and migraine are the most common neurootological conditions, all of which can trigger the anxiety disorder and panic.

Several types of these combined problems can be observed: (1) organic vestibular dysfunction with consecutive anxiety and panic; (2) established psychiatric disease with a new cochleovestibular lesion; and (3) dizziness due to panic and an independent organic lesion of the vestibular system (e.g., dizziness due to agoraphobia with compensated, previously well-known unilateral loss of function). (Szirmai et al, 2005)

The differential diagnosis can only be attained by a careful interdisciplinary way of thinking and activity, given the fact that the vestibular, neurological and psychiatric disorders-considered as pathogenic factors--are being present simultaneously in triggering the symptoms, and there can be overlaps between the certain pathological processes. (Fazekas A, 2010). Dizziness accounts for an estimated 5 percent of primary care clinic visits. The patient history can generally classify dizziness into one of four categories: vertigo, disequilibrium, presyncope, or light-headedness. The main causes of vertigo are benign paroxysmal positional vertigo, Ménière's disease, vestibular neuritis, and labyrinthitis. Many medications can cause presyncope, and regimens should be assessed in patients with this type of dizziness. Parkinson disease and diabetic neuropathy should be considered with the diagnosis of disequilibrium. Psychiatric disorders, such as depression, anxiety, and hyperventilation syndrome, can cause vague light-headedness. (Post RE & Dickerson LM., 2010)

Psychiatric diagnoses are common among patients with dizziness referred for otologic evaluation that does not show evidence of a peripheral vestibular disorder. Specific psychiatric disorders should be part of the differential diagnosis of patients who present with dizziness. (Sullivan et al, 1993)

A high degree of psychiatric disorders has repeatedly been described among patients with organic vertigo syndromes and attributed to vestibular dysfunction. According to Eckhardt-Henn's data patients with vestibular migraine and Ménière's disease showed significantly higher prevalence of psychiatric co-morbidity (MD = 57%, VM = 65%) especially with anxiety and depressive disorders, than patients with VN (22%) and BPPV (15 %) compared to normal subjects (20 %). As a consequence, a structured psychological and psychometric testing and an interdisciplinary therapy should be proceeded in cases with complex and prolonged vertigo courses, especially in patients with vestibular migraine and Ménière's disease. (Eckhardt-Henn et al, 2008)

An article by Yardley et al reviewed evidence for three mechanisms whereby psychological factors may aggravate dizziness and retard recovery from balance disorders. A common behavioural response to dizziness is to avoid activities and environments that provoke symptoms; yet, such avoidance deprives affected individuals of the exposure necessary to promote psychological and neurophysiologic adaptation. Also, anxiety arousal and hyperventilation may add to, amplify, and disinhibit the somatic symptoms induced by balance disorder. Further, attention and cognitive load may influence the central processing of information required for the perception and control of orientation (Yardley L&Redfern MS, 2001).

According to Salhofer et al's data the most prominent specific feature of migrainous vertigo was head motion intolerance. Patients with migraine showed anxiety more often and tended to have worse quality of sleep and higher depression scores. Migraine and vertigo is a risk factor for co-morbid anxiety. (Salhofer et al, 2010)

In previous studies, abnormal posturography scores under the eyes-open phase were related to high anticipatory anxiety, whereas those under the eyes-closed phase were related to phobic avoidance (Perna et al, 2001). Phobic postural vertigo (PPV) is a frequent diagnosis which can be challenging to treat. Most of these patients have psychiatric disturbances, which can cause compromised adaptive efficacy. Correlation was found between overall outcome on the Primary Care Evaluation of Mental Disorders Questionnaire and the Adaptive Operationalized Diagnostic Scale. Separate analysis revealed correlation between results of the AODS and anxiety disorders. Adaptive compromise was observed in individuals with PPV which was shown to be associated to psychiatric disorders. (Ferreira et al, 2010)

According to Brandt's data, patients with psychiatric disorders may have pathological responses on vestibular testing. Patients with anxiety may have greater sensitivity and directional preponderance in vestibular testing, while organic vestibular symptoms may precipitate consecutive panic attacks with or without agoraphobia (Brandt 2000).

Best et al (2006) didn't found correlation between an acute or chronic vestibular dysfunction and pathology on psychometric testing. Their results do not support the hypothesis that latent vestibular dysfunction or imbalance triggers anxiety disorders, above all agoraphobia. Answering the question of whether this coexistence is only coincidental, their results suggested that special vestibular syndromes—for example, vestibular migraine and Ménière's disease—may function as a trigger for a secondary somatoform disorder, but not vestibular disorders in general and especially not a subtle vestibular tone imbalance. (Best et al, 2006)

Patients with panic disorder, agoraphobia, or both are much more disabled by their dizziness than the patients with no psychiatric disorder. Anxiety and panic disorder was equally prevalent among patients with and without vestibular disease. In some cases panic disorder may provide an explanation for the dizziness, whereas in others it may be a co-morbid condition compounding the disability attributable to the vestibular disorder (Stein et al, 1994). In this study the main vestibular findings are analyzed in patients with and without anxiety disorders in few of main vestibular disorders were examined in our department.
The main vestibular disorders are benign paroxysmal positional vertigo, true Ménière's disease, the vertebrobasilar insufficiency, the vestibular neuronitis and vestibular migraine, sudden deafness with or without vestibular lesion, viral or bacterial labyrinthitis. The dizziness with headache, the Ménière's disease, the vertebrobasilar insufficiency, the vestibular neuronitis, the BPPV, and their connection with anxiety are discussed in details.

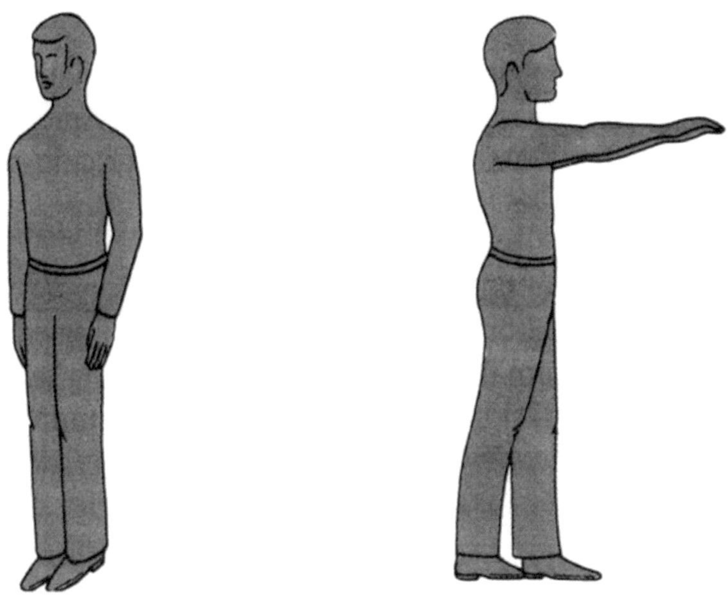

Fig. 1. Romberg and sensitized Romberg test

2. Examination methods

The examination began with the detailed case-history, and followed by the routine oto-rhino-laryngological and neurological examinations. The cochleovestibular function of all the patients was examined by separate cochlear nerve and vestibular function tests. Cochlear function tests included the pure tone audiometry, acoustic reflex threshold and decay. The vestibular tests involved statokinetic tests (Romberg, sensitized Romberg and Babinski-Weil tests) (Figure 1.); spontaneous nystagmus with Frenzel's glasses and with ENG registration as well, positional and positioning nystagmus examination using Frenzel's glasses (Figure 2.). The patients were examined by the psychiatrist before or after the vestibular examination, so anxiety disorder was diagnosed by the psychiatrist.

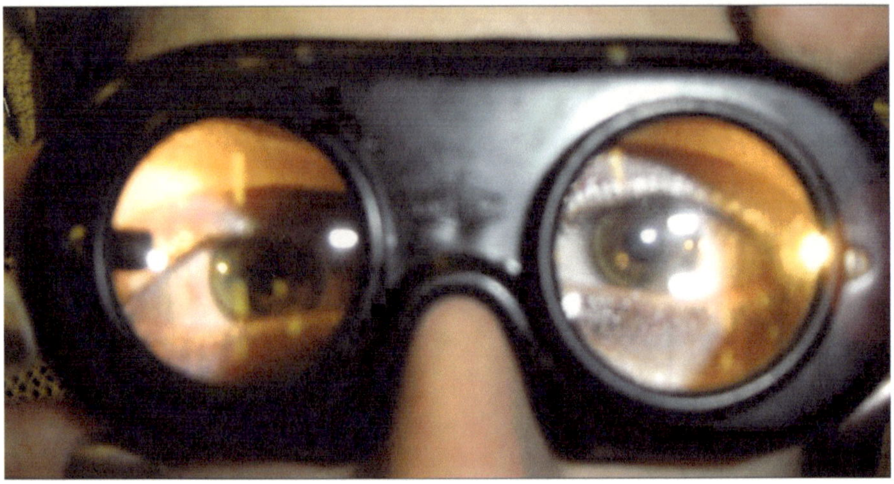

Fig. 2. Frenzel glasses

The saccadic and smooth pursuit eye movement tests were performed by a computer-based ENG system (ICS Chartr ENG® system). Finally, bithermal caloric test was carried out by the computer-based ENG (Figure 3). The caloric test aims at establishing both the absolute levels of the two lateral semicircular canals responses to standardized thermal stimuli and the relative function between the two sides. It is usually done in a standardized fashion, using either temperature to begin, conducting testing of the two sides in a defined order, and then shifting to the other temperature. A minimum of 5 minutes should be spent between the end of the nystagmic reaction and the start of the next irrigation (Noaksson et al, 1998).

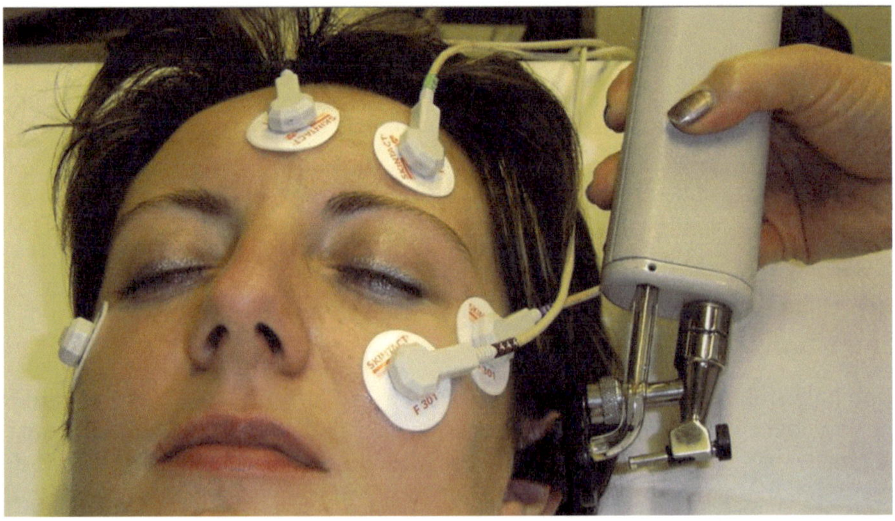

Fig. 3. Air caloric irrigation of the ear with electronystagmographic registration

The ears were irrigated with the 50C°and 25C°air insufflations, the duration of stimulation being 40 seconds. The air caloric stimulation is the routine test battery of the otoneurological department even in the cases of normal external ear canal and normal ear drum, because the air caloric system is strictly connected to the computerized ENG system. Analyzing the results of the bithermal caloric test, the computer software gives the numeric results of the average slow phase velocities (ASPV) of the caloric nystagmus. The lateral preponderance between the left and right sides, according to Jongkees' formula, was calculated (Barber&Stockwell, 1980). The directional preponderance for left and right beating nystagmus was calculated accordingly. The figure 4 shows the Jongkees formula. Caloric weakness or canal paresis is pathological, when the asymmetry is more, than 25%. Directional preponderance is pathological, when it is more than 40%. Normal range of average slow phase velocity of the caloric nystagmus with the above mentioned irrigation technique and parameters in between 20 and 35 deg/sec. The hyperreactivity (caloric nystagmus slow phase velocity is more than 40 deg/sec) often occurred in the central lesions and in anxiety disorders.

Unilateral Weakness:

$$\frac{(RW+RC)-(LW+LC)}{RW+RC+LW+LC} \times 100 = UW$$

Directional Preponderance:

$$\frac{(RW+LC)-(LW+RC)}{RW+RC+LW+LC} \times 100 = DP$$

RW=right warm, RC=right cool, LW=left warm, LC= left cool

Fig. 4. Jongkees formula

Butterfly schema- Chartr® ENG system

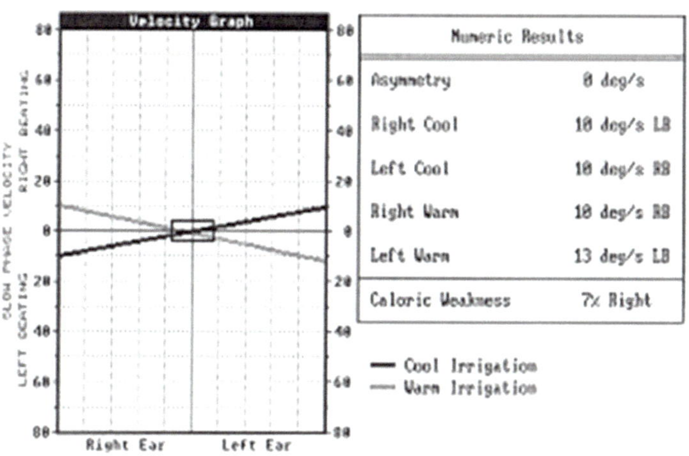

Fig. 5. Bithermal caloric test. Symmetrical, normal responsiveness

The graphic representation is the Claussen butterfly schema (Claussen C.F. & Franz B, 2006), modified by ICS Medical Corp. The figure 5 shows the normal caloric test result.
In this study the data of 700 patients with vertigo are analyzed retrospectively.

3. Patients

1249 patients were examined in the Otoneurological Department of the Semmelweis University ORL Clinic in 2010. 549 were referred because of hearing loss, tinnitus, and facial palsy, while 700 patients have vertigo or dizziness.
Some patients have vertiginous attacks with or without fluctuating hearing loss with aural fullness and tinnitus and all of these patients were sent by neurologist or their family doctor with a suspicion of Ménière's syndrome. Some patients have fluctuating vertigo with the symptoms of posterior fosse lesions, like loss of vision or drop-attacks. Some patients have sudden loss of balance, due to vestibular neuronitis. Some patients have BPPV. Some patients have migraine with vertigo. Some patients have constant imbalance or light-headedness. They are referred by neurologist or psychiatrist to confirm or exclude any type of unilateral or bilateral vestibular lesion.
The data of these 700 patients were analyzed retrospectively. The mean age of these patients was 46.2 years. (The youngest patient was 9 , the oldest was 85 years old). 45.7% of them have anxiety disorder. Panic disorder was diagnosed in 15.7% of our dizzy patients, while 11.4% have depression. More than female than male were examined in every age-group and in every disease-group. 36.8% of the male patients, while 49.0% of the female patients have anxiety disorder. The sex distribution of our patients with and without anxiety is shown on Figure 6.
The patients' diagnoses are shown on the figure 7.
Anxiety ratio is shown of figure 8.

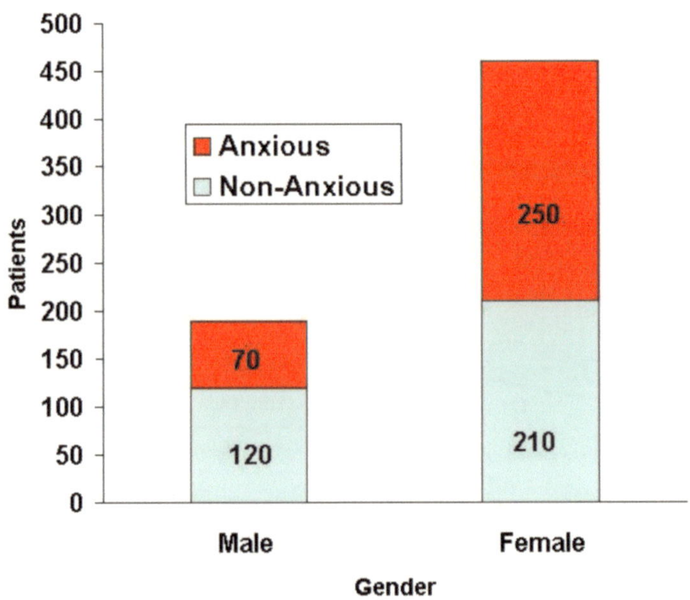

Fig. 6. Patients with and without anxiety

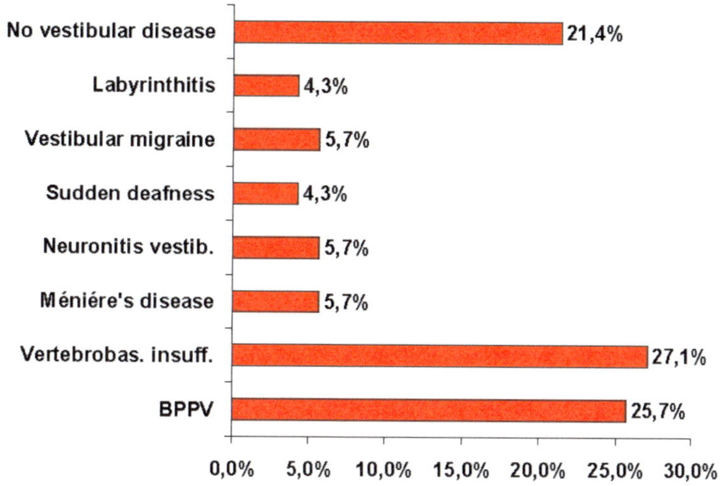

Fig. 7. Diagnoses of patients (n=700)

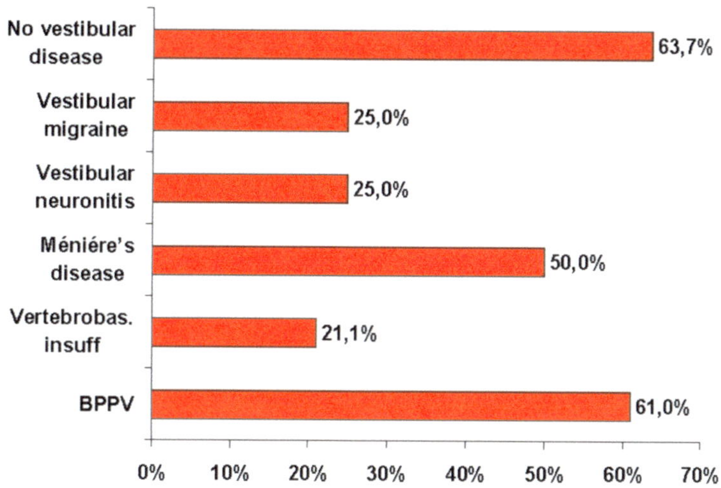

Fig. 8. Anxiety ratio in several diseases

4. Anxiety symptoms during the vestibular examination

The patients' examination starts with the detailed case history. Sometimes a patient's interpretation is redundant and can be hysterical; thus, we must listen also for the tenor or "mood" of the interpretation. The next step is to ask in a circumspect fashion about the symptoms of disease, like in a questionnaire. The doctor needs information about the patients' life style, living place and job. In our patients anxiety problems are more frequent in manual worker, and more frequent in town than in patients who are living in country. It is a time-consuming process, but very important in evaluating the connection between otoneurological disease and anxiety or sometimes depression. After this consultation but before the examination the patients often ask about the outcome of the disease, and we often must tell that we have to speak about after the examination. This fact shows the severe anxiety because of the outcome of the examination and the uncertainty of the patients.

After the case history all of our patients have audiological examination, as a part of differencialdiagnostic process of the vestibular examination. Several diseases can cause hearing loss, like Ménière's disease; in others the patients have normal hearing, like in vestibular neuronitis and BPPV. Some patients with psychiatrical disorders can aggravate the hearing loss or feels more severe than the audiometry shows. After the long audiological process we start the patient's vestibular examination. The examination of the statokinetic tests seems to be easy, but sometimes it is very difficult. The dizzy patients failed to stand up with closed eyes, or walk with closed eyes. The patients with anxiety often told during the statokinetic test examination (for example Romberg and sensitized Romberg tests, that "I cannot do it", but most of them can carry out our commands. Most of them have a problem with self-consciousness.

The spontaneous nystagmus examination can cause problems rarely, but some patients have aversion with the Frenzel's glasses ("It is too light, it is disturbing me!"). The presence of spontaneous nystagmus might show, that the patient has vestibular lesion, which is not compensated. Half of our patient with spontaneous nystagmus had anxiety disorder, half of them weren't anxious.

During the examination of positional vertigo most of the patients have aversion of motion.

Most of the patients with BPPV have a resistance to the head motion, sometimes with a stiff neck. When the patient has a long lasting recurrent BPPV, the X-ray of the neck shows a compulsion port of vertebrae. When we rotate the patient's neck, we can feel the resistance and the stiffness of the neck. After verbal persuasion we can examine the patients, meaning that the stiffness has a psychic but no neurological or rheumatologic reason. Not only in the typical BPPV, but in the central positional vertigo the patients might have aversion of motion. In our vertiginous patients with anxiety disorder positional vertigo was observed in 34.4%, while 61% of the patients with BPPV have anxiety disorder. In patients without anxiety the ratio of positional nystagmus is 23.7%. It means that all of the positional types of vertigo can generate anxiety, not only the typical BPPV. We can explain it with the disturbing effect of head movement, which can generate short oscillopsia.

The examination of the optokinetic and smooth pursuit eye movements could be tiring for the patients, but there aren't aversions to the tests.

During the caloric stimulation most of the patients with anxiety have a severe fear from the provoked vertigo. The caloric test can provoke vertigo, even in lying position which could be very severe with vegetative symptoms. If the patient have a hyporeactivity of the vestibular end organ, the vertigo is not severe, and bearable in the cases of normal vestibular responsiveness. In the cases of hyperaesthesia, hyperresponsiveness the feeling of vertigo is very unpleasant. In the patient with anxiety three type of mood can be observed during the caloric test. When the hyperresponsiveness of the vestibular end organ can be measured, the patients have severe vegetative symptoms. In these cases the uncomfortable feeling is almost normal, and based on the severe vegetative status (uncomfortable level). In patients with vegetative dystonia the vegetative symptoms are more severe, than we wait, based onto the vestibular responsiveness. In patients may have hyperreactivity with vegetative symptoms, but in patients with anxiety disorder we often see a normal or decreased responsiveness without vegetative symptoms, but more uncomfortable level told by the patients. These reactions without any vegetative symptoms can occurred in patients with anxiety; we mention it as a psychogenic reaction. Sometimes the combinations of these findings occurred. Sometimes patients are shouting and crying during the three minutes of provoked vertigo, but vegetative symptoms are missing (Figure 9). Twenty patients rejected the electronystagmographical examination after the information, that the complete ENG test might provoke vertigo four times during the caloric test.

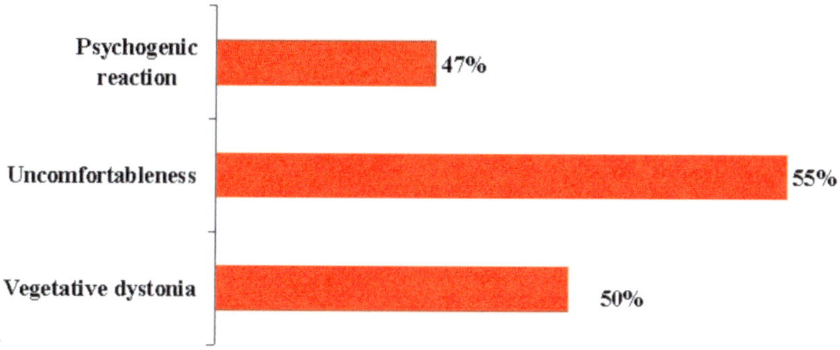

Vegetativ dystonia: Vegetative response is more increased than caloric response (doctor's opinion)

Uncomfortableness: Uncomfortable level is more severe, than the caloric reaction (patient's opinion)

Psychogenic reaction:The patient's uncomfortable level is more severe, than vegetative symptoms (doctor's opinion)

Fig. 9. Caloric test analysis

Analysis of the electronystagmographic results of the caloric weakness, and the directional preponderance are very important, which data are characteristical for the peripheral and central vestibular lesion. The ENG results are shown on figure 10.

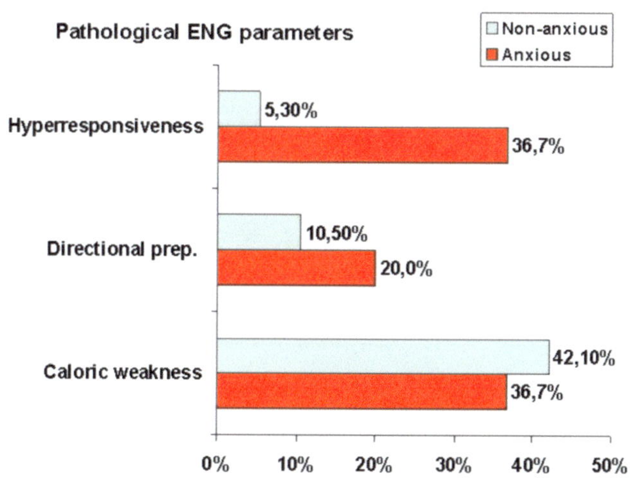

Fig. 10.

Canal paresis or caloric weakness shows, that the patient has peripheral lesion, the pathological ratio is almost the same in the anxiety and the non-anxiety groups. The directional preponderance is more frequent in the anxiety group, signalling the role of the central pathways in the pathomechanism not only in the central vestibular disorders but also in the anxiety disorders. The hypersensitivity or hyperresponsiveness of the vestibular end organ also shows the pathological function of the central vestibular pathways. Interesting and unsettled question is which the primary dysfunction was. Whether the hypersensitive vestibular system cause the motion sickness of the patients, and this motion sickness generates anxiety disorder or the anxiety disorder modulates the central vestibular pathways to give hyperactive response for the caloric stimulus. The question needs further investigations.

5. Anxiety in vestibular disorders

5.1 Headache, motion sickness and anxiety in vestibular migraine

Patients with vestibular dysfunction, migraine and/or anxiety may experience visual vertigo, whereby symptoms are provoked by disorienting visual environments (e.g. supermarkets). Patients with visual vertigo over rely on vision for balance (i.e. visually dependent). According to Pavlou et al's opinion visual vertigo significantly improves when vestibular rehabilitation incorporates exposure to optokinetic stimulation. (Pavlou et al, 2011). But when the patients have anxiety disorder, they often reject the visual stimulation and vestibular training as a therapeutical possibility.

Most of the patients with migraine have motion sickness from the early young age.

Patients with migraine frequently had abnormal caloric test responses, especially with a directional preponderance (figure 11.) In the migraine attack the patients are presumed to have hypersensitivity of the labyrinth with nausea and vomiting, (Szirmai 1997). What is the connection between the migraine, the motion sickness and the hypersensitivity of the labyrinth in the caloric test?

SP=spontaneous nystagmus, *RW=right warm, RC=right cool, LW=left warm, LC= left cool*

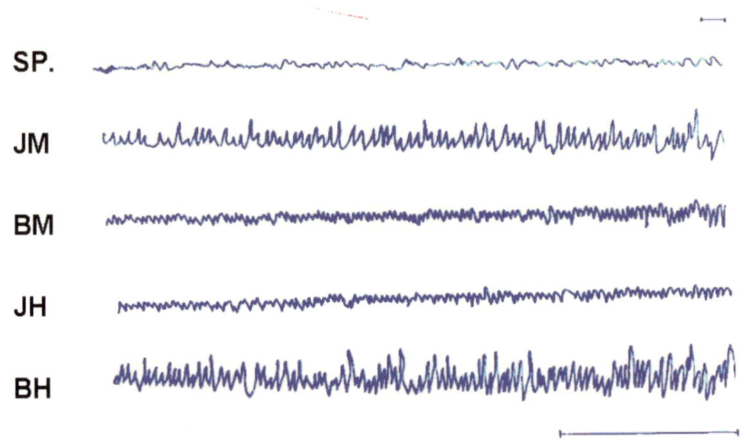

Fig. 11. Directional preponderance to the right side on electronystagmogram

25.7 % of our vertiginous patients have headache, half of them have anxiety disorders. Only 5.7% of them have vestibular migraine, the others have cervical headache or tension headache. Motion sickness was observed in 14.3% of our patients, but 90% of them has anxiety disorders. In the vestibular migraine patients group 25% of the patients have severe anxiety, but in 75% of them have motion sickness.
These data suggests that there isn't tight connection between migraine and anxiety and motion sickness. In the everyday medical experience most of the patients accept the fact, that they have motion sickness from early childhood. When the anxiety disorder develops in these patients, the motion sickness is worsened, and become more disturbing.
When the patients have migraine, they used to bear the nausea during the headache, but they cannot accept the same kind of nausea as a concomitant symptom of vertigo. It suggests that the vertigo to the higher degree than migraine can provoke anxiety disorders.

5.2 Ménière's disease

The true Ménière's disease is caused by the hydrops of the endolymph.
According to the Committee of Hearing and Equilibrium, (1995, cit. in Szirmai 2004) the classic triad is the recurrent, episodic vertigo, hearing loss, which is not always fluctuating, and the aural fullness or/and tinnitus. The criteria of the Ménière's disease at least 2 attacks, which are more than 20 minutes long , and at least once documented hearing loss.
The Ménière's disease considerably deteriorates the quality of life. During the attacks the patients may have a fear from death, especially at the beginning of the disease. Later the patients know that the symptoms will disappear after few hours.
As the attacks become more frequent, the patients have constant anticipated anxiety, thinking: „ When will the next attack come?"
The vegetative symptoms, especially the vomitus is increasing the patients' anxiety. Because of the vegetative symptoms, the patients have a feeling of uncomfortableness during the attacks. The attacks with vomiting can come unexpectedly, sometimes in an overcrowded place, or in the patients working place during a conference. Some patients have an attack at home with vomiting. Although the family is supporting them, the patients have anxiety of the situation. One of my patients told me: „ When I have an attack of Ménière's disease, and I'm laying in the bed and vomiting, my dear wife hold the pot. Although I use the toothbrush after the attack, but how can I kiss my dear wife with the same mouth? I fear of that she will disgust me! „
Later, when the patients have hearing loss, the problem is the communication with the other people. The sensorineural hearing loss and the tinnitus are very disturbing for the patients. The sensorial hearing loss with the recruitment can decrease the speech discrimination. Most of the patients cannot recognise the direction of the sounds. The patients fear from becoming ridiculous because the hearing loss and of the misunderstanding speech. Ménière patients fear loss of friends because of the communication problems. Because of the recruitment the patients have an increased sensitivity of noise. This fact can results, that patients can disturbed by several frequencies of noise and speech. Some interpersonal conflict situation can occurred because of this fact. One of my Ménière patients has a severe sensitivity of the sounds of 2000 Hz frequency. While this is one of the speech frequencies, these facts can results severe deterioration of her interpersonal connections.
Because of the recurrent attacks of vertigo and the communication problem caused by the hearing loss, the patient could have a depression or a fear from the loss of their job.
They could have problem with keeping of their living standards after becoming disabled.

Tinnitus connected to the hearing loss is very disturbing for the Ménière patients. The tinnitus is fluctuating. Before the vertiginous attack the noise and fullness in the ear is increasing, forecasting the severe attack. When the patient is anxious, or tired, the tinnitus can increasing without attack of vertigo, but this increasing of the tinnitus can provoke an anticipatory anxiety , whether the attack is coming or not. In the later phase of the Ménière's disease, the tinnitus is constant, and the patients are disturbed in falling asleep, or in listening to music, or in reading. For these patients the silence is not golden, but very disturbing. These patients could be nervous and impatient with their family, and this fact can cause conflict situation in the family and in job.

In some cases, the Ménière patients have other diseases also. The co-morbidity causes further deterioration of the quality of life, and causes difficulties in the treatment and rehabilitation (Figure 12).

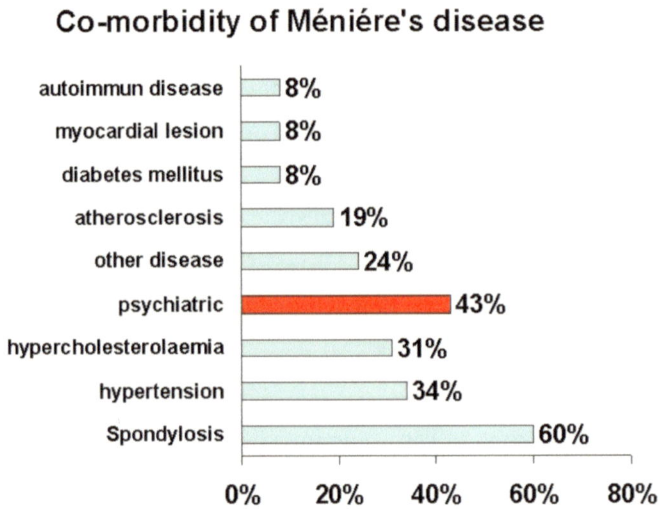

Fig. 12. Co-morbidity of Ménière's disease

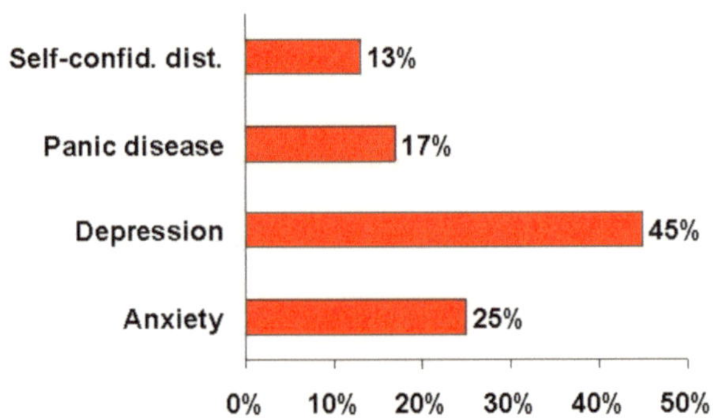

Fig. 13. Psychiatric disturbances in Ménière's disease

Patients need more pills because of the co-morbidity and sometimes the drug- interactions can cause side-effects, for example stomach-ache. In these cases the patient will stop taking medications. The psychiatric co-morbidities are one of the most important problems in the patient's rehabilitation. The Patients with Ménière's disease could have self-confidence disturbances, panic disease, depression, or anxiety disorders. The distribution of these co-existing psychiatric problems is shown in the figure 13.

5.3 Vertebrobasilar insufficiency

Vertigo, tinnitus and hearing loss occurred very frequently in the vascular posterior fossa lesions. In a slow blood flow of the temporal lobe vessels, brainstem vessels and labyrinthine artery wide range of cochleovestibular dysfunction could be observed. The evaluation of the vascular risk factors is very important in the diagnostical procedure. In the patients with vertigo, hearing loss, and tinnitus the regional slow blood flow of the brain were diagnosed by MRI, or single photon emission computer tomography. Although the blood vessels of the inner ear are invisible, but using MR and/or SPECT for the differential diagnosis in incapacitating vertigo similar to Ménière's syndrome, we can deduce for the vascular origin. Despite of the peripheral lesion of true Ménière's disease, in most of the cases of vertebrobasilar insufficiency we can diagnose central or combined vestibular lesion with ENG. (Figure 14) (Szirmai 2004).

Caloric weakness on the left side and directional preponderance to the left side
Chartr® ENG system

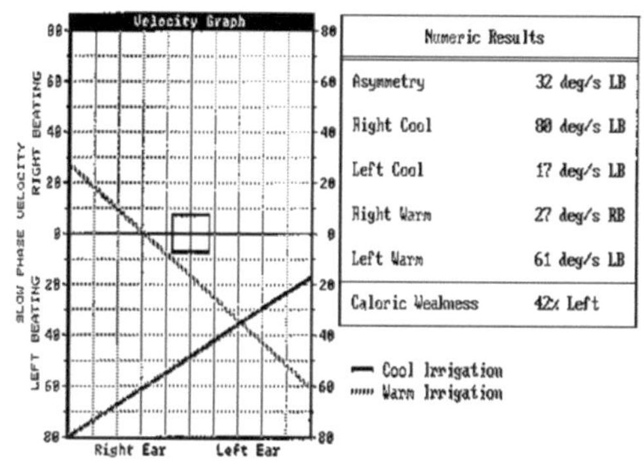

Fig. 14. Combined lesion in vertebrobasilar insufficiency

The typical symptoms of vertebrobasilar insufficiency are the rotatory vertigo provoked by head movements, with mild pain in the nuchal region, bilateral tinnitus and/or hearing loss, and drop-attacks. The vertigo can occur after head turning backwards ("upper shelves disease"). Hypertension, atherosclerosis and cervical spondylosis could be a risk factor for the disease. Most of these patients (52%) have multiple co-morbidity and risk factors (Figure 15). In 19% of the vertebrobasilar insufficiency cases the patients have psychiatric disorders previously. In our cases 21.1% of the VBI patients have consecutive anxiety disorder, and 5.3% have depression. We can evaluate fear from becoming completely deaf, and fear from the motion and public transport. Most of the patients have anxiety when they know the diagnosis, which defined as vascular disorder of the brain. They have a fear from having a stroke, becoming paralysed, or going stupid because of the slow blood flow of the brain. Most of the patients have problem with the treatment, the antiaggregation therapy with aspirin could provoke stomach-ache. When they read about dizziness in the side effect list of aspirin, some patients reject taking it. The patients have aversion of much pills, they want to stop the medical treatment. The doctors have to persuade them, that the treatment of all the risk-factors, co-morbid diseases and consecutive psychiatrical disorders are necessary.

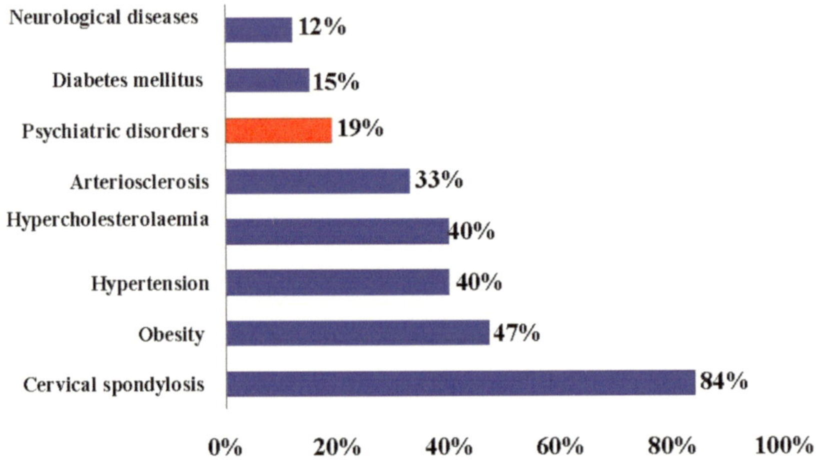

Fig. 15. Co-morbidity in vertebrobasilar insufficiency

5.4 Vestibular neuronitis

Vestibular neuronitis is a considerably frightening disorder. The sudden loss of vestibular function can cause severe, few days long rotatory vertigo with extreme severe vegetative symptoms like nausea and vomitus. The patient cannot stand up and walk. In the acute phase the patients have fear from a heart attack, or death. Dizziness or vertigo presents itself as a profound illness, giving the sensation of "imminent death". The differential diagnostic procedure is not easy; we have to exclude heart attacks, and gastroenteral disorders. The presence of spontaneous nystagmus could be helpful. When the doctor recognises, that the problem exists in the vestibular system, we can calm the patients, that their disease is not a life-threatening disease. In the acute phase of the vestibular neuronitis it seems to be enough for the patients, but later patients have to face to fact, that the recovery is a long process. Nobody dies from vertigo, but it is an illness that invalidates everybody who suffers from it preventing from carrying out a normal life, with the social consequences that it produces.

At the patients examination in the beginning of the disease we can see the harmonic vestibular syndrome, which is characteristic for the acute peripheral lesion. The patient has a severe nystagmus beating to the healthy side. If the patient can stand up, we can see deviation and tilting to the affected side. When the patient is unable to stand up, the tilting is visible in the sitting position. In the ENG we can registrate the unilateral loss of function. (Figure 16) In the first few days of disease the patient has severe vertigo and vegetative symptoms.

The severity of the vegetative symptoms depends on the sensitivity of the vestibular responsiveness. If the patients have a hyperresponsiveness, the sudden loss of the hyperreactive vestibular end-organ can cause more severe vegetative symptoms than the loss of hyporeactive one (Figure 17 and 18). The treatment could be sedative drug administration and rest in bed. Later, when the vegetative symptoms are decreased, the patients have to stop sedative drugs, and try to move. In the early phase of the recovery the patients need help. Vestibular training is necessary. Eye-movements and neck movements during the walking is advisable for the patients. In this phase the family is supporting the patient, but later, when the patients can walk, but have fear from the walk, the supporting tendency of the family could be diminished.

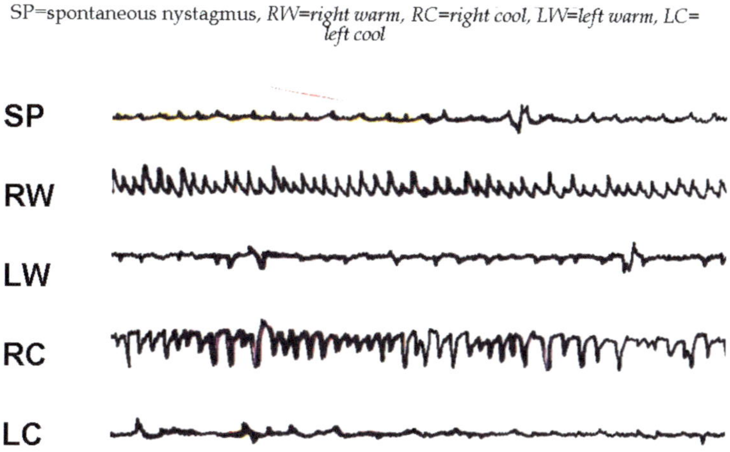

Fig. 16. Vestibular neuronitis. Caloric weakness of the left side on electronystagmogram

Later, when the patients know the diagnosis, they have anxiety from the long process of central compensation. When their vestibular status is compensated, the patients may have few minutes long oscillopsia at looking to the affected side. This oscillopsia can provoke severe anxiety and fear of motion in 25% of our patients.

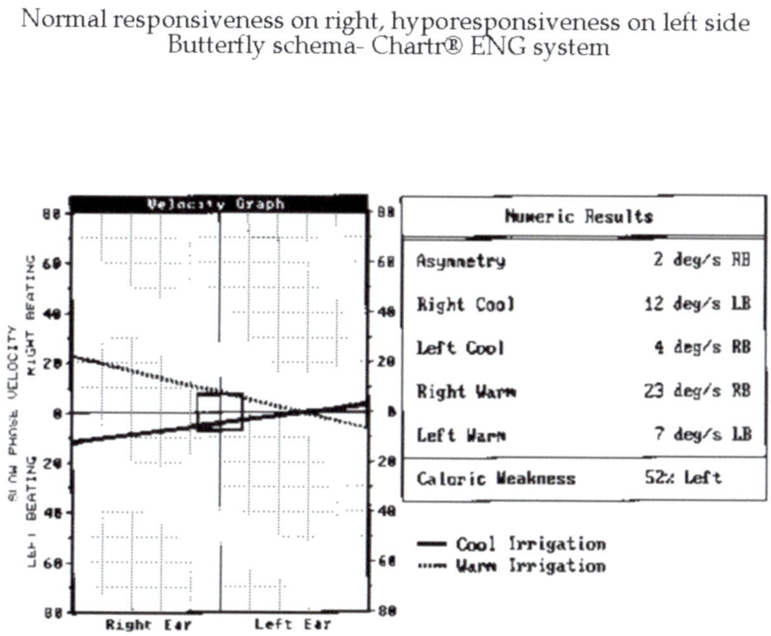

Fig. 17. Bithermal caloric test

Hyperresponsiveness on right, relative hyporesponsiveness on left side
Butterfly schema- Chartr® ENG system

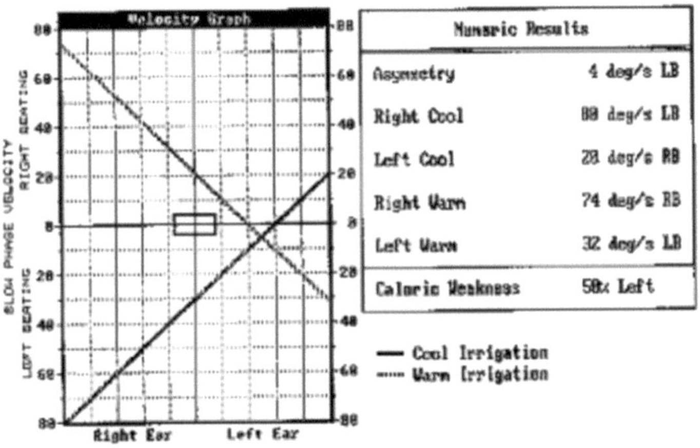

Fig. 18. Bithermal caloric test

We can avoid the anxiety of the patients, if we explain the pathomechanism of the vestibular dysfunction to the patients and teach them to keep under control their mind and give them a vestibular training program during their recovery.

5.5 Benign paroxysmal positional vertigo

Positional vertigo is caused by several central and peripheral vestibular lesions. The head or body position changing can provoke different type of positional nystagmus in central and peripheral lesions. In the central lesions the positional vertigo is direction fixed, non-fatigable. The peripheral positional nystagmus in most of the cases in direction fixed, but fatigable. The peripheral type of the positional nystagmus is often caused by canalolithiasis or cupulolithiasis. Vertiginous patients with anxiety positional vertigo were observed in 34.4%, while in patients without anxiety the ratio of positional nystagmus is 23.7%.

The disease called BPPV is a separate entity among the position- dependent types of vertigo. It might be one of the most frequent vestibular disorders, but often remained undiagnosed. The typical symptom in BPPV is the nystagmus in Dix-Hallpike manoeuvre (Figure 19.)

If we miss the Dix-Hallpike manoeuvre during the patient's examination, we will misdiagnose BPPV. Sometimes the few seconds' long vertigo results a differencialdiagnostic problems, the disease is misdiagnosed as vertebrobasilar insufficiency. This fact could result several targets for anxiety disorders: the patients have fear from vertebral artery occlusion, fear from stoke, fear from death, or being disabled. Most of patients are anxious from expectation being crazy or having anxiety disorder.

The long lasting or recurrent BPPV can provoke severe anxiety disorder, fear of motion. 61% of our patients have severe anxiety because of the recurrence of benign paroxysmal positional nystagmus.

Most of the patients with BPPV have a fear of head – motion, especially to the side of lesion. They try to avoid the head and neck movement. The result will be a stiff neck and a panic reaction after a head movement. These patients can reject the Epley manoeuvre and the vestibular training. Cognitive-behavioural therapy is an effective treatment for anxiety disorders, and vestibular rehabilitation exercises are effective for vestibular disorders. (Holmberg et al 2006). These patients have to be convinced again and again about the usefulness of vestibular training manoeuvres and they often have to use anxiolytic drugs.

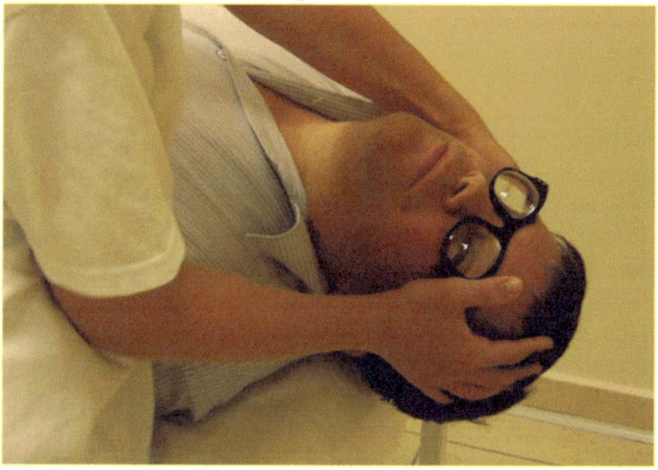

Patient's position on the table: head tilt with 45°
in hanging position. Nystagmus is observed by +18 D glasses.

Fig. 19. Dix-Hallpike manoeuvre

Some patients have anxiety disorder during the self-treatment. Few of my patients had severe anxiety because of BPPV. I have convinced them about the necessity of the training, but they have written one or more electronic letters daily to me or called me daily, whether the training technique, what they were making, was good or not.

The treatment of BPPV combined with anxiety disorder is a long lasting process and requires more empathy and patience of the doctor.

6. Anxiety disorders with dizziness without vestibular disorders

Patients with anxiety disorders could have dizziness without vestibular dysfunction.

Most of our patients have non rotatory vertigo, but constant imbalance. Patients have normal hearing and no vegetative symptoms. It seems to be very important diagnostic fact, when the patients' rotatory vertigo is organic; most of them have vegetative symptoms like nausea. During the examination the symptoms of sever anxiety are visible. Most of the young ladies with vertigo wear not normal, but elegant shoes with spike heel, while patients with vestibular dysfunction wear normal shoes. The everyday activities (shopping, working in a crowded place) are impaired because of their feeling of dizziness, while other activities like using bicycle, sports like skiing are unimpeded. Patients with organic vestibular symptoms cannot work on the latter, cannot use bike, and cannot ski, only after their complete recovery.

Analyzing the symptoms or our patients with normal vestibular system, in 67% of them generalised anxiety disorder was diagnosed. 18% of them have depression, diagnosed by psychiatrist, and 18% of them have panic disease.

Most of these patients are convinced themselves, that they have organic lesion. Most of them ask doctors again and again to send them to imaging methods (CT and MRI scan) to exclude organic lesion. ("I must have been some severe disease, because I'm suffering from dizziness.") It is very difficult to persuade them about the psychogenic reason. Few of them reject all of medical treatments and the help of psychiatrist ("I'm not crazy, I'm dizzy!"). Few of them use homeopathic drugs and several alternative ways of therapy.

7. Conclusions

The sensation of vertigo, a subjective complaint is sometimes defined as a movement illusion. Psychogenic vertigo or psychogenic superposition is relatively common in patients. To complicate the matters, vestibular dysfunctions frequently cause psychiatric illness, especially anxiety because of its incapacitating nature. The importance of the vestibular system for the internal representation of our body image accounts for the secondary psychiatric symptomatology in patients with primary vestibular disorders (Shilder, 1933, cited by Brandt, 2000).

In our experience, vertigo proved to have a bi-directional connection with psychiatric disorders. The panic disorder can be superimposed on chronic diseases with vertigo, and psychiatric patients with a cochleovestibular lesion have a diminished chance for complete recovery, and the recovery is longer. This relationship can be explained as a somatopsychic mechanism by which the vestibular symptoms provoke anxiety in the patient, who feels that the disease is a life-threatening catastrophe. Patients have severe anxiety at the beginning of the vertigo because of the uncertainty of the diagnosis. Some patients with vertigo have misdiagnosed disorder, mostly the BPPV remained undiagnosed. Undiagnosed peripheral vestibular lesion can cause psychiatric disorders, and increases somatisation tendencies in patients. In vestibular dysfunctions the mild movement of environment, like oscillopsia is often complained by patients. This feeling is very disturbing. If the doctor explains the pathophysiology of these feelings to the patients, the consecutive anxiety disorders could be avoided. If the patients don't know, what the reason of their complaints is, the vestibular symptoms can provoke anxiety. Few years after the beginning of anxiety, we can suggest based on the case history that the organic vertigo was the trigger factor of the generalised anxiety disorder. If we examine the patient in that phase, we can find normal vestibular system.

Psychogenic superposition is suggested when there is a clear dissociation between objective and subjective disequilibrium, the patients complains severe rotatory vertigo without concurrent spontaneous nystagmus. In most of these psychogenic cases the vegetative symptoms associated to acute rotatory vertigo, like nausea and vomitus are missing.

There are several controversies in the patients' handicapping in everyday life. Anxiety can cause severe problems for example the patient cannot shopping, cannot use metro because the moving steps cause motion sickness and the metro is overcrowded. On the other hand, patient can use the latter at home for working, and can make excursions with bike.

Alternatively, the psychosomatic mechanism might operate in such a way that the anxiety and panic increase vestibular responses to positional tests and caloric and rotational provocations. It can cause difficulties in the patient's examination; the patients often reject the provocative tests of the vestibular examination.

The co-existing anxiety and vertigo needs parallel treatment. Treatment possibilities include antivertiginous drugs and SSRIs, vestibular training, and psychotherapy. The vertigo treatment could be a longer process, than in non- anxious patients, and needs more empathy from the doctor. Treatment of vertigo in patients suffering from anxiety disorders requires cooperation between neurootologist and psychiatrist.

8. References

Best C, Eckhardt-Henn A, Diener G, Bense S, Breuer P, Dieterich M.: Interaction of somatoform and vestibular disorders. J Neurol Neurosurg Psychiatry. 2006 May; 77 (5): 658-64.

Barber H. O&Stockwell C. W: Manual of Electronystagmography C. V. Mosby Company, St. Louis, 1980.

Brandt T. :Vertigo Its multisensory Syndromes 2nd Edition, Springer Verlag London, 2000.

Chartr® Diagnostic Systems Operator Manual, ICS Medical Corporation, Illinois, 1994.

Claussen C.F& Franz B: Contemporary&Practical Neurootology, Solvay Pharmaceuticals, Hannover, 2006.

Eckhardt-Henn A, Best C, Bense S, Breuer P, Diener G, Tschan R, Dieterich M :Psychiatric co-morbidity in different organic vertigo syndromes. Neurol. 2008 Mar; 255(3):420-8. Epub 2008 Mar 14.

Fazekas A.: [Vertigo--comorbidity with psychiatric disorders].[Article in Hungarian] Ideggyógy Sz. 2010 Mar 30;63(3-4):113-7.

Ferreira LS, Pereira CB, Rossini S, Kanashiro AM, Adda CC, Scaff M.: Psychological assessment in patients with phobic postural vertigo. Arq Neuropsiquiatr. 2010 Apr; 68(2):224-7.

Holmberg J, Karlberg M, Harlacher U, Rivano-Fischer M, Magnusson M: Treatment of phobic postural vertigo. A controlled study of cognitive-behavioral therapy and self-controlled desensitization. Neurol. 2006 Apr; 253(4):500-6. Epub 2005 Dec 19.

Noaksson L, Schulin M, Kovacsovics B, Ledin T. Temperature Order Effects in the Caloric Reaction. Int Tinnitus J. 1998;4(1):71-73

Pavlou M, Quinn C, Murray K, Spyridakou C, Faldon M, Bronstein AM. : The effect of repeated visual motion stimuli on visual dependence and postural control in normal subjects. Gait Posture. 2011 Jan; 33(1):113-8. Epub 2010 Dec 8.

Perna G, Dario A, Caldirola D, et al. Panic disorder: The role of the balance system. *J Psychiatr Res* 35(5):279–286, 2001.

Post RE, Dickerson LM. : Dizziness: a diagnostic approach. Am Fam Physician. 2010 Aug 15; 82(4):361-8, 369.

Salhofer S, Lieba-Samal D, Freydl E, Bartl S, Wiest G, Wöber C : Migraine and vertigo--a prospective diary study. Cephalalgia. 2010 Jul;30(7):821-8. Epub 2010 Mar 12.

Stein MB, Asmundson GJ, Ireland D, Walker JR. : Panic disorder in patients attending a clinic for vestibular disorders. Am J Psychiatry. 1994 Nov; 151(11):1697-700.

Sullivan M, Clark MR, Katon WJ, Fischl M, Russo J, Dobie RA, Voorhees R.: Psychiatric and otologic diagnoses in patients complaining of dizziness. Arch Intern Med. 1993 Jun 28;153(12):1479-84.

Szirmai A. : Vestibular disorders in patients with migraine. Eur Arch Otorhinolaryngol. 1997; 254 Suppl 1:S55-7.

Szirmai Á: Ménière's syndrome: Is it a vascular lesion of inner ear? Internet-Journal Archives for Sensology and Neurootology (ASN). http://www.neurootology.org 2004.

Szirmai A , Kisely M, Nagy GY, Nedeczky Zs. , Szabados É.M. , TóthÁ: Panic disorder in otoneurogical experience International Tinnitus Journal, Vol 11, No I, 77-80, 2005.

Yardley L, Redfern MS. Psychological factors influencing recovery from balance disorders. *J Anxiety Disord* 15(1–2):107–119, 2001.

11

Significant Posturography Findings in Patients with Psychogenic Dizziness

Fumiyuki Goto[1], Kaoru Ogawa[2] and Tomoko Tsutsumi[1]
[1]*Department of otolaryngology, Hino Municipal Hospital, Tokyo*
[2]*Department of otolaryngology, Keio University, School of Medicine, Tokyo*
Japan

1. Introduction

Posturography is useful for investigating global balance performance (Kushiro & Goto, 2011). We found that anxiety affects postural perturbation in the anteroposterior axis, possibly indicating that anxiety affects the interactions between visual inputs and vestibular as well as somatosensory inputs in the maintenance of postural balance in patients complaining of dizziness (Goto et al. 2011a).

Dizziness is a common somatic complaint that can be caused by several factors including peripheral or central vestibular dysfunction. Anxiety and depression are closely related to somatic complaints, including dizziness. Patients suffering from vestibular disorders are prone to anxiety (Eagger et al., 1992), which is known to affect postural stability. Patients can present with dizziness even in the absence of any signs of organic or functional dysfunction; such patients are usually diagnosed with psychogenic dizziness. The aim of our study was to identify abnormal findings in patients with psychogenic dizziness.

Healthy subjects with high anxiety are reported to have larger sway in the anteroposterior axis (Wada et al., 2001). This characteristic disappears when the eyes are closed (Ohno et al. 2004). It is believed that anxiety affects the postural sway of the anteroposterior axis and the interactions of visual inputs with vestibular and somatosensory inputs are influenced by anxiety in healthy subjects (Wada et al. 2001). Maki and McIlroy (1996) reported that healthy subjects with elevated levels of state anxiety undergoing cognitive tasks such as mental arithmetic tend to lean forward. This observation shows that elevated levels of state anxiety cause the center of gravity to shift forward. We previously reported a clear relationship between anxiety and anteroposterior perturbations (Goto et al. 2011a).

There are several types of patients with vestibular disorders due to organic and psychogenic factors and combinations thereof. There may be some specific pattern of posturography depending on the levels of anxiety and vestibular deficits. It would be useful to know if there is a relationship between anxiety and postural sway in patients complaining of dizziness. Therefore, the relationship between the levels of anxiety and postural sway in patients complaining of dizziness was evaluated. In addition, the effect of visual input was investigated. Posturography is a useful tool for investigating the effects of various conditions (Kushiro & Goto, 2011), and we used it to evaluate postural sway. Anxiety levels were assessed by the hospital anxiety and depression scale (HADS).

2. Methods

The subjects were patients who visited Hino Municipal Hospital complaining of dizziness from January 2007 to May 2007. The average age was 51.9 ± 18.8 years (mean ± standard deviation). Before each examination, the purpose and procedure were explained and informed consent was obtained from each subject. The ethics committee of Hino Municipal Hospital approved the examinations. Examinations were carried out in accordance with the Declaration of Helsinki.

2.1 Diagnosis and psychological evaluation

To obtain a diagnosis, all patients underwent otoneurological examinations. These examinations included pure-tone audiometry, nystagmus evaluation with an infrared CCD camera, and posturography. Some patients required bithermal caloric tests, vestibular evoked myogenic potentials, auditory brain stem response, and head imaging (i.e., CT and MRI) to obtain a clinical diagnosis. In addition, the dizziness handicap inventory (DHI) and HADS (Hosaka et al. 1999) were used to evaluate the severity of dizziness and anxiety plus depression, respectively. If no apparent organic or functional abnormalities were identified from a variety of examinations, the patients was were diagnosed with psychogenic dizziness. The rest of the patients were further divided according to their anxiety level depending on the HADS score. A HADS score greater than 6 indicates that the patients had a certain level of anxiety (Hosaka et al. 1999); these patients were defined as having psychogenic + organic dizziness; if the score was less than 5, the patients were defined as having organic dizziness.

2.2 Postural sway analysis

Postural sway was measured by continuously detecting the body's center of gravity by using a force platform equipped with a data processor (Gravicorder G-6100; Anima, Tokyo, Japan). Patients were asked to stand on the platform with their feet parallel, gazing at a visual target: a black circle 17 cm in diameter on a white background fixed at a 1-m distance at eye level. Body sway was measured for 1 min with eyes open and then closed. This arrangement of the visual target produced a visual angle of 10°. The total length and area of body sway were recorded. The left–right maximum amplitude (XD) and anteroposterior maximum amplitude (YD) were also measured. From these values, the ratio of the maximum amplitude of the anteroposterior (YD) and left–right axes (XD) was calculated as YD/XD (Fig. 1). The Romberg ratio of YD/XD was calculated as the YD/XD with the eyes closed divided by that with the eyes open.

3. Results

There were 16, 25, and 13 subjects in the psychogenic, organic, and psychogenic + organic groups, respectively. The distribution of total DHI scores is shown in Fig. 2. The relationship between the ratio of maximum amplitude (YD/XD) in the eyes-open and eyes-closed conditions is shown in Fig. 3. However, there appears to be no relationship between these values. YD/XD ratios in the eyes-open and eyes-closed conditions are shown in Fig. 4. There was a statically significant difference in the YD/XD values between patients with psychogenic and organic dizziness in the eyes-open condition. However, this difference was

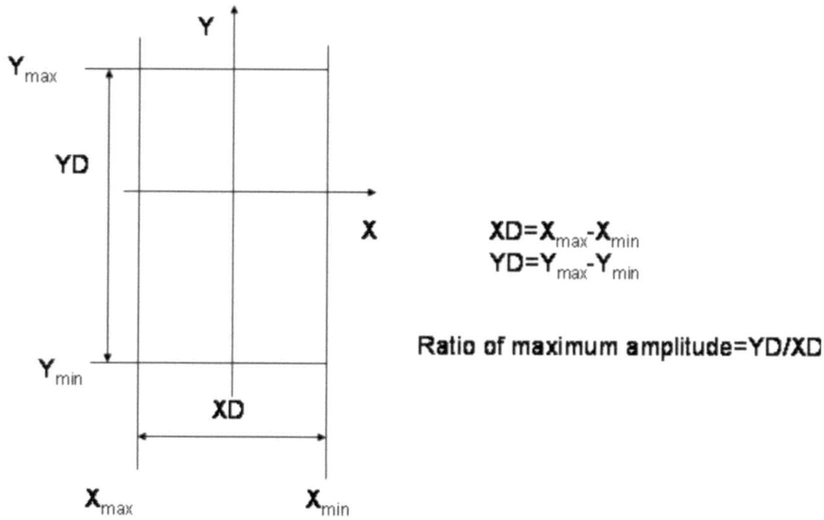

The perturbation of anterio-posterior direction is defined as Y and left-right direction is as X, respectively.

Fig. 1. The definition of the ratio of maximum amplitude (YD/XD)

not apparent in the eyes-closed condition. The Romberg ratio of YD/XD in the psychogenic group was significantly smaller than that in the organic and psychogenic + organic groups (Fig. 5). This means that the patients with psychogenic dizziness became more stable in anteroposterior direction with their eyes closed.

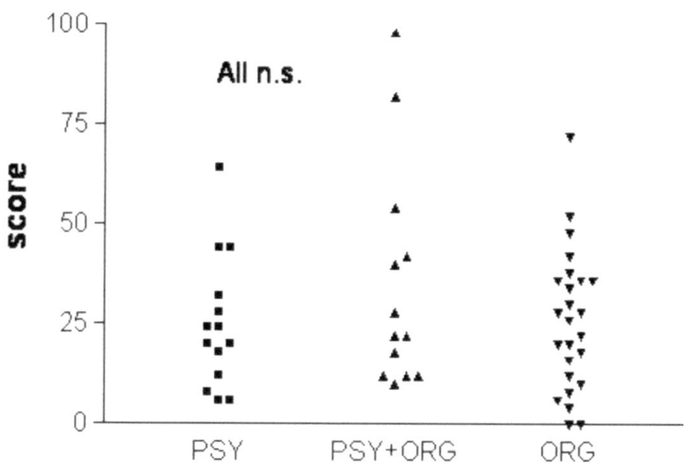

The distribution of total DHI scores is shown. There are no statistical deference in each groups. XD and YD are calculated as in figure.

Fig. 2. Dizziness handicap inventory (DHI)

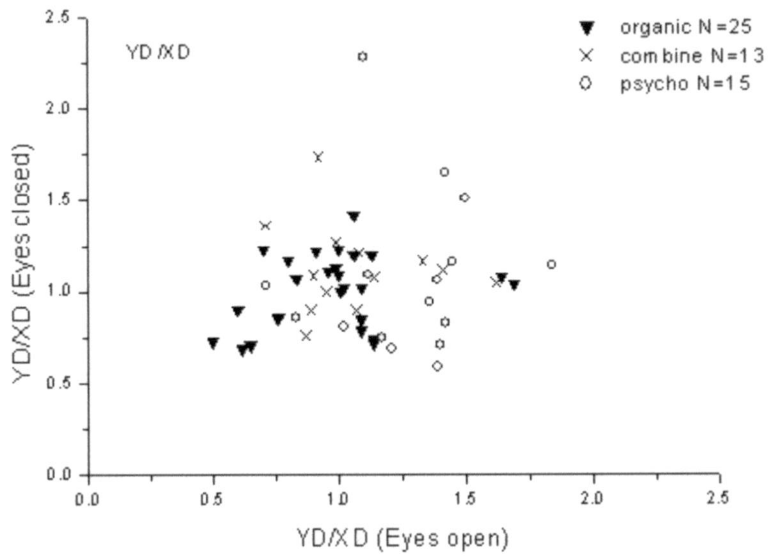

The relationship between the ratio of maximum amplitude (YD/XD) in the eyes-open and eyes-closed conditions is shown. There is no relationship between these values in both conditions.

Fig. 3. The relationship between YD/XD with eyes open and closed

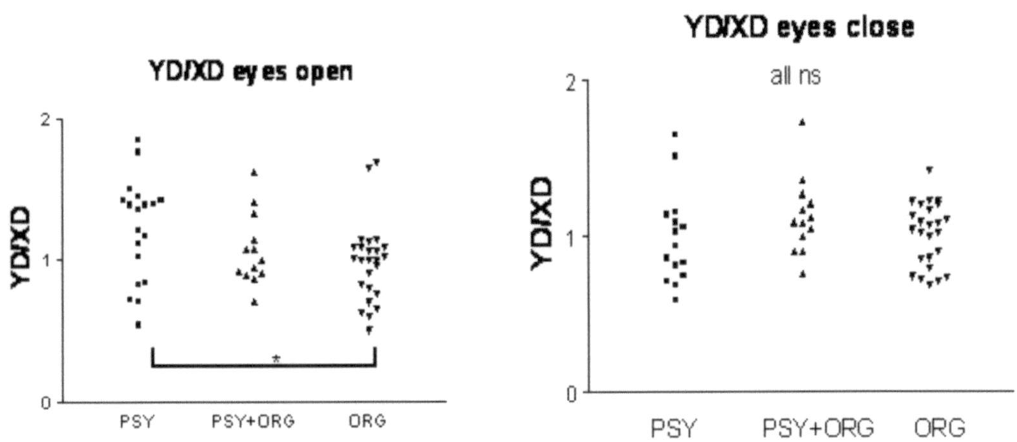

There is a statically significant difference in the YD/XD values between patients with psychogenic and organic dizziness with their eyes open. However, this difference disappears when the eyes are closed.

Fig. 4. YD/XD with eyes open and closed

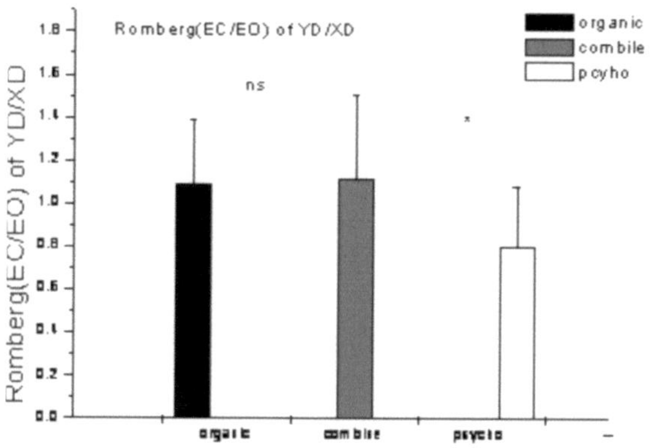

The Romberg ratio of YD/XD in psychogenic subjects was significantly smaller than that in organic or psychogenic + organic patients.

Fig. 5. The Romberg ratio (eyes closed/eyes open) of YD/XD in patients with organic, organic + psychogenic, and psychogenic dizziness

4. Discussion

We tried to identify specific posturography findings in a variety of patients complaining of dizziness. As shown in Fig. 4, our results indicate that the YD/XD value is greater in patients with psychogenic dizziness than in those with organic, and organic + psychogenic dizziness. The organic disorder itself has a significant effect on posturography results. It is believed that the effect of the organic disorder is so significant that the effect of anxiety on postural perturbation cannot be determined.

In addition, as shown in Fig. 4, the Romberg ratio was smaller in patients with psychogenic dizziness. This might be a clinical indicator of anxiety in patients with dizziness lacking organic and functional dysfunction.

Since anxiety is closely related to vertigo and dizziness, it is important to evaluate anxiety in patients reporting dizziness. This, however, is usually not easy. To obtain an accurate diagnosis, it is important to examine patients from both physical and psychiatric perspectives. Doctors in otolaryngology departments are familiar with routine physical examinations such as posturography and audiometry. However, they are not accustomed to evaluating the psychological status of patients. The only way to measure psychogenic status, including anxiety and depression, is to use self-rating questionnaires. For example, anxiety can be evaluated by the state-trait anxiety inventory (STAI), depression by the self-rating depression scale (SDS), and both anxiety and depression by the HADS, of which the latter was used in this study. Although these questionnaires are subjective measurements, it is not common to use them for evaluation. Consequently, a method for objectively evaluating anxiety would be indispensable. In both healthy subjects and patients experiencing dizziness, anxiety affects posturography in the anteroposterior direction.

If patients do not have any functional or organic abnormalities, it is a diagnostic dilemma as to why they have psychological dizziness. The diagnosis of psychological dizziness is quite important, because if the patients have it, treatment should be specially arranged. Selective serotonin reuptake inhibitors (SSRIs) and anxiolytics, including benzodiazepines, are used to treat these patients. In some cases, psychotherapy such as autogenic training can be successfully used to control anxiety (Goto et al. 2011b).

In a previous study, we found that anxiety affects the postural perturbation in the anteroposterior axis and that this trend disappears when the eyes are closed. Power spectrum analysis clearly demonstrates that the effect of visual input on vestibular and somatosensory inputs is affected by anxiety.
In the present study, we found that the Romberg ratio of YD/XD is significantly smaller in patients with psychogenic dizziness. The Romberg ratio of YD/XD might be a potential clinical indicator of anxiety in patients with dizziness who lack organic and functional dysfunction.

5. Conclusions

Our results indicate that anxiety affects postural perturbations in the anteroposterior axis and that the Romberg ratio of YD/XD might be a potential clinical indicator of anxiety in patients with dizziness and without organic or functional dysfunction. This research sheds new light on the mechanisms of dizziness and initiates the development of novel, promising diagnostic strategies.

6. Acknowledgments

This research was supported in part by research funds from MOA, HEALTH SCIENCE FOUNDATION on 2011.

7. References

Eagger, S.; Luxon, L.M.; Davies, R.A.; Coelho, A. & Ron, M.A. (1992). Psychiatric morbidity in patients with peripheral vestibular disorder: a clinical and neuro-otological study. *Journal of Neurology Neurosurgery & Psychiatry*, Vol. 55, 5,pp. 383-387, 00223050

Goto, F.; Kabeya, M.; Kushiro, K., Tsutsumi; T. & Hayashi, K. (2011a). Effect of anxiety on antero-posterior postural stability in patients with dizziness. *Neuroscience Letters*, Vol. 487, pp. 204-206, 0304-3940

Goto, F.; Nakai, K. & Ogawa, K. (2011b) Application of autogenic training in patients with Meniere disease. *European Archives of Oto-rhino-laryngology* Feb 18 ,0937-4477

Hosaka, T.; Awazu, H.; Aoki, T.; Okuyama, T. & Yamawaki, S. (1999). Screening for adjustment disorders and major depression in otolaryngology patients using the hospital anxiety and depression scale. *International Journal of Psychiatry in Clinical Practice*, Vol. 3, pp. 43-48, 1365-1501

Kushiro, K. & Goto, F. (2011). Effect of masticating chewing gum on postural stability during upright standing. *Neuroscience Letters*, Vol. 487, pp. 196-198, 0304-3940, 0304-3940

Maki, B.E. & McIlroy, W.E. (1996). Influence of arousal and attention on the control of postural sway. *Journal of Vestibular Research*, Vol. 6, 1,pp. 53-59, 0957-4271

Ohno, H.; Wada, M.; Saitoh, J.; Sunaga, N. & Nagai, M. (2004). The effect of anxiety on postural control in humans depends on visual information processing. *Neuroscience Letters*, Vol. 364, 1,pp. 37-39, 0304-3940

Wada, M.; Sunaga, N. & Nagai, M. (2001). Anxiety affects the postural sway of the antero-posterior axis in college students. *Neuroscience Letters*, Vol. 302, 2-3,pp. 157-159, 0304-3940

12

Anxiety Disorders in Epilepsy

Ozalp Ekinci
Antakya State Hospital of Child Care, Hatay
Turkey

1. Introduction

Epilepsy is a heterogeneous entity with enormous variation in etiology and clinical features and is defined as two unprovoked seizures of any type (Waaler et al., 2000). Epilepsy is one of the most common neurological disorders in pediatric and adult population (Moshé et al., 2011). Research in the past 20 years showed that the patients with epilepsy commonly have coexisting psychiatric conditions including mood disorders, anxiety disorders, psychotic disorders and attention deficit hyperactivity disorder (Garcia Morales et al., 2008; Waaler et al., 2000; Ekinci et al., 2009). Historically, psychiatric disorders in epilepsy have been considered a consequence of psychosocial disturbance due to poor adaptation to a chronic disease with stigma (Thome Souza et al., 2004). However, recent studies indicates that there is a bidirectional relationship between epilepsy and psychiatric disorders. This relationship may be conceptualized as an epiphenomena rather than cause-consequence factors (Kanner, 2011; Thome Souza et al 2004).

2. Anxiety disorders in epilepsy

Among the psychiatric comorbidites in epilepsy, anxiety disorders are highly frequent and have a profound influence on the quality of life of epilepsy patients (Kanner et al., 2010; Beyenburg et al., 2005; Choi-Kwon et al., 2003; Johnson et al., 2004; Tellez-Zenteno et al., 2007). Several studies have reported elevated rates of panic attacks, panic disorder, obsessive compulsive disorder (OCD), social anxiety disorder and generalized anxiety disorder (GAD) in adult patients with epilepsy as compared with the general population (Piazzini et al., 2001; Issacs, 2004; Baker at al., 2005; Marsh & Rao 2002; Vazquez & Devinsky 2003).

2.1 DSM-IV anxiety disorders

The DSM-IV defines 11 different types of anxiety disorders. Generalized anxiety disorder presents with (GAD) a disabling and persistent worry that is free-floating and present much of the time for at least 6 months. Somatic or vegetative symptoms such as increased fatigue, insomnia, difficulty with concentration, and sleep problems are commonly seen in GAD. Panic attacks are defined by sudden and severe paroxysmal episodes of anxiety of typically sudden onset and short duration. A frequency of more than one attack per week for a period of at least 1 month is in the diagnostic criteria of panic disorder. Obsessive-compulsive disorder (OCD) is characterized by recurrent unwanted, intrusive and stressing thoughts or images often allied with compulsive actions (American Psychiatric Association, 1994).

2.2 The prevalence and the phenomenology of anxiety disorders in epilepsy

The differences in the methodology of the studies have affected the consistency of prevalence rates of anxiety disorders in epilepsy (Williams et al., 2002; Ekinci et al., 2009). The avaliable data indicates a prevalence somewhere between 14% and 78% (Wittchen et al., 2002; Vasquez & Devinsky, 2003; Kanner et al., 2001) in adults and somewhere between 16% and 48% in children and adolescents (Ettinger et al., 1998; Williams et al., 2003; Caplan et al., 2004; Alwash et al., 2000).

It is important to note that the special features of anxiety disorders in epilepsy have not been studied sufficiently in clinical and community studies. Therefore, it's largely unknown if the current diagnostic instruments for anxiety disorders perform adequately in this special population. Because of the complex nature of epilepsy, the phenomenology of anxiety disorders may be different than in the general population, which can make it difficult to isolate symptoms to a single DSM-IV-TR diagnosis. For example, the fear of unexpected seizures in special places may lead to a variant of agoraphobia. In children, the fear of having a seizure can be associated with anxiety about separation from the parents or home. The fear of embarrassment about having a seizure in public may also lead to a variant of social phobia and result in isolation of the patient from social activites (Ekinci et al., 2009; Beyenburg et al., 2005). It is also important to highlight that DSM-IV-TR criteria require the absence of a physiological condition when considering symptoms in anxiety disorders (DSM IV, 1994). However, experimental studies suggest that kindling mechanisms and the recurrent epileptic stimulation of the amygdala may predispose patients with epilepsy to interictal anxiety (Depaulis et al., 1997). Because of this, it would be reasonable to consider an alternative classification system for epilepsy-related anxiety that accounts for the different manifestations of anxiety in individuals with epilepsy. For instance, some individuals experience anxiety in response to the stress of the condition (i.e., reactive) or whereas others because of a preexisting propensity for anxiety (i.e., endogenous) (Ekinci et al 2009). Beyenburg et al. in his comprehensive review offer phenomenologic suggestions about the types of anxiety disorders in epilepsy (Beyenburg et al., 2005).

3. Associated factors of anxiety disorders in epilepsy

Multiple factors have been found to be associated with anxiety symptoms and/or DSM IV anxiety disorders in patients with epilepsy. In this chapter, the factors associated with anxiety disorders in epilepsy are grouped in five categories including: Neurobiological factors, psycholocial factors, epilepsy related factors, age of the patients and the medication related factors.

3.1 Neurobiological factors

There is neurobiological evidence for the possible common pathophysiological mechanisms of anxiety symptoms and epileptic seizures. This theory is mainly based on the observation that epileptic activity in certain areas of the brain directly causes paroxysmal anxiety, usually in the form of panic (Chapouthier & Venault, 2001; Trimble & Van Elst, 2003). The amygdala seems to be a particularly important structure for the production of anxiety symptoms and epileptic discharges in temporal lobe epilepsy (Beyenburg et al., 2005). In correlation with this hypothesis, patients with temporal lobe epilepsy and ictal anxiety symptoms have been found to have a reduced amygdala volume (Cendes et al., 1994). Neurotransmitter systems are also suggested be related with the link of anxiety disorders and epilepsy. The role of GABA receptors and neurotransmitters including serotonin, dopamine and noradrenaline in both epilepsy and anxiety disorders indicate another pathophysiological similarity between the two disorders (Beyenburg et al., 2005; Lydiard, 2003; Charney, 2003).

3.2 Psychological factors

Psychological factors, such as the unpredictability of seizures, the fear of death, feeling of poor control over seizures, and perceived stigma likely predispose some epilepsy patients to anxiety (Pellock, 2004; Jacoby et al., 2005; Beyenburg et al., 2005). Misinformation or insufficient information about the disorder also seems to be related to increased anxiety (Ekinci et al., 2009; Couldridge et al., 2001). Lower levels of epilepsy knowledge were found to be significantly related to higher levels of social anxiety, higher levels of depression, and lower levels of self-esteem (Baker et al., 2005).

3.3 Epilepsy related factors

Previous studies linked some epilepsy related factors with anxiety symptoms. Higher seizure frequency has been found to be associated with anxiety disorders in some adult studies (Jacoby et al., 1996). In the case of children and adolescents, most of the literature supports a direct relationship between increased seizure frequency and anxiety disorders (Williams et al., 2003; Ettinger et al., 1998; Kessler et al 2001; Oguz et al 2002; Alwash et al., 2000; Adeewuya et al., 2005). In adults, the risk of anxiety disorders appears to be higher in focal (especially temporal lobe) than in generalized epilepsies (Garcia Morales et al., 2008; Goldstein & Harden, 2000; Vasquez & Devinsky 2003; Marsh & Rao, 2002, Piazzini et al., 2001). Anxiety disorders were found to be linked with the seizures originated from left temporal lobe but this is not entirely consistent in the literature (Andelman et al., 2001). In children and adolescents, the contribution of seizure type to anxiety disorders appears to be much less clear. Most of the studies have failed to demonstrate a relationship between seizure type and risk of anxiety [Williams et al., 2003; Ettinger et al., 1998; Oguz et al., 2002; Pianta & Lothman, 1994). Epilepsy surgery is also reported to be related with the development of anxiety symptoms. Transient anxiety symptoms have been reported after following temporal lobe surgery for epilepsy (Ring et al., 1998).

3.4 Age as a factor

The age of the patient and the age of seizure onset were examined as associated factors for anxiety disorders in epilepsy. In adult patients, first-onset epilepsy in late life is shown to be linked with higher levels of anxiety (Baker et al., 2001). However, in children and adolescents, most of the studies do not support a relationship between age at seizure onset and increased risk of anxiety (Williams et al., 2003; Ettinger et al., 1998; Pianta et al., 1994; Oguz et al., 2002). In pediatric population, older age has been found to be a significant risk factor for anxiety. Adolescents with epilepsy are considered to be at higher risk for anxiety than younger children (Oguz et al., 2002; Williams et al., 2003). There are several possible explanations for this relation. Adolescents have a greater cognitive capacity than children to understand and question the unpredictable and poorly controlled nature of the seizure disorder. This can, in turn, potentiate anxiety and contribute to negative emotional responses. Morever, with the significant social demands and challenges, adolescence is unique among the other phases of development. Peer relationships are central to the teenage experience and the risk of having a seizure at school or in a social activity with friends is a severe threat to an adolescent's ability to successfully achieve the developmental milestones for this age. This can result in significant problems with self-esteem and potential social isolation, thus increasing the likelihood of anxiety in various forms (Ekinci et al., 2009).

3.5 The possible role of antiepileptic drugs

Most of the previous studies have demonstrated that antiepileptic drug (AED) polytherapy is associated with increased risk of anxiety disorders (Mula & Sanders 2007; Williams et al., 2003; Ettinger et al., 1998; Oguz et al., 2002; Adeewuya et al., 2005). This increased risk can occur as a side effect of the AEDs or as a function of complications related to AED withdrawal. However, it is unclear whether there is a direct causal relationship between AED polytherapy and anxiety. It is also possible that the need of using AED polytherapy may reflect the the intractability of the seizure disorder.

4. Treatment of anxiety disorders in epilepsy

4.1 Psychosocial interventions

For the optimal management of anxiety disorders in epilepsy, an essential component is the adequate explanation of the condition (Couldrigde et al., 2001; Kendal et al., 2004). The degree of information requested may vary relatively between patients and families in different socioculturel levels. A comprehensive psychoeducation can be best achieved with the availability of professional specialists including nurses (Beyenburg et al., 2005).

Regular psychiatric and/or psychological consultation that involves developmentally appropriate methods of approach is important. Among the psychosocial approaches, cognitive behavioural therapy (CBT) may potentially serve as a treatment option both for anxiety symptoms and also for the optimal seizure control (Ekinci et al., 2009; Goldstein et., al 2003; Spector et al., 1999; Engelberts et al., 2002). CBT has been found to be effective in adult patients with epilepsy who have agoraphobia and OCD (Newsom-Davis et al., 1998). A more recent study showed CBT as an acceptable and promising treatment option for the patients with epilepsy and comorbid anxiety symptoms (Macrodimitri et al., 2011).

4.2 Medical treatment

A limited number of studies have focused on the pharmacotherapy of anxiety disorders in epilepsy to date. The available research have revealed that the SSRI group antidepressants appear to be safe and effective treatment options (Scicutella & Ettinger, 2002; Schmitz, 2002; Kanner et al., 2000; Jobe & Browning, 2005). The possible psychiatric and/or therapeutic effects of AED also deserve attention. Some AED including valproate, gabapentin, tiagabine and vigabatrine have been reported to anxiolytic effects and have been used with varying success in the treatment of anxiety disorders in adult studies (Johannessen Landmark, 2008; Kinrys et al., 2003; Blanco et al., 2003, Pande et al., 2000,2003; Rosenthal, 2003). Several hypotheses and suggestions have been made for why some AEDs have anti-anxiety effects (Ketter et al., 1999). There is some evidence that the past history and family history of psychiatric disorders may increase the risk of psychiatric side effects with AEDs (Mula &

Monaco, 2007; Marsh & Rao, 2002). It is suggested that the AEDs that attenuate glutamate excitatory neurotransmission (e.g., lamotrigine) may cause neurotransmitter activation that leads to an increase in anxiety and GABAergic AEDs may serve to decrease anxiety (e.g., barbiturates, benzodiazepines, valporate, tiagabine, gabapentin and vigabatrin) (Ketter et al., 1999; Mula & Monaco, 2007). Beyond this theoretical explanation, there are no placebo-controlled studies on the anxiolytic effects of AEDs in adults or pediatric patients with epilepsy. Nevertheless, based on the extant literature thus far, it is reasonable to consider choosing an AED with anxiolytic potential in a patient with epilepsy who also has a comorbid anxiety disorder. (Scicutella & Ettinger, 2002; Beyenburg et al., 2005; Mula & Monaco 2007).

5. The differential diagnosis of seizures and anxiety disorders

It is important to note that this chapter mainly discusses the anxiety disorders in patients with epilepsy which are unrelated with seizure events. This type of anxiety is defined as interictal anxiety. However, patients with epilepsy can also experience increased levels of anxiety at different stages of the seizure events, such as preictally, ictally, or postictally. Ictal anxiety is defined as anxiety symptoms during the seizure event. Ictal anxiety is known to be associated with focal seizures of temporal origin, particularly when there is amygdalar involvement (Marsh & Rao 2002; Vasquez & Devinsky 2003). Anxiety as a postictal phenomenon refers to the anxiety symptoms shortly after a seizure or a cluster of seizures (Kanner et al., 2004). This type of anxiety may be associated with dysphoria or depressive symptoms (Kanner & Palac, 2000). Postictal anxiety symptoms similar to those in panic attacks can be observed in temporal lobe epilepsy and less frequently in extratemporal lobe epilepsies (Beyenburg et al., 2005). The differential diagnosis of seizure-related events is sometimes problematic for the clinicians since such events may be misled by panic attacks that present like complex partial seizures (Bernik et al., 2002). Differentiating symptoms that are more suggestive of a seizure include motor automatisms, alterations in consciousness, the possible presence of an aura and postictal confusion (Vasquez & Devinsky 2003; Scicutella & Ettinger, 2002). In addition, panic attacks usually last several minutes whereas seizures are usually more brief. The exception to this, of course, is seizures that secondarily generalize or progress to status epilepticus (Ekinci et al., 2009). Complicated cases may warrant further investigation with EEG, Video EEG monitoring, and/or brain imaging studies (Handal et al., 1995).

6. Suggestions and future research

When compared with depression, less attention has been focused on anxiety disorders in epilepsy. The factors that have been suggested for the increased risk of anxiety disorders in epilepsy are reviewed in Figure 1. For the management of this disabling comorbidity, different strategies including psychosocial, behavioral and medicational interventions are found to be helpful. However, for an effective management, gaining optimal seizure control must be the first step. Without total seizure control, complete treatment of anxiety symptoms is considered unlikely (Ekinci et al., 2009; Beyenburg et al., 2005). Further research is needed to better examine the specific phenomenology of anxiety disorders in patients with epilepsy in order to guide clinicians about when psychiatric referrals are needed.

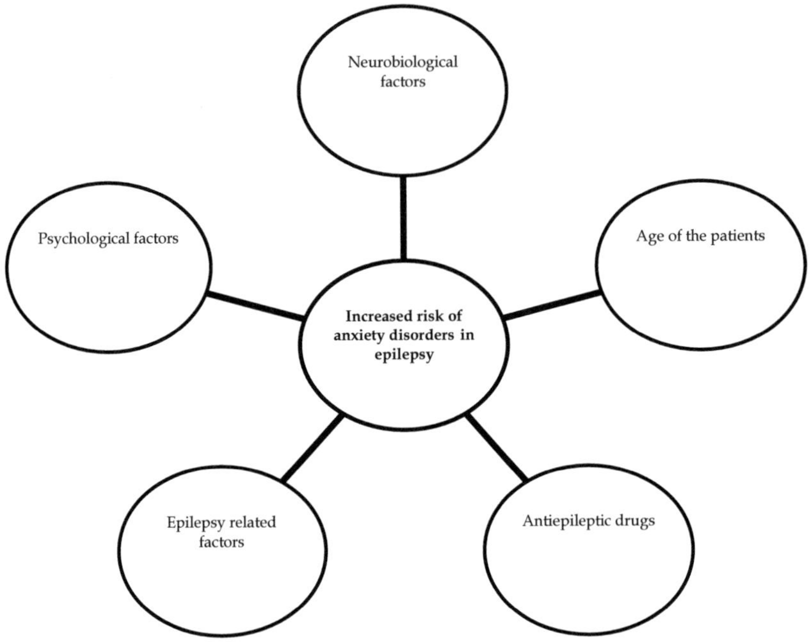

Fig. 1. Overview of the factors associated with increased risk of anxiety disorders in patients with epilepsy

Neurobiological factors: The role of of amygdala and GABA receptors
Unpredictability of seizures, the fear of death, feeling of poor control over seizures and the perceived stigma
Epilepsy related factors: Higher seizure frequency, focal epilepsy types (especially temporal lobe epilepsy) and epilepsy surgery (especially after temporal lobe surgery)
Age of the patients: In adults, later onset of epilepsy. In pediatric population, older age
Role of antiepileptic drugs (AED): AED polytherapy and the effects of spesific AED on anxiety symptoms

7. Conclusion

Anxiety symptoms, either in the form of the DSM- IV diagnoses or single symptoms, are frequenty experienced in patients with epilepsy. Morever, anxiety in epilepsy is not simply a reactive emotional response to epilepsy or just a feature of the seizures. The current literature indicates that anxiety disorders are frequent comorbid conditions of epilepsy in children, adolescents and adults. The worries of the patients about having accidents, losing control and social embarrassment may be associated with an underdiagnosed or untreated anxiety disorder. Comprehensive and effective management of anxiety symptoms can be accomplished by a psychiatrist and/or psychologist, particularly when a the patients' condition is more severe and/or refractory. The collaboration between different disciplines, including the psychiatry and neurology specialists, offers the best hope for early identification and treatment of anxiety disorders in epilepsy. Because of the potentially severe impact of anxiety disorders on the quality of life in patients with epilepsy, anxiety symptoms should be screened and treated early in this special population.

8. References

Adewuya, A.O. & Ola, B.A. (2005). Prevalence of and risk factors for anxiety and depressive disorders in Nigerian adolescents with epilepsy. Epilepsy Behav, 6, 3, 342–7.

Alwash, R.H.; Hussein, M.J. & Matloub FF. (2000). Symptoms of anxiety and depression among adolescents with seizures in Irbid, northern Jordan. Seizure, 9, 6, 412–6.

American Psychiatric Association. (1994). Diagnostic and statistical manual of mental disorders—fourth edition, text revision (DSM-IV-TR). Washington, DC.

Andelman, F.; Fied, I. & Neufeld, M.Y. (2001). Quality of life self-assessment as a function of lateralization of lesion in candidates for epilepsy surgery. Epilepsia, 42, 4, 549–55.

Baker, G.A.; Jacoby, A.; Buck, D.; Brooks, J; Potts, P. & Chadwick, D.W. (2001). The quality of life of older people with epilepsy: findings from a UK community study. Seizure, 10, 2, 92–9.

Baker, G.A.; Spector, S.; McGrath, Y. & Soteriou, H. (2005). Impact of epilepsy in adolescence. a UK controlled study. Epilepsy Behav, 6, 4, 556–62.

Bernik, M.A.; Corregiari, F.M. & Braun, I.M. (2002). Panic attacks in the differential diagnosis and treatment of resistant epilepsy. Depress Anxiety, 15, 4, 190–2.

Beyenburg, S.; Stoffel-Wagner, B. & Bauer J, et al. (2001). Neuroactive steroids and seizure susceptibility. Epilepsy Res, 44, (2-3), 141–53.

Charney ,D.S. (2003). Neuroanatomical circuits modulating fear and anxiety behaviors. Acta Psychiatr Scand, (Suppl. 417), 38–50.

Blanco, C.; Schneier, F.R. & Schmidt, A (2003). Pharmacological treatment of social anxiety disorder: a meta-analysis. Depress Anxiety, 18, 1, 29–40.

Caplan, R.; Siddarth, P. & Gurbani, S. et al. (2005). Depression and anxiety disorders in pediatric epilepsy. Epilepsia, 46, 5, 720–30.

Cendes, F.; Andermann, F. & Gloor, P. et al. (1994). Relationship between atrophy of the amygdala and ictal fear in temporal lobe epilepsy. Brain, 117, 4, 739–46.

Chapouthier, G.; Venault, P. (2001). A pharmacological link between epilepsy and anxiety? Trends Pharmacol Sci, 22, 491–3.

Couldridge, L.; Kendall, S. & March, A. (2001). A systematic overview—a decade of research: the information and counselling needs of people with epilepsy. Seizure, 10, 8, 605–14.

Depaulis, A.; Helfer, V.; Deransart, C. & Marescaux, C. (1997). Anxiogeniclike consequences in animal models of complex partial seizures. Neurosci Biobehav Rev, 21, 767–74.

Engelberts, N.H.; Klein, M.; Kasteleijn-Nolst Trenite, D.G.; Heimans, J.J. & Van der Ploeg, H.M. (2002). The effectiveness of psychological interventions for patients with relatively well-controlled epilepsy. Epilepsy Behav, 3, 420–6.

Ettinger, A.B.; Weisbrot, D.M. & Nolan, E.E., et al. (1998). Symptoms of depression and anxiety in pediatric epilepsy patients. Epilepsia, 39, 595–9.

García-Morales, I.; De la Peña Mayor, P. & Kanner, A,M. (2008). Psychiatric comorbidities in epilepsy: identification and treatment. Neurologist, Nov, 14(6 Suppl 1), 15-25.

Goldstein, M.A. & Harden CL. (2000). Epilepsy and anxiety. Epilepsy Behav, 1, 228–34.

Goldstein, L.H.; McAlpine, M.; Deale, A.; Toone, B.K. & Mellers, J.D. (2003). Cognitive behaviour therapy with adults with intractable epilepsy and psychiatric comorbidity: preliminary observations on changes in psychological state and seizure frequency. Behav Res Ther, 41, 447–60.

Handal, N.M.; Masand, P. &Weilburg, J.B. (1995). Panic disorder and complex partial seizures: a truly complex relationship. Psychosomatics, 36, 498–502.

Jacoby, A.; Snape, D. & Baker, G.A. (2005). Epilepsy and social identity: the stigma of a chronic neurological disorder. Lancet Neurol, 4, 171–8.

Jobe, P.C. & Browning, R.A. (2005). The serotonergic and noradrenergic effects of antidepressant drugs are anticonvulsant, not proconvulsant. Epilepsy Behav, 7, 602–19.

Johannessen Landmark, C. (2008). Antiepileptic drugs in non-epilepsy disorders: relations between mechanisms of action and clinical efficacy. CNS Drugs, 22, 27–47.

Jones, R.; Rickards, H. & Cavanna, A.E. (2010). The prevalence of psychiatric disorders in epilepsy: a critical review of the evidence. Funct Neurol, 25, 191-4.

Johnson, E.K.; Jones, J.E.; Seidenberg, M. & Hermann, B.P. (2004). The relative impact of anxiety, depression, and clinical seizure features on health-related quality of life in epilepsy. Epilepsia. 2004, 45, 544-50.

Kanner, A.M. (2011). Depression and epilepsy: A bidirectional relation? Epilepsia. Jan;52 Suppl 1:21-7. doi: 10.1111/j.1528-1167.2010.02907.x.

Kanner, A.M.; Barry, J.J.; Gilliam, F.; Hermann, B. & Meador, K.J. (2010). Anxiety disorders, subsyndromic depressive episodes, and major depressive episodes: do they differ on their impact on the quality of life of patients with epilepsy? Epilepsia, 51, 1152-8.

Kanner, A.M. & Palac, S. (2000). Depression in epilepsy: a common but often unrecognized comorbid malady. Epilepsy Behav, 1, 37–51.

Kanner, A.M.; Soto, A. & Gross-Kanner, H. (2004). Prevalence and clinical characteristics of postictal psychiatric symptoms in partial epilepsy. Neurology, 62, 708–13.

Kendall, S.; Thompson,D. & Couldridge, L. (2004). The information needs of carers of adults diagnosed with epilepsy. Seizure, 13, 499–508.

Kessler, R.C.; Avenevoli, S. & Merikangas K. (2001). Mood disorders in children and adolescents: an epidemiologic perspective. Biol Psychiatry, 49, 1002–14.

Ketter, T.A.; Post, R.M. & Theodore, W.H. (1993). Positive and negative psychiatric effects of antiepileptic drugs in patients with seizure disorders. Neurology, 53(Suppl. 2), 53–67.

Kinrys, G.; Pollack, M.H.; Simon, N.M.; Worthington, J.J.; Nardi, A.E. & Versiani, M. (2003). Valproic acid for the treatment of social anxiety disorder. Int Clin Psychopharmacol, 18, 169–72.

Lydiard, R.B. (2003). The role of GABA in anxiety disorders. J Clin Psychiatry, 64, (Suppl. 3), 21–7.

Marsh, L. & Rao V (2002). Psychiatric complications in patients with epilepsy: a review. Epilepsy Res, 49:11–33.

Macrodimitris, S.; Wershler, J. & Hatfield, M., et al. (2011). Group cognitive-behavioral therapy for patients with epilepsy and comorbid depression and anxiety Epilepsy Behav. 20, 1, 83-8.

Moshé, S.L.; Perucca, E.; Wiebe, S. & Mathern, G.W. (2011). The International League Against Epilepsy at the threshold of its second century: year 1. Epilepsia, 52,1, 185-7. doi: 10.1111/j.1528-1167.2010.02922.x.

Mula, M.; Pini, S. & Cassano, G.B. (2007). The role of anticonvulsant drugs in anxiety disorders: a critical review of the evidence. J Clin Psychopharmacol, 27, 263–72.

Mula, M. & Monaco, F. (2009). Antiepileptic drugs and psychopathology of epilepsy: an update. Epileptic Disord, 11, 1, 1-9.

Newsom-Davis, I.; Goldstein, L.H. & Fitzpatrick, D. (1988). Fear of seizures: an investigation and treatment. Seizure, 7, 101–6.

Issacs, K.L.; Philbeck, J.W.; Barr, W.B.; Devinsky, O. & Alper, K. (2004). Obsessive-compulsive symptoms in patients with temporal lobe epilepsy. Epilepsy Behav, 5, 569–74.

Oguz, A.; Kurul, S. & Dirik, E. (2002). Relationship of epilepsy-related factors to anxiety and depression scores in epileptic children. J Child Neurol, 17, 37–40.

Pande, A.C.; Crockatt, J.G. & Feltner, D.E. et al (2003). Pregabalin in generalized anxiety disorder: a placebo-controlled trial. Am J Psychiatry 160, 533–40.

Pande, A.C.; Pollack, M.H. & Crockatt, J. et al. (2000). Placebo-controlled study of gabapentin treatment of panic disorder. J Clin Psychopharmacol 20, 467–71.

Pellock, J.M. (2004). Defining the problem: psychiatric and behavioral comorbidity in children and adolescents with epilepsy. Epilepsy Behav 5(Suppl.), 3–9.

Pianta, R.C. & Lothman, D.J. (1994). Predicting behavior problems in children with epilepsy: child factors, disease factors, family stress, and child–mother interaction. Child Dev, 65, 1415–28.

Piazzini, A.; Canevini, M.P.; Maggiori, G. & Canger, R. (2001). Depression and anxiety in patients with epilepsy. Epilepsy Behav, 2, 481–9.

Ring, H.A.; Moriarty, J. & Trimble, M.R. (1998). A prospective study of the early postsurgical psychiatric associations of epilepsy surgery. J Neurol Neurosurg Psychiatry 64, 5, 601604.

Rosenthal, M. (2003). Tiagabine for the treatment of generalized anxiety disorder: a randomized, open-label, clinical trial with paroxetine as a positive control. J Clin Psychiatry, 64, 1245–9.

Schmitz, B. (2002). Antidepressant drugs: indications and guidelines for use in epilepsy. Epilepsia, 43(Suppl. 2), 14–8.

Scicutella, A. & Ettinger, A.B. (2002). Treatment of anxiety in epilepsy. Epilepsy Behav, 3(Suppl. 5), 10–2.

Spector, S.; Tranah, A.; Cull, C. & Goldstein, L.H. (1999). Reduction in seizure frequency following a short-term group intervention for adults with epilepsy. Seizure, 8, 297–303.

Tellez-Zenteno, J.F.; Patten, S.B.; Jetté, N.; Williams, J. & Wiebe, S. (2007). Psychiatric comorbidity in epilepsy: a population-based analysis. Epilepsia. 2007, 48, 12, 2336-44.

Thome-Souza, S.; Kuczynski, E. & Assumpção, Jr F., et al. (2004). Which factors may play a pivotal role on determining the type of psychiatric disorder in children and adolescents with epilepsy? Epilepsy Behav, 5, 988–94.

Trimble, M.R. & Van, Elst, L.T. (2003). The amygdala and psychopathology studies in epilepsy. Ann NY Acad Sci, 985, 461–8.

Vazquez, B. & Devinsky, O. (2003). Epilepsy and anxiety. Epilepsy Behav, 4(Suppl. 4), 20–5.

Waaler, P.E.; Blom, B.H.; Skeidsvoll, H. & Mykletun, A. (2000). Prevalence, classification, and severity of epilepsy in children in western Norway. Epilepsia, 41, 7, 802-10.

Williams, J.; Steel, C. & Sharp, G.B. et al. (2003). Anxiety in children with epilepsy. Epilepsy Behav, 4, 729-32.

Wittchen, H.U.; Kessler, R.C.; Beesdo, K.; Krause, P.; Hofler, M. & Hoyer, J. (2002). Generalized anxiety and depression in primary care: prevalence, recognition, and management. J Clin Psychiatry, 63(Suppl. 8), 24-34.

13

Disabling Osteoarthritis and Symptomatic Anxiety: Impact and Implications

Ray Marks
Departments of Health, Physical Education & Gerontological Studies and Services
City University of New York, York College and Health and Behavior Studies
Columbia University, Teachers College, New York
USA

1. Introduction

Psychological conditions, such as anxiety, are highly prevalent among adults in general, and among adults with a variety of medical disorders (Fava et al., 2010) and chronic physical conditions, in particular (Sareen et al., 2006; Scott et al., 2007). Anxiety, which may commonly take the form of panic attacks or generalized anxiety, is also frequently associated with depression (Burns et al., 2010; Scott et al., 2007), worse subjective physical health (Paukert et al., 2010), and chronic conditions such as arthritis (Sareen et al., 2006).

This chapter describes the literature and research evidence concerning the nature of anxiety, its prevalence among aging adults, and the impact of comorbid and/or concurrent anxiety symptoms among adults with moderate to severe osteoarthritis, a highly prevalent and painful disabling joint disease. It also highlights the implications of anxiety in the context of osteoarthritis and advocates for improved efforts to identify and treat concomitant anxiety among adults with this condition, regardless of disease stage.

To achieve these aims, the author reports data embedded in the PubMed, Scopus, Science Citation and PsychInfo data bases, as well as data extracted from records of 1,000 hip osteoarthritis surgical candidates. Divided into three parts, this evidence is used to describe the clinical syndromes of anxiety and osteoarthritis, to highlight the implications of the presence of preexisting comorbid anxiety, comorbid anxiety and depression, as well as state anxiety in adults diagnosed as having osteoarthritis, and to argue for more routine screening of anxiety among cases with osteoarthritis.

2. Anxiety and anxiety disorders

Anxiety, a generic term encompassing several common mental health disorders is a psychological syndrome associated with excess fear, and worry. Varying from mild to severe, anxiety disorders are common, costly public health problems that can affect as many as 24.9% of adults over their lifetime (Kessler et al., 1994), and can occur independently, as well as in association with many chronic health conditions (Ying et al., 2010). In addition, anxiety, which is an emotional reaction associated with a heightened state of arousal (Scopaz et al., 2009), is often associated with high rates of medically unexplained syndromes and the excessive utilization of health care resources. As well, anxiety disorders are strongly associated with low levels of physical health and life quality (Medlowicz & Stein, 2000), as well as high levels of physical disability and functional limitations (Brenes et al., 2005). Anxiety, is also found to play a role in influencing the functional ability of persons with arthritis (Hill et al., 2007), plus the frequency and extent of athletic and sports injuries (Lavallee & Flint, 1996), a strong precursor of future osteoarthritis.

Occurring in at least 5-10% of medically ill or primary care patients (Fava et al., 2010), including those with depression (Kroenke et al., 2010), anxiety can contribute to the fear-avoidance process that can adversely impact health outcomes in people with musculoskeletal conditions (Scopaz et al., 2009). Compared to a prevalence rate for depression of 7.2% in the general population, social anxiety occurred 7% of the time, panic disorder, 4.6% of the time, and generalized anxiety disorder occurred 3.4% of the time (Wiltink et al., 2010). Indeed, despite the fact that anxiety is often overlooked in medical settings when compared to depression, anxiety disorders and their adverse health effects in adults with chronic health conditions can be demonstrated to be as great as those identified for depression (Roy-Byrne et al., 2008).

Several current researchers have consequently posed strong arguments in favor of heightened efforts to screen for the presence of an anxiety disorder in the context of primary care and related settings. In addition, some have stressed the further importance of identifying and correctly diagnosing the type(s) of anxiety syndrome (s) that prevail. In addition, most current reports stress the importance of effectively intervening to minimize the progression of anxiety disorder syndromes, all of which can have an extremely negative impact on the affected individual, including their ability to work and to carry out commonplace activities of daily living (Roy-Byrne et al., 2008; www.medicalnewstoday/info/anxiety, 2010)

In terms of classifying anxiety disorders, which are neurotic disorders where the symptom of anxiety is present or is the predominant feature (Davies & Craig, 2010), two chief categories have been delineated, namely, trait and state anxiety. Trait anxiety refers to the presence of a long-lasting disorder of excessive emotional arousal, which can get worse if not treated (National Institutes of Health, 2009). Commonly termed the generalized anxiety disorder or GAD, this well-established diagnostic disorder is associated with excessive worry about a variety of non-specific situations that are perceived as threatening. Panic disorder, another form of anxiety, is more closely related to a specific extrinsic threat and frequently occurs episodically in response to this identifiable stimulus. While both forms may have a genetic origin, suggesting they are not readily amenable to intervention, both may prevail as learned responses as a result of certain life experiences and exposures and may hence be modifiable (Thompson, 1993). Post-traumatic syndrome, obsessive-compulsive disorder, phobias, social anxiety disorder, and separation anxiety disorder are other forms of anxiety that may prevail among adult populations, and alone or in combination with other forms of anxiety and/or health conditions, all can interfere with work, school, social and work relationships, and the adoption and adherence to health-enhancing behaviors.

Moreover, since many forms of anxiety are accompanied by physical symptoms such as pain and heart palpitations, breathlessness, hyperventilation, headaches, nausea, tiredness, and tension, tremor, parasthesia, irritability, and gastrointestinal disturbances (Tyrer, 1984), the presence of an anxiety disorder can significantly influence one's physical health status in an adverse manner. Physical illnesses, in turn, can readily precipitate psychological distress in the form of state anxiety, a transitory emotional state of apprehension, especially prevalent among older adults (Paukert et al., 2010). Moreover, the presence of such a transitory state of anxiety, may indicate the underlying presence of GAD in the geriatric medically ill patient, and according to Wetherell et al. (2010) should not be discounted simply as a by-product of medical illnesses or depression, because left untreated, could significantly heighten the severity of the prevailing health condition(s). A persistent state of transitory anxiety can also serve as a precursor for subsequent depression (VanDyke et al., 2004).

Because all anxiety disorders have such an immense personal and social cost, the ability to accurately measure these states is crucial. Among the validated inventories described in the literature for detecting and classifying the presence, type, and magnitude of anxiety are: the Structured Clinical Interview for DSM-IV (SCID) and Diagnostic Criteria for Psychosomatic Research (DCPR) (Fava et al., 2010); the Beck Anxiety Scale (Ozcetin et al., 2007), the Generalized Anxiety Disorder (GAD) Scale (Kroenke et al. 2010; Wetherell et al., 2010); the Brief Symptom Inventory-18, Mini International Neuropsychiatric Interview; the Anxiety Disorders Interview Schedule (Wetheral et al., 2010); the Hospital Anxiety and Depression Scale (HADS) (Axford et al., 2010); the Hopkins Symptom Checklist (Brennes et al., 2005); The Zung Depression and Anxiety Inventory (Salafi et al., 1991), The Mental Health Inventory (Smith & Zautra, 2008), the State Trait Anxiety Inventory (Montin et al., 20070, and the Spielberger State and Trait Anxiety Inventory (Giraudet-Le Quintrec et al., 2003). It should be noted though that while all of these instruments provide measures of the extent of anxiety, they have often been used without specification of their circumstances, all use self-report and commonly differ in terms of the particular form of anxiety that is included (McCracken et al., 1996).

However, using the DSM-IV inventory, studies have shown a significant linear relationship between the presence of anxiety and depressive disorders and the presence of medically unexplained physical symptoms, and more medical symptoms in adults with chronic medical illnesses (Katon et al., 2007). In addition, among most common medical disorders, pain is as consistently associated with anxiety as objective disease indicators are (Katon et al.). Potential causes and predictors of anxiety in addition to medical illnesses and pain include: genetics, the environment, including the physical, psychological and dietary environment, trauma (National Institutes of Health, 2009), obesity and a high fat diet (Van Der Kraan, 2010), being female, having low perceived health and high levels of disability (Wu et al., 2002), and possible brain biochemistry abnormalities. Potential determinants of excess disability due to anxiety may include: suboptimal physical activity levels, benzodiazepine and psychotropic medication usage, and insufficient levels of social support (Brenes et al., 2005).

3. Osteoarthritis

Osteoarthritis, a highly prevalent chronic health condition affecting many older adults commonly results in progressively destructive changes in one or more joints and its surrounding tissues. Often associated with other chronic health conditions, most commonly, cardiovascular diseases and obesity, the disease produces varying degrees of chronic and acute pain, plus disability. The disease specifically limits the ability to function physically, as well as the chances of experiencing a high life quality (Montin et al., 2007).

Although often described solely as a physically disabling syndrome, amenable largely to pharmacologic interventions (Tallon et al., 2000), a reasonable body of research shows behavioral conditions such as anxiety can occur at rates of up to 50% among osteoarthritis cases (Mella et al., 2010). In addition, the importance of identifying and acknowledging this possibility is supported by recent evidence showing adults with knee osteoarthritis report considerable anxiety (Tallon et al., 2000), and tend to have poorer function if they exhibit high rather than low anxiety rates (Scopaz et al., 2009). The osteoarthritic patient with high anxiety levels is also found to experience higher disability rates than those with lower anxiety levels (Creamer et al., 2000). At the hip, where the disease affects 3/100 men and women between 55-74 years of age (Whittle et al., 1990), it is anticipated that existential anxiety (Gustafsson et al., 2010) and/or comorbid anxiety and depression are likely to co-exist (Ying et al., 2010), and contribute to its severity (Scott et al., 2007). Yet interventions to minimize anxiety have traditionally played a very limited role in the case management process for this condition.

Indeed, despite the immense impact of osteoarthritis on the national health expenditures of the United States (Weinberger et al., 1989), very little specific information about the role of anxiety and poor psychological health on the magnitude of the disability experienced by adults with this condition exists, when compared to the plethora of research on the physical problems accompanying the disease. In addition, reports that do exist are conflicting. For example, while one highlighted a need for an evaluation of mental health status at time of surgery for purposes of maximizing functional status following hip replacement surgery (Bischoff et al., 2004), another found no immediate impact on this (Caracciolo & Giaquinto, 2005).

To provide a more comprehensive understanding of this topic than is presently available, all relevant papers published between 1976 and Jan 2011 in the major data bases were extracted and reviewed. In addition, related data from this researcher's clinical observations were scrutinized. These data were specifically explored to examine if pain, the problem of most significance to people with osteoarthritis, is significantly heightened by the presence of excessive anxiety as observed early on by Lunghi et al. They were also explored to identify if higher levels of anxiety are likely to be associated with higher degrees of functional impairment among this patient population as discussed by Lunghi et al.

3.1 Key research findings

In support of the findings by Lunghi et al. Summers et al. who examined cases of primary hip or knee osteoarthritis using outpatient department computer lists showed higher levels of state anxiety were significantly correlated with higher pain scores on all dimensions of the McGill Pain Questionnaire, except the evaluation dimension. In addition, high levels of trait anxiety were significantly associated with higher levels of affective pain and pain intensity scores. State anxiety was also significantly and positively correlated with all measures on the Sickness Impact Profile Inventory, and high levels of trait anxiety were associated with greater functional impairment on several of the Sickness Impact Profile subscales, and the overall score. This research was consistent with findings by Salafi et al. (1991) who examined the relationship between disability and psychological variables of anxiety and depression among 61 women with symptomatic knee osteoarthritis. Using an anxiety inventory, and a pain and disability index, they found disability and pain correlated with the degree of psychological involvement.

Similarly, a more recent paper that focused on psychological factors and their relation to osteoarthritis pain in a sample of 266 cases with hip and/or knee osteoarthritis, revealed a strong association between worsened measures of mental health and pain and risk of pain flares (Wise et al., 2009). This finding was consistent with work by Creamer et al. who examined the relationship of anxiety and depression among cases with knee osteoarthritis and found anxiety as assessed using the trait section of the Speilberger State Trait Anxiety

Inventory was associated with self-reported disability as measured using the Western Ontario Measurement Assessment tool (Creamer et al., 2000).

While Creamer et al. felt it was unclear from their cross-sectional study whether anxiety is a risk factor for subsequent disability or whether disability is, itself, a reason why subjects become more anxious, anxiety could provoke the onset of degenerative joint changes if after an acute injury for example, pain and fear triggered anxiety and movement limitations that lead to loss of muscle bulk, generalized deconditioning and loss of confidence. Although only prospective studies can potentially clarify this issue, anxiety can foster injury (Lavallee and Flint, 1996), and injury can lead to osteoarthritic joint damage. Especially in the context of total hip replacement for severe hip osteoarthritis where many candidates have previously fallen and fractured their hips, it seems patients who demonstrate declining, rather than improved functional ability following this procedure, may do so as a result of factors related to their mental health status, rather than their physical status (Badura-Brzoza et al., 2008). In this regard, Rolfson et al. (2009) found pre-operative anxiety/depression was a strong predictor of pain relief and patient satisfaction, in that those who were less anxious had less pain and were more satisfied with the surgical procedure and its outcome. Similarly, Badura-Brzoza et al. (2009) who conducted a longitudinal investigation concerning the relation between some psychological and psychiatric factors and their influence on health-related quality of life in 102 patients after total hip replacement, found trait anxiety was significantly associated with postoperative mental as well as physical performance.

Likewise, Smith and Zautra (2008) who examined the effects of anxiety on pain in women with osteoarthritis and rheumatoid arthritis found anxiety was related to elevations in current and forthcoming pain estimates, suggesting anxiety is important in explaining the progression of the disease, and in provoking a fear of participating in those physical activities that are essential for minimizing overall disability. In particular, when studying the differential effects of depression and anxiety on pain, it was noted that the effects were nearly twice as large for anxiety compared to depression, suggesting the mechanism of action is unique, and needs much more emphasis in the clinical arena than is presently evidenced.

These data were further substantiated by Axelrod et al. (2010) who undertook to ascertain the prevalence of anxiety and depressive disorders in an outpatient population with osteoarthritis. This group also examined the interrelationships between the severity of the disease, pain, disability, and depression, using the Hospital Anxiety and Depression Scale (HADS), along with a structured clinical interview. Among the 54 patients studied, the majority of whom were women, the prevalence of clinically significant anxiety and/or depression was 40.7%. In addition, this group found pain correlated with the prevailing anxiety and depression scores and disability was greater in patients with a combined depression and anxiety history.

3.2 Additional research findings

Since anxiety can undoubtedly contribute to a poor treatment response, if unrecognized and/or untreated (Katon et al., 2007), we recently elected to conduct a retrospective review of the available records of 1,000 hip osteoarthritis surgical candidates to ascertain whether anxiety is a prevalent feature of this condition, and if so, what implications, if any, does the presence of anxiety have for this population. Additional data on medical comorbidities, pain, and function before surgery, and discharge destination after surgery, which is a proxy for functional achievement was also extracted. As outlined in a previous publication (Marks, 2009), the peri-operative data showed approximately nine percent (92 cases) of the cohort had a prior mental health disorder, and among these patients, 5.5% (44 cases) reported Trait Anxiety histories, alone or in combination with Trait Depression. Among the 112 cases reporting either the presence of Trait Anxiety and/or State Anxiety, 9 cases reported having both of these conditions, and a further 9 with Depression histories reported State Anxiety. However, most of the 90 cases experiencing State Anxiety had no prior anxiety history (See Table 1).

	Depr Hx	Dep+SA	Dep/Anx Hx	TA	SA	SA+ TA
N	50	9	20	22	90	9
%	5	0.9	2.0	2.2	9.0	0.9

Abbreviations: Dep=depression; Hx=history; SA=state anxiety; TA=trait anxiety

Table 1. Distribution of mental health status of 92 cases with pre-existing Depression and/or Anxiety and 90 reporting State Anxiety among 1,000 hip osteoarthritis cases requiring hip replacement related surgery and percentage of these cases in each observed diagnostic category.

When analyzed further to examine the implications of the presence of anxiety on the presentation of the surgical patients' health status, more women than men with hip osteoarthritis were found to suffer from either trait depression and anxiety, trait anxiety, and/or state anxiety ($p < 0.001$), and those with depression and anxiety histories tended to be more impaired before surgery in terms of numbers of blocks they were able to walk than those with no mental health condition (See Table 2).

Condition	N	Mean	SEM	F	p
Depression+Anxiety	17	2.94	.9	1.94	.12
Trait Anxiety	22	4.05	1.1		
Otherwise Healthy	40	5.04	.8		
State Anxiety	29	3.14	.5		

Table 2. Table showing mean and standard error of the mean (SEM) numbers of blocks walked prior to surgery as reported by 108 cases with different categories of mental health status about to undergo hip surgery for hip osteoarthritis related problems.

In addition, those with concomitant depression and anxiety histories also tended to recover more slowly than those with no such history ($p < 0.001$) and had higher levels of pain on a visual analogue scale than those with anxiety alone or those with no such history ($p < 0.008$) (See Table 3).

From the data reviewed, it was also shown that those with anxiety histories tended to be heavier on average than those with no anxiety history with body mass indices of 28.5±8.0 compared to 27.2±3.9, respectively, and on average most had at least one comorbid health condition, even though the sub-group representing those with a Trait Anxiety history tended to be younger than those with depression, those with no anxiety or depression history, and those exhibiting State Anxiety (58.1±11.9 versus 62.5±10.7, 62.5±11.5 and 64.6±12.5 years of age, respectively).

By contrast, those patients expressing State Anxiety tended to be slightly older than the average otherwise healthy patient, and not surprisingly therefore, this subgroup presented with higher numbers of comorbid illnesses on average than those with Trait Anxiety or No Anxiety (1.6 versus 1.22 versus 0; $p < 001$).

Condition	N	Day 1 Post Surgery	Day 3 Post Surgery	Extent of Improvement	% Change
Depression +Anxiety	17	7.5+13.1	74.5+65.9	67	90
Trait Anxiety	18	9.8+18.5	68.7+48.6	58.9	85
Otherwise Healthy	37	13.5+21.7	116.2+65.6	102.7	112
State Anxiety	19	50.9+45.4	70.6+44.1	19.7	27
p		0.001	0.046		

Table 3. Table showing Day 1 and Day 3 recovery rates in distance walked in feet after surgery for 91 cases with hip osteoarthritis as assessed by analysis of variance.

In terms of discharge destination, a surrogate functional measure of outcome, the discharge site correlated with the presence or absence of an anxiety history, and in a comparative subsample analysis, 25% of 42 cases with an anxiety history were discharged to Rehabilitation Centers, compared to 10.6 percent of 47 cases with no pre-existing anxiety history (p < 001).

Finally, the State Anxiety perceptions expressed by patients prior to surgery were highly variable even though several broad categories or several themes could be identified among these as outlined in Table 4.

In addition to the variety of issues perceived as threatening to several cases of hip osteoarthritis undergoing surgery who had had no prior background history of anxiety, among patients who expressed feelings of anxiety before their surgery and who had either a pre-existing anxiety or depression history, there were the following comments:

2 cases said they were generally anxious about surgery

1 case said they were very nervous about surgery

1 other case said they were anxious about rehabilitation and scarring

1 further case said they were very anxious and despondent over pain and immobility to walk and care for grandchildren

Finally, one said they were anxious about experiencing excessive pain and had a fear of the hospital.

Thus no specific pattern of fears or anxiety were evident, and clearly some were worried about pending events, and some were more apprehensive over future events.

4. Implications of anxiety in the context of osteoarthritis

Osteoarthritis is a common painful disease affecting many older adults. Associated with functional limitations and pain, the problem of major concern to patients, the disease is often progressive and requires extensive self-management.

Although there is no hard evidence the assessment and treatment of anxiety will reduce the burden of osteoarthritis, it is the author's view that the aforementioned research provides a fairly solid argument for intervening to prevent and treat both trait and state anxiety that may detrimentally handicap a patient's ability to maximize their own health. That is, as outlined by Summers et al. (1988), there is little doubt that psychological factors such as the presence of anxiety and/or anxiety and depression are of significance in pathogenesis of osteoarthritis, and are especially likely to influence pain and the degree of functional impairment experienced by this patient group, both negatively and significantly (Hochberg

Types of Anxiety Expressed	Examples and Numbers of Patients Experiencing these Feelings
General anxiety	*"Anxious to get condition corrected"-1* *"I feel very anxious"-3* *"I feel anxious and want to speak to a nurse"-1*
Pain and mobility	*"I am anxious about pain"-4* *"I am anxious because I can't convey information about pain"* -1 *"1 am anxious about whether pain will go away"* – 1
Surgery	*"I am anxious about surgery in view of age"* – 1 *"I am anxious about recovery and surgery going well -2"* *"Anxious about work after surgery"* - 2 *"Worried operation will have complications"* -1 *"Anxious about operation"* -1 *"I am feeling anxious and nervous about the surgery"-14*
Other	*"Anxious about medications and food"* – 1 *"Anxious about surgery and history of phlebitis"* – 1 *"Anxious because of dependency for activities of daily living"* - 1 *"Anxious about physical limitations"* – 1 *"Anxious about limited function-walking and shopping"* -1 *"Anxious about physical condition"* -1 *"Anxious about being released to early"* -1 *"Anxious about extent of disability"* -1
Anxious about post-operative situation	*"Very worried about post-operative pain"*-1 *"Anxious and scared about surgery and ability to move around afterwards"*-2 *"Anxious about returning to normal"* -1

Table 4. Table showing a selected variety of anxiety perceptions and their sub-themes as expressed by adults undergoing hip joint surgery for hip osteoarthritis before surgery.

et al., 1989). More specifically, psychological factors, such as anxiety, which is amenable to intervention, can potentially predict early warning signs of hypertension/heart disease, a common comorbid condition observed in people with osteoarthritis that increases the prevailing disability quite considerably (Marks & Allegrante, 2002; Weinberger et al., 1989). Moreover, as argued by Summers et al. (1988) variables such as anxiety may have a negative impact on the adult with osteoarthritis, because anxiety may reduce pain tolerance, thus contributing to an ongoing cycle of inactivity and further pain.

Not surprisingly, Davis et al. (1992) who examined the associations of various health indicators and the psychological well-being of adults with and without radiographic knee osteoarthritis found psychological well-being and health status were consistently associated with knee pain, regardless of whether the individual had evidence of radiographic knee osteoarthritis or not. That is, self-reported knee pain correlated significantly with the presence of psychological distress, rather than visible joint destruction, a finding also noted for 61 women with knee osteoarthritis by Salafi et al. (1991) and by Creamer et al. (2000).

Similarly Van Baar et al. (1998) found that after controlling for other characteristics, the psychological characteristics of patients with osteoarthritis, contributed as much as the more traditional kinesiological measures to the patient's disability.

These findings of Van Baar et al. (1998) were consistent with those of Sareen et al. who examined the relationship between comorbid anxiety disorders and the presence of various physical conditions. This group found the presence of anxiety was associated with poorer levels of physical functioning, and past 30-day disability scores due to physical problems. It was concluded that anxiety disorders are independently associated with several physical conditions including arthritis, and as such can significantly impact quality of life and disability, and perceived barriers to care (Weinberger et al., 1989). Not unexpectedly, a related prospective study by Dieppe et al. (2000) found adults with osteoarthritis examined over an eight year period generally had a poor outcome with high levels of physical disability, as well as anxiety, and a high level of healthcare resource utilization, especially if they had knee osteoarthritis.

The high rate of anxiety symptoms in people with osteoarthritis, and its strong negative correlation with their functional scores (Ozcetin et al., 2007) is not unexpected given its association with both pain and with obesity (Witlink et al., 2010), and avoidance behaviors (Scopaz et al., 2009). Indeed allied research shows obesity, a highly prevalent condition observed among adults with osteoarthritis can significantly increase the risk for mental illness, and the finding that the cohort studied by Marks (2007) tended to show higher body mass indices in those with anxiety histories supports this relationship. Moreover, as discussed by Chan et al. (2008), adults with mental illnesses, including anxiety, obesity and one or more physical illness, such as osteoarthritis, are more likely to be impaired than those without any mental illnesses.

New evidence from an animal model of arthritis, further suggests arthritis is likely to be accompanied by both heightened anxiety responses, as well as a locomotor impairment in its early phases (Skulova et al., 2010), thus stressing the importance of early treatment of osteoarthritis, in general to allay reactive anxiety that can trigger movement avoidance, loss of muscle bulk, generalized deconditioning and loss of confidence (Creamer et al., 2000). Strengthening this argument is evidence from several clinical studies that reveal that negative affective states, such as anxiety, are strongly associated with pain, disability and poor life quality among people with osteoarthritis (e.g., Creamer et al., 2000; Keefe et al., 2002; Ozcetin et al., 2007), and level of pain and pain-related fear are correlated with functional limitations (Heuts et al., 2004). Anxiety and depression can also co-exist among adults with osteoarthritis and this could have an even greater influence on their ability to function physically than those with only one of these conditions, as identified by Axelrod et al. (20010).

This link between anxiety, pain, and disability in people with osteoarthritis, which was also observed by Marks (2007) in almost 9.5% of end-stage hip osteoarthritis cases suggests ample numbers of adults with disabling osteoarthritis may have mood and/or anxiety disorder histories that may often go undetected or overlooked in the treatment schedule being offered. An equal number may exhibit prevailing symptoms of emotional distress that may occur simultaneously or independently, either before or after surgery, or both, as well, and this can magnify pre-operative osteoarthritis disability and slow the post-operative recovery process (Badura-Brzoza et al., 2008), thus strengthening the case for preventing and treating anxiety in adults with osteoarthritis at all disease stages. Indeed, even though surgery for osteoarthritis is usually successful, it has been observed that even the presence of moderate trait anxiety can significantly impair the hip osteoarthritis surgical candidates health quality of life both before, as well as after surgery (Montin et al., 2007), even though this is often believed to return the patient to optimal function. The cumulative effect of anxiety on osteoarthritis outcomes is conceptualized in Figure 1.

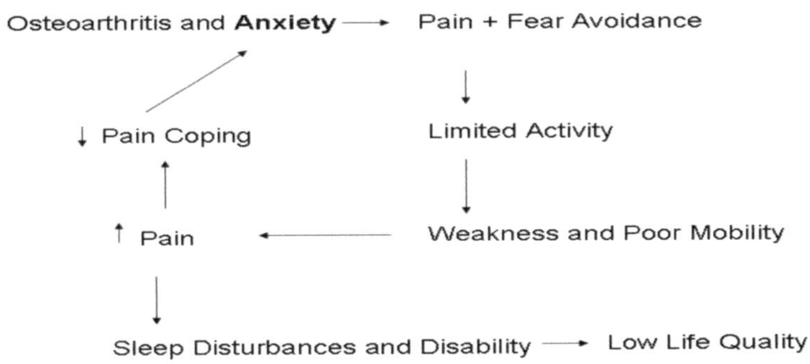
Osteoarthritis and Anxiety
Pain + Fear Avoidance
↓ Pain Coping
Limited Activity
↑ Pain
Weakness and Poor Mobility
Sleep Disturbances and Disability
Low Life Quality

Fig. 1. Schematic representation of problems heightened by anxiety among cases with osteoarthritis.

Unfortunately, as Memel (2000) argued more than 10 years ago, general practitioners and other health providers have commonly lacked knowledge about either the importance of and/or the need to assess and treat the presence of anxiety in their osteoarthritis patients, even though data to this effect has prevailed. This need to enhance screening efforts and foster optimal psychological health among cases with osteoarthritis is becoming increasingly clear however, as outlined in Table 5 and Figure 1 above.

Additionally, data by Vrizekolk et al. (2010) provide further support for the importance of examining and diagnosing the presence of an anxiety related syndrome among cases with osteoarthritis, as well as among the general primary care population of adults. This group, who examined the psychological health status of patients with a variety of rheumatic conditions including osteoarthritis, found 64 percent of the sample met criteria for psychological distress at baseline. Although treatment improved this, 69 percent still experienced elevated distress levels and maladaptive illness cognitions after rehabilitation. These data are not surprising given findings that clearly show adults with trait anxiety are likely to experience worse outcomes than those who are not anxious, as well as higher pain levels, poorer coping behaviors, lower levels of physical activity participation, lower levels of social support, and poor sleep patterns, which in turn, could increase their pain and disablement experience adversely (Dekker et al., 2009; Khuwaje et al., 2010; Louie et al., 2010., Montin et al., 2007).

Moreover, since distinctive anxiety disorder subtypes prevail among adults with osteoarthritis, the specific type of anxiety disorder may contribute differentially or incrementally to the overall health related situation, plus the extent and rate of recovery, and may hence require specific, rather than the more common generic intervention approaches. In addition, to support and promote optimal health outcomes for the individual osteoarthritis sufferer, recent findings by Burns et al. (2010) suggest there may be advantages to assessing and categorizing any prevailing anxiety into either a distress or a fear disorder. This is because they found the generalized anxiety or distress disorder was associated with elevated anxiety symptoms during and after treatment. In contrast, fear disorders (i.e., panic disorder, agoraphobia, social phobia, specific phobia) were linked to depression. It could thus be of interest to examine these two specific anxiety-associated subcategories among cases of osteoarthritis, and as Burns suggests develop interventions to specifically target the type of prevailing distress observed.

Authors	Study procedures	Key findings
Axford et al. (2010)	54 cases with lower limb OA were studied	Anxiety is common in OA and is related to pain and disability
Badura-Brzoza et al. (2008)	Longitudinal study of 103 cases undergoing hip replacement surgery	Total hip replacement outcomes are influenced by trait anxiety
Creamer et al. (2000)	Cross-sectional study of 69 knee OA cases	Disability was associated with anxiety
Montin et al. (2007)	Longitudinal study hip OA cases before + after surgery	Pre-operative trait anxiety predicted health quality of life before and after surgery
Salmon et al. ((2001)	Longitudinal study of 102 cases undergoing hip Replacement surgery	Recovery at follow-up was slower in those with greater anxiety
Smith & Zautra, (2008)	88 cases of women with OA were studied	Anxiety was related to elevations in current and future pain at twice the rate for depression

Table 5. Overview of key findings linking anxiety to osteoarthritis outcomes over the past decade.

Furthermore, since a reasonable proportion of adults with both severe disabling osteoarthritis and GAD may be abusing addictive chemical substances to overcome their anxiety and/or pain (Alegria et al., 2010), this phenomenon should be specifically sought and treated accordingly, because this situation can significantly increase the chances of excess disability (Patten et al., 2006). Other evidence suggests that if either or both of these behavioral syndromes are not clearly distinguished, and adequately treated, their presence could result in higher levels of pain, slower recovery rates at follow-up if surgery is indicated (Salmon et al., 2001), more intense disease activity, and lower health quality of life than is desirable (James et al., 2005; Montin et al., 2007).

In sum, as outlined in Table 5, sufficient past and emerging evidence supports the view that in addition to examining the physical status of adults in routine clinical settings, primary care providers should go beyond their usual medical history to identify and diagnose the presence of psychological symptoms such as anxiety among their osteoarthritis patients. Those with low perceived health, those in pain, those who are overweight, those who have comorbid conditions, and those with high disability levels who are female should be especially targeted to avoid the adverse impact of anxiety on their health outcomes (Wu et al., 2002).

Similar assessments of the patient's needs and characteristics conducted in the context of the surgical setting, followed by tailored and targeted interventions with follow-up visits to re-examine their levels of anxiety with validated tests would also be highly desirable as outlined by Montin et al. (2007). Here again, women in the higher age categories, those with trait anxiety histories who are more likely to experience state anxiety (Montin et al., 2007), those who are overweight, those who exhibit excessively high anxiety levels (Daltroy et al., 1998), as well as those using narcotics should be specifically targeted. Available treatment options include the use of video information (Ayral et al. 2002), serotonin-reuptake inhibitors (Wu et al., 2002), benzodiazepines applied in therapeutic doses, pre-operative education (Bondy et al., 1999; Giraudet-Le Quintrec et al., 2003; Lin et al., 1997), guided imagery (Montin et al., 2007), anxiety management (Feeney, 2004), social rehabilitation (Badura-Brzoza et al., 2008), and Cognitive Behavioral Therapy (Davis al., 2010) and the mode of intervention should take into account the diagnostic category and its severity.

Indeed, it seems imperative to do this for two reasons. First, because research shows adults with osteoarthritis who are found to suffer from trait anxiety are likely to experience worse outcomes than those who are not anxious, as well as higher current and future pain levels, poorer coping behaviors, lower levels of physical activity participation, lower levels of social support, and poor sleep patterns, which in turn, could increase their pain and disablement experience adversely (Dekker et al., 2009; Khuwaje et al., 2010; Louie et al., 2010., Montin et al., 2007; Smith & Zautra, 2008). Second, pre-operative state anxiety, which is associated with post-operative state anxiety is a significant predictor of pain among patients undergoing knee or hip replacements (Feeney (2004), and those who exhibit state anxiety are also likely to recover more slowly after surgery in the absence of intervention.

5. Conclusion

Anxiety is a serious health condition that may impact the extent of a chronic medical condition (Katon et al., 2007), as well as life quality and the ability to function optimally. Similarly, osteoarthritis, a progressive joint disease associated with pain and disability among aging adults (Hochberg et al., 1989, 1995) has been linked to a poor health outcome and excessive usage of health resources. Commonly described as a physical problem, premorbid or state-related affective comorbid conditions such as anxiety, which significantly increases the progression of disability among older adults (Brenes et al., 2005) may similarly influence osteoarthritis disease outcomes adversely. In particular, anxiety is commonly associated with poor adherence to self-care regimens and increased symptom burden and these factors can provoke or exacerbate osteoarthritis progression as suggested by findings of Katon et al. (2007). Not surprisingly, although often neglected in the context of primary care, an increasing body of emerging data shows consistent evidence of pre-morbid and/or concurrent psychiatric health conditions in sub-populations of adults with one or more medical diagnoses such as osteoarthritis that should be diagnosed and treated accordingly (Keefe et al., 2002). In addition, those with anxiety disorder histories appear to experience a lower life quality (Hopman-Rock et al., 1997), higher rates of pain and disability (Axford et al., 2010), and a lower ability to recover rapidly after joint replacement surgery when compared to their non-affected counterparts, plus less satisfaction with their intervention.

Yet, in the case of osteoarthritis, it is more common than not for practitioners to focus on the physical aspects of the disease and its medical management rather than on its psychological correlates, and thus no efforts may be forthcoming to implement anxiety reducing treatments that could positively affect functional outcomes later on. This specific situation may need to be remediated at the training level because it may be that primary care providers are unaware of the current research in this area showing psychosocial factors such as anxiety, which can predate the disease or can result from the condition, can determine the extent of the disability that arises over time. They may also be unaware of the methods of assessing anxiety clinically, and of the diverse modes of intervention that can alleviate anxiety. They may also assume that the level of anxiety that may prevail in cases with osteoarthritis of one or more joints is simply to be expected. Similarly adults with arthritis may be reticent to express their fears, thus remaining untreated.

Nonetheless, as outlined by Abrams et al. (2010) and Kim et al. (2010), because anxiety is an important health variable as far as increasing premature mortality and morbidity rates among the older chronically ill and disabled adult, especially the female osteoarthritis patient who is overweight and in the higher age range (Montin et al., 2007), psychometric tests for anxiety should be routinely applied, and those at risk should be treated accordingly, rather than overlooked, in both clinical and surgical settings (Axford et al., 2010). Other evidence shows that even if pain-relieving surgery is undertaken, patients with anxiety may not respond as well to surgery as those with no anxiety (Salmon et al., 2001), and their complexity of care may be increased (Montin et al., 2007), especially if cases with mixed anxiety states and or/anxiety and depression are not identified.

Indeed, the identification and accurate diagnosis of the presence of anxiety, plus the timely implementation of appropriate interventions to alleviate or minimize anxiety, might not only improve upon current health related outcomes, but might also serve to lower health service utilization and costs associated with the overall management of progressively disabling osteoarthritis. Moreover, timely intervention that maximizes function might also reduce symptoms of hypertension and heart disease and asthma caused by psychological distress, as well as any tendency to excess body weight, and pain that independently contributes to osteoarthritis disability. As well, the need for joint replacement surgery may be reduced or delayed by incorporating effective behavioral and psychological approaches into conservative treatment plans (Keefe et al., 2002). Finally, people with advanced osteoarthritis may benefit from joint replacement surgery to a greater extent than those treated solely in the biomedical model-if at the time of hospital referral - those with anxiety histories and those who express pre-surgical anxiety are identified, and precautions are taken to offset these risks as discussed by Giraudet-Le Quintrec et al. (2003).

In the interim, given that anxiety is commonly associated with chronic physical conditions such as osteoarthritis (Scott et al., 2007; Wu et al., 2002), and that anxiety may contribute to pain, pain-related fears and negative functional outcomes (Heuts et al., 2004), as well as indirectly to some forms of osteoarthritis as a result of injury (Lavallee & Flint, 1996), there is clearly a strong to prevent anxiety where this can be predicted, as well as a strong imperative to identify anxiety where it exists, and as to clearly characterize its specific nature, and better understand its etiology and temporal dimensions, in order to intervene effectively in the context of this disease. To this end Hill et al. (2007) emphasized that physicians need to recognize as well as address the significant additional negative impact anxiety can render on the patients' physical well being. In addition, Dorr and Chao (2007), who found that the pre-surgical emotional state of the patient undergoing joint replacement surgery affected their feelings of satisfaction after surgery, advocated for appropriate pre-operative education to allay any unwarranted negative impact. In addition, Dorr and Chao advocated for the implementation of an active physical therapy program individualized for the abilities and goals of the patient, rather than pharmaceutical approaches to aid recovery post-surgery. They also stressed the need for surgeons to understand the expectations of the patient, and to direct them to realistic goals, in order to allow patients to exceed their expectations.

In addition to this, to offset excess state or situational anxiety and/or distress in the surgical setting, there is a need to carefully examine the nature of the threat being perceived by those with clear state anxiety, as these issues vary widely, and cannot be dealt with in a uniform way. To this end, more research conducted on patients with different forms of osteoarthritis, more research to clarify the distinction between depression and anxiety, and anxiety and fear, and its relationship to osteoarthritis, plus more efforts to uncover the types of anxiety that most influence key features of the condition is clearly indicated. A greater ability to minimize pain experienced as a result of osteoarthritis pathology through non-pharmacologic management strategies is also indicated to reduce reactive anxiety states and their adverse effects on the existing disease process and its functional outcomes. As well, more careful study of the differential effects of depression and anxiety, the link between anxiety, obesity, and osteoarthritis pain, as well as heart disease and osteoarthritis, plus training clinicians and support staff to recognize and diagnose anxiety disorders and to tailor their treatments in light of their diagnoses is highly recommended. The use of both pharmacologic as well as non-pharmacologic strategies that can successfully target the mechanisms underlying the prevailing problem is strongly indicated as well (Smith & Zautra, 2008).

It is recognized this multi-pronged approach of routinely examining psychological variables including anxiety among patients with osteoarthritis, trying to minimize pain, while intervening as indicated to minimize the adverse effect of anxiety on functional outcomes might increase medical costs, as well as provider time initially. However, cost savings and vastly improved health outcomes including physical health, social functioning, and increased health-related quality of life are predicted in the long term (Katon et al., 2007). Indeed, as outlined by Hill et al. (2007) and Perrucio et al. (2011), because optimal mental well-being is critical for maximizing conservative as well as replacement surgery outcomes for patients with osteoarthritis, an exclusive focus on physical health that leads to missed opportunities for recognizing and successfully enhancing opportunities to improve the patient's overall health status, will not only increase economic costs, but the immense social costs of the disease, as well.

6. References

Abrams, T.E., Vaughan-Sarrazin, M., Rosenthal, G.E., (2010) Influence of psychiatric comorbidity on surgical mortality. *Archives of Surgery*, Vol. 145, pp: 947-953.

Alegría, A.A., Hasin, D.S., Nunes, E.V., Liu, S.M., Davies, C., Grant, B.F., Blanco, C. (2010) Comorbidity of generalized anxiety disorder and substance use disorders: results from the National Epidemiologic Survey on Alcohol and Related Conditions. *Journal of Clinical Psychiatry*, Vol. 71, pp: 1187-1195.

Ayral, X., Giequere, C., Duhalde, A., Boucheny, D/. Dougados, M., (2002) Effects of video information on preoperative anxiety level and tolerability of joint lavage in knee osteoarthritis. *Arthritis and Rheumatism*, Vol. 15, pp: 380-382.

Axford, J., Butt, A., Heron, C., Hammond, J., Morgan, J., Alavi, A., Bolton, J., Bland, M., (2010) Prevalence of anxiety and depression in osteoarthritis: use of the Hospital Anxiety and Depression Scale as a screening tool. *Clinical Rheumatology*, Vol. 29, pp: 1277-1283.

Badura-Brzoza, K., Zajac, P., Kasperska-Zajac, A., Brzoza, Z., Matysiakiewicz, J., Piegza, M., Hese, R., Rogala, B., Semenowicz, J., Koczy, Bogdan. (2008) Anxiety and depression and their influence on the quality of life after total hip replacement: preliminary report. *International Journal of Psychiatry in Clinical Practice,* Vol.12, pp. 280-284.

Badura-Brzoza, K., Zajac, P., Brzoza, Z., Kasperska-Zajac, A., Matysiakiewicz, J., Piegza, M., Hese, R.T., Rogala, B., Semenowicz, J., Koczy, B. (2009) Psychological and psychiatric factors related to health-related quality of life after total hip replacement -preliminary report. *European Psychiatry*, Vol. 24, pp: 119-124.

Bischoff-Ferrari, H.J., Lingard, E.A., Losina, E., Baron, J.A., Roos, E.M., Phillips, C.B., Mahamed, N. N., Bareett, Katz, J.N., (2004) Psychosocial and geriatric correlates of functional status after total hip replacement. *Arthritis and Rheumatism,* Vol. 51; pp: 829-835.

Bondy, L.R., Sims, N., Schroeder, D.R., Offord, K.P., & Narr, B.J., (1999) The effect of anaesthetic patient education on preoperative patient anxiety. Regional Anesthesia and Pain Medicine, Vol. 24, pp: 158-164.

Brenes, G.A., Guralnik, J. M., Williamson, J. D., Fried, L.P., Simpson, C., Simonsick, E.M., Penninx, B.W.J.H , (2005) The influence of anxiety on progression of disability. Journal of the American Geriatric Society, Vol. 53, pp: 34-39.

Burns, M.N., Siddique, J., Fokuo, J.K, Mohr, D.C., (2010) Comorbid anxiety disorders and treatment of depression in people with multiple sclerosis. Rehabilitation Psychology, Vol. 55, pp: 255-262.

Caracciolo, B., Giaquinto, S., (2005) Self-perceived distress and self-perceived functional recovery after recent total hip and knee arthroplasty. Archives of Gerontology and Geriatrics, Vol. 41, pp: 177-181.

Chan, S., Sambamoorthi, U., Rust, G., (2008) Co-occurring mental illness and health care utilization and expenditures in adults with obesity and chronic physical illness. Disease Management, Vol. 11, pp: 153-160.

Creamer, P., Lethbridge-Cejku, M., Hochberg, M.C., (2000) Factors associated with functional impairment in symptomatic knee osteoarthritis. Rheumatology, Vol. 39: pp: 490-496.

Daltroy, L.H., Morlino, C.I., Eaton, H.M., Poss, R., Liang, M.H., (1998) Preoperative education for total hip and knee replacement patients. Arthritis Care and Research, Vol. 11, pp: 469-478.

Davies, T., Craig, T.K., (2010) ABC of Mental Health. John Wiley and Sons, United Kingdom.

Davis, M.A., Ettinger, W.H., Neuhaus, J.M., Barclay, J.D., Segal, M.R., (1992) Correlates of knee pain among US adults with and without radiographic knee osteoarthritis. Journal of Rheumatology, Vol. 19, pp: 1943-1949.

Davis, L., Barlow, D.H., Smith, L., (2010) Comorbidity and the treatment of principal anxiety disorders in a naturalistic sample. Behavior Therapy, Vol. 41, pp; 296-305.

Dekker, J., Van Dijk, G.M., Veenhof, C., (2009) Risk factors for functional decline in osteoarthritis of the hip. Current Opinion in Rheumatology, Vol. 21, pp: 520-524.

Dieppe, P., Cushnaghan, J., Tucker, M., Browning, S., Shepstone, L., (2000) The Bristol 'OA5000 study': progression and impact of the disease after 8 years. Osteoarthritis Cartilage, Vol. 8, pp: 63-68.

Dorr, L.D., Chao, L, (2007). The emotional state of the patient after total hip and knee arthroplasty. Clinical Orthopedics and Related Research,Vol. 463, pp:7-12

Fava, G.A., Porcelli, P., Rafanelli, C., Mangelli, L., Grandi, S., (2010) The spectrum of anxiety disorders in the medically ill. Journal of Clinical Psychiatry, Vol. 71, pp: 910-914.

Feeney, S.L., (2004) The relationship between pain and negative affect in older adults: anxiety as a predictor of pain. Journal of Anxiety Disorders, Vol. 18, pp: 733-744.

Giraudet-Le Quintrec, J.S., Coste, J., Vastel, L., Pacualt, V., Jeanne, L., Lamas, J.P., et al., (2003) Positive effect of patient education for hip surgery: a randomized trial. Clinical Orthopedics and Related Research, Vol. 414, pp: 112-120.

Gustafsson, B.A., Ekman, S-L., Ponzer, S., Heikkila, K., (2010) The hip and knee replacement operation: an extensive life event. Scandinavian Journal of Caring Sciences, Vol. 24, pp: 663-670.

Heuts, P.H., Vlaeyen, J.W., Roelofs, J., de Bie, R.A., Aretz, K., van Weel, C., van Schayck, O. C., (2004) Pain-related fear and daily functioning in patients with osteoarthritis. Pain, Vol. 110, pp: 228-235.

Hill, C.L., Gill, T., Taylor, A.W., Daly, A., Grande, E.D., Adams, R. J., (2007) Psychological factors and quality of life in arthritis: a population based model. Clinical Rheumatology, Vol. 26, pp: 1049-1054.

Hochberg, M.C., Lawrence, R.C., Everett, D.F., Cornoni-Huntley, J., (1989) Epidemiological associations of pain in osteoarthritis of the knee: data from the National Health and Nutrition Examination Survey and the National Health and Nutrition Examination-I epidemiologic follow-up survey. Seminars in Arthritis and Rheumatism, Vol. 18, pp: 4-9.

Hochberg, M.C., Kasper, J., Williamson, J., Skinner, A., Fried, L.P., (1995) The contribution of osteoarthritis to disability: preliminary data from the woman's Health and Aging Study. Journal of Rheumatology, Vol. 43, pp: S16-18.

Hopman-Rock, M., Kraaimaat, F. W., Bijlsma, J.W., (1997) Quality of life in elderly subjects with pain in the hip or knee. Quality of Life Research, Vol. 6, pp. 67-76.

James, N., Miller, C.W., Brown, K.C., Weaver, M., (2005) Pain disability among older adults with arthritis. Journal of Aging & Health, Vol. 17, pp: 56-69.

Katon, W., Lin, E.H.B., Kroenik, K., (2007) The association of depression and anxiety with medical symptom burden in patients with chronic medical illness. General Hospital Psychiatry, Vol. 29, pp. 147-155.

Keefe, F.J., Smith, S.J., Buffington, A.L., Gibson, J., Studts, J.L., Caldwell, D.S., (2002) Recent advances and future directions in the biopsychosocial assessment and treatment of arthritis. Journal of Consulting Clinical Psychology, Vol. 703, pp: 640-655.

Kessler, R.C., McGonagle, K. A., Zhao, S., Nelson, C.B., Hughes, M., Eshleman, S, Wittchen, H-U., Kendler, K.S. (1994) Lifetime and 12-month prevalence of DSM-R psychiatric disorders in the United States: results from the National comorbidity Survey. Archives of General Psychiatry, Vol. 51, pp. 8-19.

Khuwaja, A.K., Lalni, S., Dhanani, R., Azam, I.S., Rafique, G., White, F., (2010) Anxiety and depression among outpatients with type 2 diabetes: a multi-centre study of prevalence and associated factors. Diabetology METAB Syndrome, Vol. 2, pp: 72:

Kim, S.H., Kang, S., Kim, Y.M., Kim, B.G., Seong, S.J., Cha, S.D., Park, C.Y., Yun, Y.H., (2010) Prevalence and predictors of anxiety and depression among cervical cancer survivors in Korea. International Journal of Gynecology and Cancer, Vol. 20, pp: 1017-1024.

Kroenke, K., Spitzer, R.L., Williams, J.B., Löwe, B., (2010). The Patient Health Questionnaire Somatic, Anxiety, and Depressive Symptom Scales: a systematic review. General Hospital Psychiatry, Vol. 32, pp: 345-359.

Lavallee, L., Flint, F., (1996) The relationship of stress, competitive anxiety, mood state, and social support to athletic injury. Journal of Athletic Training, Vol. 31, pp. 296-299.

Lin, P. C., Lin, L.C., Lin, J.J., (1997) Comparing the effectiveness of different educational programs for patients with total knee arthroplasty. Orthopedic Nursing, Vol. 16, pp: 43-49.

Lunghi, M.E., Miller, P.M., McQuillan, W.M., (1978) Psycho-social factors in osteoarthritis of the hip. Journal of Psychosomatic Research, Vol. 22, pp: 57-63.

Louie, G.H., Tektonidou, M.G, Caban-Martinez, A.J., Ward, M.M., (2010) Sleep disturbances in adults with arthritis: prevalence, mediators, and subgroups at greatest risk. Arthritis Care Research, Vol. 63: pp: 247-260.

Marks, R., Allegrante, J.P., (2002) Comorbid disease profiles of adults with end-stage hip osteoarthritis. Medical Science Monitor, Vol. 8, pp: 305-309.

Marks R., (2009) Comorbid depression and anxiety impact hip osteoarthritis disability. Disability & Health, Vol. 2, pp: :27-35.

McCraken, L.M., Gross, R. T., Aikens, J., Carnrike, C.L.M., (1996) The assessment of anxiety and fear in persons with chronic pain: a comparison of instruments. Behavior Research and Therapy, Vol. 34, pp: 927-933.

Mella, L.F., Bertolo, M.B., Dalgalarrondo, P., (2010) Depressive symptoms in rheumatoid arthritis. Rev Bras Psiquiatr, Vol. 32, pp: 257-263.

Memel, D.S., Kirwan, J.R., Sharp, D.J., Hehir, M., (2000) General practitioners miss disability and anxiety as well as depression in their patients with osteoarthritis. British Journal of General Practice, Vol. 15, pp: 645-648.

Mendlowicz, M. V., Stein, M. B., (2000) Quality of life in individuals with anxiety disorders. American Journal of Psychiatry, Vol. 157, pp. 669-682.

Montin, L., Leino-Kilpi, H., Katajisto, J., Lepisto, J., Kettunenen J., Suominenen T., (2007) Anxiety and health-related quality of life of patients undergoing total hip arthroplasty for osteoarthritis. Chronic Illness, Vol. 3, pp. 219-227.

National Institutes of Health. Anxiety Disorders. NIH Publication No. 09 3879. U.S. Department of Health and Human Services, Wa, DC., 2009.

Ozcetin, A., Ataoglu, S., Kocer, E., Yazici, S., Yildiz, O., Ataoglul, A., Icmeli, C., (2007) Effects of depression and anxiety on quality of life of patients with rheumatoid arthritis, knee osteoarthritis and fibromyalgia syndrome. West Indian Medical Journal, Vol. 56, pp. 122-129.

Patten, S.B., Williams, J.V.A., JianLi, W. (2006) Mental disorders in a population sample with musculoskeletal disorders. BMC Musculoskeletal Disorders, Vol. 7, pp: 37-10.

Paukert, A.L., Pettit, J.W., Kinik, M.E., Wilson, N., Novy, D.M., Rhoades HM et al., (2010) The roles of social support and self-efficacy in physical health's impact on depressive and anxiety symptoms in older adults. Journal of Clinical Psychology Medical Settings, Vol. 17, pp: 387-400.

Perruccio, A.V., Davis, A.M., Hogg-Johnson, S., Badley, E.M., (2011) The importance of self-rated health and mental well-being in predicting health outcomes following total joint replacement surgery for osteoarthritis. Arthritis Care and Research, Mar 18. doi: 10.1002/acr.20467.

Rolfson, O., Dahlberg, L.E., Nilsson, J.A., Malchau, H., Garellick, G. (2009) Variables determining outcome in total hip replacement surgery. Journal of Bone and Joint Surgery, Vol. 91, pp: 157-161.

Roy-Byrne, P.P., Kessler, R.C., Goodwin, R.D., Lydiard, B., Katon, W. (2008) Anxiety disorders and comorbid medical illness. General Hospital Psychiatry, Vol. 30, pp: 208-225.

Salaffi F, Cavalieri F, Nolli M, Ferraccioloi, G., (1991) Analysis of disability in knee osteoarthritis. Relationship with age and psychological variables but not with radiographic score. Journal of Rheumatology, Vol. 8, pp. 1581-1586.

Salmon P, Hall GM, Peerbhoy D., (2001) Influence of the emotional response to surgery on functional recovery during 6 months after hip arthroplasty. Journal of Behavioral Medicine, Vol. 24, pp: 489-502.

Sareen J, Jacobi F, Cox BJ, Belik SL, Clara I, Stein MB., (2006) Disability and poor quality of life associated with comorbid anxiety disorders and physical conditions. Archives of Internal Medicine, Vol. 166, pp: 2109-2116.

Scopaz, K.A., Piva, S.R., Wisniwski, S, Fitzgerald, G.K., (2009) Relationship of fear, anxiety, and depression with physical function in patients with knee osteoarthritis. Archives of Physical Medicine and Rehabilitation, Vol. 90, pp: 1866-1973.

Scott, K.M., Brufaerts, R., Tsang, A., Ormel, J., Alonso, J., Angermeyer, M.C. et al., (2007) Depression-anxiety relationships with chronic physical conditions: results from the World Mental Health surveys. Journal of Affective Disorders, Vol. 103, pp:113-120.

Skurlova, M., Stofkova, A., Jurcovicovam, J. (2010) Anxiety-like behavior in the elevated-plus maze tests and enhanced IL-1, Il-6, NADPH oxidase-1, and iNOS mRNAs in the hippocampus during early stage of adjuvant arthritis in rats. Neuroscience Letters, Oct 20.

Smith, B. W., Zautra, A.J., (2008) The effects of anxiety and depression on weekly pain in women with arthritis. Pain, Vol. 138, pp: 354-361.

Summers, M.N., Haley, W.E., Reveille, J.D., Alarcón, G.S. (1988) Radiographic assessment and psychologic variables as predictors of pain and functional impairment in osteoarthritis of the knee or hip. Arthritis and Rheumatism, Vol. 31, pp: 204-209.

Tallon, D., Chard, J., Dieppe, P., (2000) Exploring the priorities of patients with osteoarthritis of the knee. Arthritis Care and Research, Vol. 13, pp: 312-319.

Turk, D.C., (2002) A diathesis-stress model of chronic pain and disability following traumatic injury. Pain Research Man, Vol. 71, pp. 9-19.

Thompson, R.F., (1993) The brain: a neuroscience primer, Second Edition. W.H. Freeman and Company, United States.

Van Der Kraan, P.M., (2010) Osteoarthritis and a high-fat diet: the full 'OA syndrome' in a small animal model. Arthritis Research and Therapy, Vol. 12, pp. 130.

Weinberger, M., Tierney, W. M., Booher, P. (1989) Common problems experienced by adults with osteoarthritis. Arthritis Care and Research, Vol. 2, pp: 94-100.

What is anxiety? Anxiety symptoms and causes. Retrieved from www.medicalnewstoday/info/anxiety, January 9, 2010.

Wu, L.R., Parkerson, G.R., Doraiswamy, P.M., (2002) Health perception, pain, and disability as correlates of anxiety and depression symptoms in primary care patients. Journal of the American Board of Family Practitioners, Vol. 15, pp: 183-190.

Turk, D. C., (2002) A diathesis-stress model of chronic pain and disability following traumatic injury. Pain Research and Management, Vol. 71, pp: 9-19.

Tyrer, P., (1984) Classification of anxiety. British Journal of Psychiatry, Vol. 144, pp: 78-83.

Van Baar, M.E., Dekker, J., Lemmens, J.A., Oostendorp, R.A., Bijlsma, J.W., (1998) Pain and disability in patients with osteoarthritis of hip or knee: the relationship with articular, kinesiological, and psychological characteristics. Journal of Rheumatology, Vol. 25, pp:125-133.

Van der Kraan, P.M., (2010) Osteoarthritis and a high-fat diet: the full 'OA syndrome' in a small animal model. Arthritis Research and Therapy Vol. 12, pp: 130.

VanDyke, M. M., Parker, J.C., Smarr, K. L., Hewett, J. E., Johnson, G. E., Slaughter, J. R., Walker, Se. E., (2004) Anxiety in rheumatoid arthritis. Arthritis and Rheumatism, Vol. 51, pp. 408-412.

Vriezekol, J., Eijsbouts, A., Evers, A., Stenger, A., Van Den Hoogen, F., Van Lankveld, W., (2010) Poor psychological health status among patients with inflammatory rheumatic diseases and osteoarthritis in multidisciplinary rehabilitation: need for a routine psychological assessment. Disability Rehabilitation, Vol. 32, pp: 836-844.

Wetherell, J.L., Ayers, C.R., Nuevo, R., Stein, M.B., Ramsdell, J., Patterson, T.L., (2010) Medical conditions and depressive, anxiety, and somatic symptoms in older adults with and without generalized anxiety disorder. Aging Mental Health, Vol. 14, pp: 764-768.

Whittle, J., Steinberg, E.P., Anderson, G.F., Herbert, R., Hochberg, M.C., (1990) Incidence of and indications for total hip replacement among elderly Americans. Arthritis and Rheumatism, Vol. 3, S: 139.

Wiltink, J., Beutel, M. E., Ojeda, F.M., Wild, P. S., Munzel, T., Blankenberg, S., Michal, M., (2010) Prevalence of distress, comorbid conditions and well being in the general population. Journal of Affective Disorders, Nov. 22

Wise, B.L., Niu, J., Zhang, N., Jordan, J.M., Choy, E., Hunter, D.J., (2009) Psychological factors and their relation to osteoarthritis pain. Osteoarthritis and Cartilage, pp: 883-887.

Ying, D.G., Jiang, S., Yang, H., Zhu, S., (2010) Frequency of generalized anxiety disorder in Chinese primary care. Postgraduate Medicine, Vol. 122, pp: 32-38.

14

The Association Between Chronic Back Pain and Psychiatric Disorders; Results from a Longitudinal Population-Based Study

Hedda van 't Land, Jacqueline Verdurmen, Margreet ten Have,
Saskia van Dorsselaer and Ron de Graaf
Netherlands Institute of Mental Health and Addiction, Utrecht
The Netherlands

1. Introduction

Chronic back pain is a common pain condition; it results in significant personal, social and occupational impairment, role disability and health care utilization.[30, 34, 9, 32, 24]
Epidemiologic studies have found that chronic back pain is comorbid with psychiatric disorders, other chronic pain conditions (migraine, arthritis, headache) and chronic psychical conditions.[26, 15, 30, 5, 13] Most of the published studies regarding the assocation between chronic back pain and psychiatric disorders focus on the association with major depression.[30, 5, 21, 22, 4] It is found that the prevalence of major depression among persons with chronic pain is about 2-3 times higher than among pain-free individuals.[18] A study conducted by Von Korff et al. (2005) showed that chronic back pain is also significantly associated with mood, anxiety (except agoraphobia without panic) and alcohol abuse and dependence disorders.[30] A recent international study conducted by Tsang et al. (2008) found that various chronic pain conditions (headache, back or neck pain, arthritis or joint pain) are associated with depression-anxiety spectrum disorders both in developed and developing countries.[29]
Although an association between chronic back pain and psychiatric disorders has been repeatedly demonstrated, little is known about the temporal relationship between the two, as most studies are based on clinical samples and cross-sectional data.[6] Fishbain et al. (1997) analysed 40 studies addressing the temporal relationship between generic pain and major depression. However, no firm conclusions could be drawn as most of these studies differed in study design, methods and definition to identify depression.[11] Fishbain et al. (1997) stated that more support was found for the hypothesis that pain precedes depression, although some of the selected studies found depression to be a predictor of first onset pain.[22, 31, 4, 16, 3, 20] The aims of the present study are:

1. To assess cross-sectionally the association between chronic back pain and various mood, anxiety and substance use disorders;
2. To assess longitudinally the temporal relationship between chronic back pain and psychiatric disorders.

2. Material and methods

Sampling procedure

Data from NEMESIS were used. NEMESIS (see[2], for a detailed description of the objectives of this study) is a population-based study with repeated measurements among the same subjects in 1996 (T_0), 1997 (T_1) and 1999 (T_2). A stratified, random sampling procedure was utilized. First, a sample was drawn from 90 Dutch municipalities, stratified by urbanicity and sufficiently distributed over the 12 provinces of the Netherlands. Post office registers were used to draw a sample of private households (addresses). The number of households selected in each municipality was in proportion to its population. One respondent in each household was selected randomly, according to whose birthday was most recent, on the condition that he or she was between 18 and 65 years of age and sufficiently fluent in Dutch. To maximize the response and to compensate for any seasonal influences, the initial data collection phase was spread over the entire period from February to December, 1996. At baseline, a total of 7076 people (response rate of 69.7%) were interviewed. Informed consent was obtained for the interview. All participants in the baseline interview (T0) were approached for the follow-up waves, one year (T1) and three years (T2) after T0. Of the 7076 participants at baseline, 5618 subjects (response 79.4%) were available for re-interview at T_1 and 4796 subjects (response of T_1 subjects: 85.4%) at T_2. The ethics committee of the Netherlands Institute of Mental Health and Addiction approved these procedures. The subjects well reflected the Dutch population in terms of gender, civil status and degree of urbanization.[14] Only the 18-24 age group was underrepresented.
Loss of subjects in the second or subsequent waves of longitudinal data collection can be selective. Therefore, it was examined whether nonresponders at T_1 and T_2 differed from responders at T_1 and T_2 on the presence of psychiatric disorders or chronic back pain at T_0. After adjustment for demographic variables, a 12-month chronic back pain at T_0 did not increase the probability of loss to follow-up between T_0 and T_1 nor between T_0 and T_2 (OR= 1.00, CI= 0.81-1.22; OR= 1.09, CI= 0.91-1.30). After adjustment for demographic variables, any 12-month psychiatric disorder at T_0 only slightly increased the probability of loss to follow-up between T_0 and T_1 as well as between T_0 and T_2 (OR=1.20, CI=1.04-1.38; OR=1.29, CI=1.15-1.46)[14]

Instruments

Psychiatric disorders

The Diagnostic and Statistical Manual of Mental Disorders (DSM-III-R) Axis I psychiatric disorders were diagnosed with the computerised version of the Composite International Diagnostic Interview (CIDI version 1.1;[27]). The CIDI is a structured interview, developed by the World Health Organization, based on the Diagnostic Interview Schedule (DIS) and the Present State Examination (PSE), and administered by trained interviewers. The CIDI has good test-retest reliability[35] and validity[10] for all psychiatric disorders examined in NEMESIS. The following classes and seperate diagnoses of psychiatric disorders were measured: mood disorders (major depression, dysthymia, bipolar disorder); anxiety disorders (obsessive compulsive disorder, generalized anxiety disorder, simple phobia, social phobia, agoraphobia, and panic disorder); substance use disorders (alcohol abuse, alcohol dependency, drug abuse, drug dependency).

Chronic back pain and other somatic illnesses

Chronic back pain and other somatic illnesses were assessed at two waves (T_0 and T_2) by means of a questionnaire listing 31 chronic somatic conditions divided over different somatic classes, in line with the classification used in the National Comorbidity Survey Replication (NCS-R)[30]: asthma, chronic pain conditions (arthritis, migraine, chronic back pain), cardiovascular disease (high blood pressure, heart attack, stroke), digestive disease (stomach ulcer, intestinal/abdominal disorders, gallbladder, liver disease, cirrhosis), sensory impairment, diabetes, chronic cystitis (kidney punch, kidney disease, chronic bladder infection), thyroid gland diseases, other (sinusitis, epilepsy, dizziness, skin disease, cancer, multiple sclerosis, Parkinson's disease, myalgic encephalomyelitis, severe injury, HIV/AIDS).

Self-report was used to ascertain chronic back pain (and other physical illnesses). Subjects were asked whether they had chronic back pain in the prior 12 months (at T_0) or 24 months (at T_2), lasting longer than three months. Different studies indicate that self-report on the presence of chronic diseases have a moderate to high agreement with medical records.[25, 19, 17]

Sociodemographic variables

The following sociodemographic variabes were measured at T_0: gender; age (18-24, 25-34, 35-44, 45-54, 55-64); highest completed level of education (primary vocational, lower vocational, secondary-middle vocational, higher vocational, academic); living conditions (living with partner with or without children, parent living alone, living alone, living with parents, living with other people); urbanicity (very low, low, average, high, very high); employment status (employed, housewife or houseman, student, unemployed, disabled, retired, other).

Statistical analyses

To assess cross-sectional comorbidity between chronic back pain and 12-month psychiatric disorders (research question 1), logistic regression analysis was used generating odds ratios (ORs) and 95% confidence intervals (CI). Data were used of the first wave (T_0; n=7076).

To examine whether having chronic back pain increases the risk of developing a psychiatric disorder (research question 2), 3-year incidence figures of psychiatric disorders were calculated. For this analysis, subjects were selected without lifetime psychiatric disorder at T_0. Again, logistic regression analysis was used to calculate the association between chronic back pain and later onset of psychiatric disorders.

To examine whether having a psychiatric disorder elevates the risk of developing chronic back pain (research question 2), 2-year incidence figures of chronic back pain were calculated at T_2. At T_1, no somatic illnesses (including chronic back pain) were assessed. Therefore, only 2-year incidence figures could be calculated (at T_2 subjects were asked whether they experienced chronic back pain that lasted longer than three months in the preceding 24 months). For this analysis, subjects without diagnosis of chronic back pain at baseline (T_0) were selected. Again, logistic regression analysis was performed to calculate the association between classes of psychiatric disorders (mood disorders, anxiety disorders and substance use disorders) and later onset of chronic back pain. The sample sizes were too small to study the association between individual psychiatric disorders and later onset of chronic back pain.

Adjustment of statistical analyses was necessary as chronic back pain is associated with various socio-demographic factors and other somatic illnesses, such as arthritis, migraine, cardiovascular diseases.[26,15,30,5,13] In the first step, all analyses were adjusted for sociodemographic variables (age, gender and education; Model 1); in the second step additionally for employment status, living conditions and the dichotomous (yes/no) variable 'any other somatic illness than chronic back pain' (Model 2), ruling out that any relationship found between chronic back pain and psychiatric disorders was mediated by any of the somatic illnesses listed above in the paragraph 'chronic back pain and other somatic illnesses'. Significance was set at the two-sided 0.05 level. All calculations were performed using STATA 8.0 statistical software.[28] The appropriate statistical weight was employed in all analyses to ensure the data were representative of the national population. Weighted data can cause problems in estimating variances, standard errors and corresponding tests and confidence intervals. Therefore, STATA[28] was applied, using the Taylor series linearization method.

3. Results

Sociodemographic variables

The 12-month prevalence estimate of chronic back pain was 8.2%. More women than men had chronic back pain (9.4% were female and 7.1% male; p< 0.001). The rate of chronic back pain increased with age. Lower educational level, parent living alone and being unemployed were also related to higher prevalence estimates of chronic back pain.

		Chronic back pain (n=631) %	p-value
Gender	Male	7.1	<0.001
	Female	9.4	
Age	18-24	3.6	<0.001
	25-34	4.9	
	35-44	8.7	
	45-54	10.8	
	55-64	14.2	
Educational level	Primary, basic vocational	16.9	<0.001
	Lower secondary	10.4	
	Higher secondary	6.9	
	Higer professional, university	4.8	
Urbanicity	Very low	7.7	
	Low	8.2	
	Average	8.8	
	High	8.1	
	Very high	8.3	
Living conditions	Living with partner	9.0	<0.001
	Parent living alone	10.4	
	Living alone	7.5	
	Living with parents	2.9	
	Living with other people	6.9	
Employment	Employed	6.3	<0.001
	Housewife/man	12.9	
	Student	2.2	
	Unemployed/ disablement	17.6	
	Retired/other	12.6	

Table 1. Sociodemographic variables of Dutch adults with chronic back pain (n=7076)

Chronic back pain and comorbid psychiatric disorders

Comorbidity between chronic back pain and psychiatric disorders was first assessed cross-sectionally. Chronic back pain and any psychiatric disorder appeared to be significantly associated, as shown by the adjusted odds in both models (Table 2).

Psychiatric disorder	Chronic back pain (n=631)	No chronic back pain (n=6445)	Model 1 I		Model 2 II	
	%	%	OR	95% CI	OR	95% CI
Mood disorder	11.8	7.3	1.64***	1.25-2.14	1.42*	1.08-1.88
Anxiety disorder	19.5	11.8	1.69***	1.34-2.12	1.52**	1.20-1.92
Substance use disorder	8.5	8.9	1.56*	1.07-2.28	1.53*	1.05-2.23
Any psychiatric disorder	29.7	22.7	1.59***	1.31-1.94	1.44***	1.18-1.75
Two or more psychiatric disorders	12.6	7.3	1.82***	1.37-2.41	1.58**	1.18-2.12

I Adjusted for age, gender and educational level.
II Adjusted for age, gender, educational level, urbanicity, household composition, employment status, any other somatic illness than chronic back pain (see paragraph 'chronic back pain and other somatic illnesses' for detailed description).
* $p<0.05$; ** $p<0.01$; *** $p< 0.001$

Table 2. Association between chronic back pain and psychiatric disorders in the Dutch adult population (12-month prevalence estimates, Odds ratios and 95% confidence intervals)

Looking at the classes of psychiatric disorders, the adjusted odds for mood disorder, anxiety disorder and substance use disorder were also significant in both models. Additional analyses (not in table) demonstrated that for the following individual psychiatric disorders in both models the association was significant: obsessive compulsive disorder (Model 2: OR=3.62; CI=1.51-8.69), generalised anxiety (Model 2: OR=3.13; CI=1.71-5.74), simple phobia (Model 2: OR=1.38;CI=1.03-1.84 in model 2), dysthymia (Model 2: OR=1.85;CI=1.23-2.79) and alcohol abuse (Model 2: OR=1.92; CI=1.11-3.32).

Temporal relationship

The temporal relationship between chronic back pain and psychiatric disorders was assessed longitudinally. Results showed that subjects with chronic back pain had an elevated risk of developing any psychiatric disorder in both models (Table 3). In both models it was found that the risk of developing a mood or anxiety disorder was significantly higher among subjects with chronic back pain. Additional analyses (not in table) showed that for the individual psychiatric disorders in both models the risk was significant for obsessive compulsive disorder (Model 2: OR=3.36; CI=1.05-10.7), major depression (Model 2: OR=2.49; CI=1.73-3.59) and simple phobia (Model 2: OR=1.88; CI=1.20-2.94).

	Chronic back pain %	No chronic back pain %	Odds ratio's and 95% confidence interval			
			Model 1 I		Model 2 II	
			OR	95% CI	OR	95% CI
Mood disorder[III]	11.4	5.1	2.14***	1.63-3.57	2.37***	1.60-3.52
Anxiety disorder	9.8	5.3	1.80**	1.17-2.79	1.74*	1.13-2.67
Substance use disorder	3.3	3.9	1.23	0.62-2.41	1.20	0.60-2.41
Any psychiatric disorder	20.0	10.7	2.28***	1.57-3.32	2.25***	1.54-3.28

I Adjusted for age, gender and educational level.
II Adjusted for age, gender, educational level, urbanicity, household composition, employment status, any other somatic illness than chronic back pain (see paragraph 'chronic back pain and other somatic illnesses' for description).
III The incidence rate for a diagnostic grouping involves the first onset of any disorder from that grouping in subjects who had never had any disorder in that grouping before the first assessement. The incidence rate for the separate disorders involves the first onset of that disorder irrespective of whether the subjects in question had ever had any other disorder from the same grouping. This explains why the rates for some groupings come out lower than the rates for some of the separate disorders within them.
* p<0.05; ** p<0.01; *** p< 0.001

Table 3. Three-years incidence of psychiatric disorders among Dutch adults with and without chronic back pain

To examine whether having a psychiatric disorder elevates the risk of developing chronic back pain, 2-year incidence figures were calculated among subjects with and without psychiatric disorders. Results showed that the risk of developing chronic back pain was significantly higher among subjects with an anxiety disorder in both models (Table 4).

	Chronic back pain %	Odds ratio's and 95% confidence interval			
		Model 1 I		Model 2 II	
		OR	95% CI	OR	95% CI
No mood disorder	5.3	1		1	
Mood disorder	6.0	1.13	0.62-2.05	1.16	0.64-2.13
No anxiety disorder	5.0	1		1	
Anxiety disorder	7.9	1.62*	1.02-2.59	**1.65***	1.03-2.64
No Substance use disorder	5.3	1		1	
Substance use disorder	5.1	1.09	0.57-2.05	1.17	0.61-2.21
No psychiatric disorder	5.0	1		1	
Any psychiatric disorder	6.6	1.39	0.96-2.02	1.43	0.98-2.08

I Adjusted for age, gender and educational level.
II Adjusted for age, gender, educational level, urbanicity, household composition, employment status, any other somatic illness than chronic back pain (see paragraph 'chronic back pain and other somatic illnesses' for description).
* p<0.05; ** p<0.01; *** p< 0.001

Table 4. Two-years incidence of chronic back pain among Dutch adults with and without a 12-month psychiatric disorder.

4. Discussion

This article provides the first longitudinal population-based assessment of the temporal relationship between chronic back pain and mood, anxiety and substance use disorders. The study also adds to current knowledge on cross-sectional associations between chronic back pain and psychiatric disorders.

The key findings of this study are that persons with chronic back pain are more likely to have mood, anxiety and alcohol abuse disorder. These results add to the growing body of knowledge that chronic back pain is associated not only with depression but also with anxiety and alcohol abuse disorder.[30, 7]

Secondly, regarding the temporal relationship this study provides empirical support for both the consequence (chronic back pain precedes the development of psychiatric disorders) and the antecedent hypothesis (anxiety disorders precede the development of chronic back pain). Regarding the consequence hypothesis, it was found that pre-existing chronic back pain not only elevates the risk of developing a mood disorder (major depression[6, 5, 11]), but also of other psychiatric disorders, such as obsessive-compulsive disorder and simple phobia. Regarding the antecedent hypothesis, it was found that anxiety disorders predict new onset chronic back pain.

In interpreting these results, first several strengths and limitations of this study need to be considered. The present study has important advantages over other studies. Until recently, research in this field focused exclusively on the association between chronic back pain and depression. Our study has a much broader scope, by focusing on mood disorders, anxiety disorders and substance use disorders. In addition, a valid and reliable instrument (CIDI) was used measuring DSM-III-R Axis I psychiatric disorders. Also a limitation of this study needs to be considered: the ascertainment of chronic back pain on self-report. It was not feasible to abstract medical records or to conduct a medical assessement to determine whether chronic back pain was present or absent. As noted earlier, results indicate that self-report has a moderate to high agreement with medical records on the presence of chronic diseases.[25, 19, 17] Another limitation is that no information on pain severity and duration of the chronic back pain was collected. Consequently, exceeding the scope of this study is the estimation of duration and pain severity-specific curves for subjects with chronic back pain in relation to psychiatric disorder onset rates.

This study provides empirical support for both the consequence and the antecedent hypothesis. It remains unclear, however, which causal mechanisms underly the temporal relationship between the two. Various explanations may be put forward for the antecedent hypothesis; having an anxiety disorder may lead to physical symptoms such as pain due to increased physiological arousal.[16] In addition, people with anxiety disorders may be more likely to somatize their psychological symptoms, with somatization being the mediating variable, as a way of expressing their general distress by reporting pain.[7] Regarding the consequence hypothesis, it has been assumed that chronic pain of any type rather than chronic back pain specifically may be a generic risk factor in the development of psychiatric disorders.[6] In this study, however, all statistical analyses were adjusted for two other chronic pain conditions than chronic back pain: arthritis and migraine. After this adjustment, the temporal relationship between chronic back pain and psychiatric disorders remained significant, in the sense that pre-existing chronic back pain precedes the development of psychiatric disorders. It therefore does not seem plausible to assume that chronic pain of any type would serve as a mediating variable underlying the temporal relationship between chronic back pain and psychiatric disorders. A third hypothesis can be put forward presuming that chronic back pain and certain psychiatric disorders share the same pathogenesis; prior research has for example identified neurochemical links between depression and chronic pain in the sense that both serotonin and norepinephrine appear to play a role in the pathogenesis of both chronic pain and depression.[11,6] A fourth hypothesis to be tested is whether chronic back pain and certain psychiatric disorders may share a common risk factor, such as psychological stress. Contemporary models portray low back pain as a sensory-affective response, involving physiological, cognitive, and behavioral components.[34] More research is needed to explore the relationship between chronic back pain/generic pain and psychiatric disorders in depth, by adressing the causal mechanisms that may be involved. It needs for example to be examined whether allevation of pain helps to ameliorate psychiatric symptoms and likewise whether relief of psychiatric symptoms improves pain.[1]

Our findings are important to care providers treating patients with chronic back pain and to clinical care givers treating people with anxiety disorders. As the combination of depression and pain is associated with worse outcomes than either condition alone, it is important to recognize psychiatric disorders in clinical and primary care settings.[1] Care providers should be aware of the co-occurrence of chronic back pain and psychiatric disorders, of the elevated risk patients with chronic back pain have of developing mood and anxiety disorders and of the elevated risk people with anxiety disorders have to develop chronic back pain. Dual treatment of both chronic back pain and psychiatric disorders is needed to improve pain outcomes. Currently, there is a lack of recommendations for valid screening scales for psychiatric disorders and psychiatric treatments appropriate for people with chronic pain conditions. This study underscores the necessity that valid screening tools for psychiatric disorders should to be made available and that guidelines should be developed to inform caretakers how to treat patients with chronic back pain and psychiatric disorders.

5. Acknowledgements

The NEMESIS study was supported by the Ministry of Health Welfare and Sports of the Netherlands.

6. References

[1] Bair MJ, Robinson RL, Katon W, Kroenke K. Depression and pain comorbidity: a literature review. Arch Intern Med 163:2433-45, 2003.

[2] Bijl RV, Ravelli A, Van Zessen G. Prevalence of psychiatric disorder in the general population: results of The Netherlands Mental Health Survey and Incidence Study (NEMESIS). Soc Psychiatry Psychiatr Epidemiol 33:587–95, 1998.

[3] Carroll LJ, Cassidy JD, Coté P. Depression as a risk factor for onset of an episode of troublesome neck and low back pain. Pain 107:134-139, 2004.

[4] Croft PR, Papageorgiou AC, Ferry S, Thomas E, Jayson MI, Silman AJ (1995). Psychologic distress and low back pain. Evidence from a prospective study in the general population. Spine 20:2731-7, 1995.

[5] Currie SR, Wang J. Chronic back pain and major depression in the general Canadian population. Pain 107:54-60, 2004.

[6] Currie SR, Wang J. More data on major depression as an antecedent risk factor for first onset of chronic back pain. Psychological Medicine 35:1275-1282, 2005.

[7] Dersh J, Polatin PB, Gatchel RJ. Chronic pain and psychopathology: research findings and theoretical considerations. Psychosomatic Medicine 64:773-786, 2002.

[8] Deyo RA, Rainville J, Kent DL. What can the history and physical examination tell us about low back pain? JAMA 268:760-765, 1992.

[9] Engels CC, Von Korff M, Katon WJ. Back pain in primary care: predictors of high health-care costs. Pain 65:197-204, 1996.

[10] Farmer AE, Jenkins PL, Katz R, Ryder L. Comparison of CATEGO-derived ICD-8 and DSM-III classifications using the CIDI in severely ill subjects. Brit J Psychiatr 158:177–182, 1990.

[11] Fishbain DA, Cutler R, Rosomoff HL, Rosomoff RS. Chronic pain-associated depression: antecedent or consequence of chronic pain? A Review. The Clinical Journal of Pain 13: 116-137, 1997.

[12] Frymoyer JW. Quality: An international challenge to the diagnosis and treatment of the disorders of the lumbar spine. Spine 18:2147-2152, 1993.

[13] Gureje O, Von Korff M, Simon GE, Gater R. Persistent pain and well being: a World Health Organization Study in primary care. J Am Med Assoc 280:147-151, 1998.

[14] Graaf R de, Bijl RV, Smit F, Ravelli A, Vollebergh WAM. Psychiatric and sociodemographic predictors of attrition in a longitudinal study: the Netherlands Mental Health Survey and Incidence Study (NEMESIS). Am J Epidemiol 152:1039-47, 2000.

[15] Hestbaek L. Leboef-Yde C, Manniche C. Is low back pain part of a general health pattern or is it a seperate and distinct entity? A critical review of comorbidity with low back pain. Journal Manipul Physiol Ther 26:243-252, 2003.

[16] Hotopf M, Mayou R, Wadsworth M, Wessely S. Temporal relationships between physical symptoms and psychiatric disorder. British Journal of Psychiatry 173: 255-261, 1998.

[17] Kehoe R, Wu S-Y, Leske MC, Chylack LT. Comparing self-report and physician reported medical history. American Journal of Epidemiology 139:813-818, 1994.

[18] Kessler RC, Ormel J, Demler O, Stang PE. Comorbid mental disorders account for the role impairment of commonly occurring chronic physical disorders: results from the National Comorbidity Survey. Journal of Occupational and Environmental Medicine 45: 1257-1266, 2003.

[19] Kriegsman DM, Penninx BW, Van Eijk JT, Boeke AJ, Deeg DJ. Self-reports and general practitioner information on the presence of chronic diseases in community dwelling elderly. Journal of Clinical Epidemiology 49:1407-1417, 1996.

[20] Larson SL, Clark MR, Eaton WW. Depressive disorder as a long-term antecedent risk factor for incident back pain: a 13-year follow-up study from the Baltimore Epidemiological Catchment Area Sample. Psychological Medicine 34: 211-219, 2004.

[21] Magni G, Caldeiron C, Rigatt-Luchini S, Merksey H. Chronic musculoskeletal pain and depressive symptoms in the general population. An analysis of the 1st National Health and Nutrition Examination Survey Data. Pain 43: 299-307, 1990.

[22] Magni G, Marchetti M, Moreschi C, Merksey H, Luchini SR. Chronic musculoskeletal pain and depressive symptoms in the National Health and Nutrition Examination. I. Epidemiologic follow-up study. Pain 53: 163-8, 1993.

[23] McDowell I, Newell C. Measuring Health: A guide to rating scales and questionnaires (2nd ed., rev.). New York: Oxford University Press, 1996.

[24] Nachemson AL. Newest knowlegde of low back pain. A critical look. Clin Orthop 279: 8-20, 1992.

[25] NCHS. Evaluation of National Health Interview Survey diagnostic reporting. Vital and Health Statistics 2:120:1-116, 1992.

[26] Raspe A, Matthis C, Heon-Klin V, Raspe H. Chronic back pain: more than pain in the back. Findings of a regional survey among insurees of a workers pension insurance fund. Rehabilitation 42:195-203, 2003.

[27] Smeets RMW, Dingemans PMAJ. Composite International Diagnostic Interview (CIDI), version 1.1. WHO: Amsterdam, 1993.

[28] StataCorp. Stata Statistical Software, release 7.0. College Station, TX: Stata Corporation, 2001.

[29] Tsang A, Von Korff M, Lee S, Alonso J, Karam E, Angermeyer MC, Borges GL, Bromet EJ, De Girolamo G, Graaf R de, Gureje O, Lepine JP, Haro JM, Levinson D, Oakley Browne MA, Posada-Villa J, Seedat S, Watanabe M. Common chronic pain conditions in developed and developing countries: gender and age differences and comorbidity with depression-anxiety disorders. Journal of Pain 9: 883-891, 2008.

[30] Von Korff M, Crane P, Lane M., Miglioretti DL, Simon G, Saunders K, Stang P, Brandenbrug N, Kessler R. Chronic spinal pain and physical-mental comorbidity in the United States: results from the National Comorbidity Survey Replication. Pain 2005; 113:331-339.

[31] Von Korff M, Le Resche L, Dworkin SF. First onset of common pain symptoms: a prospective study of depression as a risk factor. Pain 55:251-258, 1993.

[32] Von Korff M., Ormel J, Keefe F, Dworkin SF (1992). Grading the severity of chronic pain. Pain 50:133-149, 1992.

[33] Ware JE, Sherbourne CD. The MOS 36-item Short Form Health Survey (SF-36): I. Conceptual framework and item selection. Medical Care 30:473-483, 1992.

[34] Vowles KE, Zvolensky MJ, Gross RT, Sperry JA. Pain-Related Anxiety in the Prediction of Chronic Low-Back Pain Distress. Journal of Behavioural Medicine 72:77- 89, 2004.

[35] Wittchen H. Reliability and validity studies of the WHO-Composite International Diagnostic Interview (CIDI): a critical review. J Psychiatr Res 28:57–84 24, 1994.

Part 4

Therapy of Anxiety Disorders

15

The Differential Impact of Expectancies and Symptom Severity on Cognitive Behavior Therapy Outcome in Panic Disorder with Agoraphobia

Theodora E. Katerelos[1], Claude Bélanger[1,2,3], Michel Perreault[1,2,3]
Ghassan El-Baalbaki[1] and John Pecknold[2,3]
[1]*Department of Psychology, University of Quebec in Montreal*
[2]*Douglas Mental Health University Institute*
[3]*Department of Psychiatry, McGill University*
Montreal, Quebec
Canada

1. Introduction

Cognitive behavior therapy (CBT) is the treatment of choice for panic disorder with agoraphobia (PDA). Numerous studies have been conducted on the short- and long-term effectiveness of CBT. Treatment effectiveness could range as low as 25% and as high as 90% (e.g., Barlow et al. 1989; Black et al., 1993; Fava et al., 1995; Margraf et al., 1993; Öst & Westling, 1995; Shear et al., 1994; Taylor et al., 1996). Nevertheless, most studies have concluded that CBT appears to be the most effective treatment to date in reducing panic-related symptomatology in the short- and long-term (Clark et al., 1994; Craske et al., 1991; Fava, et al., 1995). However, some clients continue to experience anticipatory anxiety and avoidance following CBT (Clark et al., 1994; Craske et al., 1991; Klosko et al., 1990). Brown and Barlow (1995) conducted a long-term outcome study using stringent criteria for treatment efficacy. Although the treatment had produced substantial improvements, their findings revealed that only 20.6% of their sample could be considered as treatment success after two years. One of their recommendations for future studies was to examine predictors of treatment response. Following up on these recommendations, the present study aims to determine why some clients do not respond to CBT or only show partial benefits.

Outcome studies have examined the impact of different client variables such as motivation, personality traits, socio-demographic characteristics, diagnosis, and intelligence to name a few. The important role of client variables in psychotherapy has been confirmed in numerous studies since the 1940's (see Garfield, 1986 and Lambert & Assay, 1984). Highlen and Hill (1984) conducted an extensive review on the effects of psychotherapy and concluded that client characteristics are the most important and influential factors relating to treatment outcome and to long-term improvement (Highlen & Hill, 1984).

Several variables listed by Highlen and Hill (1984), have been important in predicting treatment outcome and long-term improvement in PDA. For instance, the severity of agoraphobic avoidance and depressed mood have been detected as predictors in the maintenance of panic attacks (Keijsers et al., 1994). Comorbidity has also been a determining factor that predicts poorer outcome in PDA after cognitive-behavior therapy and pharmacologic treatment have been administered (Keijsers et al., 1994; Pollack et al.,1994; Pollack et al., 1993). The use of "safety behaviors" has been found to reduce the effectiveness of exposure (Wells et al., 1995). Safety behaviors may include both behaviors and objects that are designed to help patients prevent their feared consequences from coming true. Such behaviors may include carrying water, chewing gum, listening to the radio, standing near a wall (in case one experiences symptoms of dizziness), and other similar behaviors that help them cope with their symptoms. Finally, anxiety sensitivity, an expectancy variable, has been associated with poorer outcome and relapse in patients with PDA (Keijsers et al., 1994; Reiss, 1991; Reiss et al., 1986; Schmidt et al.,1997).

Individuals with PDA live in anticipation or expectation of the next panic attack and may restructure their lifestyle in response to this anticipation. Panic disorder patients will anticipate with fear that their bodily sensations associated with panic attacks will result in harmful psychological, somatic or social consequences (Craske & Barlow, 1993). Anxiety sensitivity is this belief that the experience of anxiety will cause them harm. (Reiss, 1991; Reiss et al., 1986). Anxiety sensitivity arose out of research conducted on motivation to avoid feared objects, situations or physical symptoms (Reiss, 1991). From this research, Reiss' expectancy theory (Reiss, 1991; Reiss & Havercamp, 1996; Reiss et al., 1986) emerged which proposed that fear is composed of two distinct factors: expectations (what one expects will happen to him/her) and sensitivities (why one is afraid of the expected occurrence). According to this theory, individuals may hold danger expectancies (e.g., "I expect to get bitten by that dog"), expectations of being socially evaluated ("I expect others to laugh at me") and anxiety expectancies (e.g., "I expect to have a panic attack if I go on the subway"). With regards to sensitivity, individuals may possess sensitivities regarding injury (e.g., "I expect to die from an infection if the dog bites me"), social evaluation (e.g., "I expect to turn red if they laugh at me") and anxiety (e.g., "I expect to have a heart attack if I panic"). While expectations and sensitivities vary from one individual to another, they seem to be particularly elevated in individuals with panic disorder (e.g., Reiss, 1991; McNally, 1992; Taylor et al., 1992). The above studies reviewed on expectancies indicate that they may be important contributors to PDA development, especially with respect to anxiety sensitivity (Reiss et al., 1986; Schmidt et al., 1997).

Expectancy theory further postulates that anxiety expectancy stems from learned experiences that a given stimulus will generate anxiety or fear (Reiss & McNally, 1985). Nevertheless, a person need not experience anxiety in a particular situation in order to anticipate it. Certain situations may come to be associated with fear or anxiety after an individual has witnessed someone having a panic attack. Conversely, it is believed that anxiety sensitivity may be developed through learned experiences (Donnell & McNally, 1990) and inherited through biological factors (Reiss & McNally, 1985). For instance, although Donnell and McNally (1990) found that participants with high anxiety sensitivity were more likely to have experienced both a personal and family history of panic, two-thirds had never suffered a panic attack. In addition, findings from a retrospective study on the origins of anxiety sensitivity suggested that participants with high levels of anxiety sensitivity may have learned to catastrophize about the occurrence of bodily symptoms through parental reinforcement of sick-role behavior related to physical symptoms rather than anxiety-related symptoms (Watt et al., 1998). Schmidt and colleagues (1997) also revealed that anxiety sensitivity predicts the development of panic and other anxiety symptoms independent of history of panic and trait anxiety. Thus, anxiety sensitivity is not considered a consequence of experiencing a panic attack, but rather a predisposing bio-psycho-social factor to developing panic. This suggests that an individual who experiences a panic attack but does not develop panic disorder may not have the biological markers nor the psychological and social attributes to developing panic disorder. This is somewhat consistent with Clarke's (1986) cognitive model of panic that posits that the development and maintenance of panic arise from a fear that bodily sensations will lead to harmful consequences.

Several studies have demonstrated that a greater association exists between anxiety expectancy and avoidance behavior, rather than with the occurrence of panic attacks and avoidance (e.g., Cox et al., 1995; Cox et al., 1991; Craske et al., 1988; Whittal & Goetsch, 1997). As expectation of panic increases, so does avoidance. This finding is also supported by Craske and Barlow's (1988) hypothesis suggesting a greater relationship between avoidance behavior and anxiety expectancy.

Treatments aimed at diminishing the expectation of anxiety may also be effective in reducing the amount of fear actually experienced by the individual (e.g., Kirsch et al., 1983). For instance, Kirsch and colleagues (1983) succeeded in diminishing the amount of fear experienced in snake phobic patients through systematic desensitization and through an expectancy modification procedure. They concluded that the level of fear experienced by individuals with a snake phobia varies as a function of anxiety expectancy. Southworth and Kirsch (1988) also found that when the expectations of the occurrence of anxiety are reduced, patients with agoraphobia experienced less fear. These findings suggest that when clients expect to experience anxiety and they do not after several sessions of exposure, their fear ultimately diminishes. Changing expectations may have a direct impact on symptoms.

Earlier studies on the effects of expectancies on outcome mostly focussed on prognostic expectations (i.e., the probability of a therapeutic success) that clients have when they enter into treatment (e.g., Frank, 1959; Goldstein & Shipman, 1961; see Goldstein, 1962; Piper & Wogan, 1970). However, in a review on psychotherapy, Perotti and Hopewell (1980) concluded that although expectancy effects are important in various interventions including systematic desensitization, pre-treatment expectations have little effect. Measuring expectations both at pretherapy and during the early treatment phase may not only provide information on whether clients can change their expectations but it may also shed some light on the impact these cognitive shifts have on outcome. After several sessions of therapy, expectations may shift towards a positive direction if clients perceive improvement or they may shift towards a negative direction if no benefits are noticed (Weiner, 1982).

The research on panic disorder with agoraphobia has established the importance of expectancies in the development and maintenance of PDA (Ehlers, 1995; Maller & Reiss, 1992; Schmidt et al., 1997; Watt et al., 1998). However, there is a paucity of data examining the differential effects of distinct types of expectancies (i.e., anxiety expectancy and sensitivity, avoidance expectancy) on initial severity and outcome of PDA using a cognitive-behavioral treatment. Studies examining possible predictors in treatment outcome have determined that pre-symptom severity has an impact, especially pre-treatment agoraphobic avoidance and longer duration (e.g., Basoglu et al., 1994; de Beurs et al., 1995; Williams, & Falbo, 1996). However, no study to our knowledge has examined the differential impact of symptom severity and expectancies on cognitive-behavior therapy outcome of panic disorder with agoraphobia. Examining the relative contribution of these variables may foster a greater understanding as to why some PDA clients show partial or no response to CBT. This may enable therapists to better prepare their treatment plan.

There were several objectives to this study. First, we examined the impact of different types of expectancies on pre-treatment symptom severity. Expectancies that were examined included anxiety sensitivity, anxiety expectancy and prognostic expectancy as measured by avoidance expectancy (i.e., expectancy of avoidance at the end of treatment). Symptom severity was measured in terms of frequency of catastrophic cognitions during a panic attack, degree of fear of symptoms already experienced during a panic attack, panic symptomatology, avoidance, and by depressive symptoms. It was predicted that the severity of baseline expectancy would be associated with baseline symptom severity. Second, we examined the impact of the initial treatment phase scores in contrast to baseline scores on outcome. With respect to symptoms, our hypothesis is consistent with theories on in-session change in cognitive-behavior therapy that suggest that shifts in symptoms during sessions are better predictors of outcome than pretreatment severity (see Muran et al., 1995). We predicted that initial treatment phase symptom scores would be better predictors of outcome than baseline scores. With respect to expectancies, it was hypothesised that early treatment phase scores would be better predictors of outcome than baseline. After being exposed to several components of therapy, it is assumed that participants will adjust their expectations to be more consistent with the information received in the first few sessions. Finally, we examined the contribution of expectancies above and beyond the contribution of symptoms on the outcome of PDA following a cognitive-behavior therapy.

2. Method

2.1 Participants

The sample consisted of 49 participants (14 males, 35 females) with a principal DSM-IV (Diagnostic and Statistical Manual of Mental Disorders, 4th ed.; American Psychiatric Association, 1994) diagnosis of panic disorder with agoraphobia. Sixteen participants dropped out from pre- to post-treatment. Eleven males and 22 females completed the study. The mean age of the initial sample was 39.3 years (SD = 11.19; range: 19 - 65 years) and the mean education level was 11.6 years (SD = 3.06). The average number of years of marriage or cohabitation was 12.3 years (SD = 11.98). There were 71.5% of the participants who were either married or cohabiting, 22.4% were single, 2% were separated or divorced and 2% were widowed. Most participants (n = 31; 63.3%) were taking psychoactive medication for their panic attacks. Twenty-three participants were recruited from two specialised outpatient anxiety disorder clinics in Montreal: the Douglas Hospital Anxiety Clinic (n = 8) and the Centre for Intervention for Cognitive Behavioral Therapy at Louis-H. Lafontaine Hospital (n = 15). The remaining participants were recruited from advertisements in the local newspapers (n=26).

Patients included in the study met the following criteria: (a) a primary DSM-IV diagnosis of PDA assigned by one of the psychiatrists; (b) a primary diagnosis of PDA with a clinical severity rating of 4 or above on a scale ranging from 0 (none) to 8 (very severely disturbing-disabling), established by administering the Anxiety Disorders Interview Schedule for DSM-IV, Lifetime Version (ADIS-IV-L; DiNardo, Brown, & Barlow, 1994), (c) a secondary DSM-IV axis I diagnosis with an assigned ADIS-IV-L clinical severity rating which ranges from moderate to severely disabling (i.e., 4 to 6) and consists of a rating of 2 or more levels lower than the PDA rating, (d) age between 18 and 65 years, and (e) at least a mean of 1 panic attack per week in the 3 weeks prior to participation in the assessment. Exclusion criteria included: (a) the presence of substance-related, psychotic and bipolar disorders and any organic brain conditions as evaluated by the psychiatrists; and, (b) the presence of any unstable medical condition considered by the evaluating psychiatrist to be mistaken for anxiety symptoms (e.g., thyroid disorders, asthma, cardiovascular diseases, etc).

The average duration of PDA was 13 years (SD = 10.4; range: 1 - 40 years). Secondary diagnoses as assessed by the psychiatrists and the ADIS-IV-L included other anxiety disorders, hypochondriasis and affective disorders. Twenty-four patients also met criteria for one or more of the following secondary diagnoses ranging from moderate (i.e., 4) to severely disabling (i.e, 6): generalized anxiety disorder (n = 13), dysthymia (n = 4), social phobia (n = 3), post traumatic stress disorder (n = 3), specific phobia (n = 2), obsessive compulsive disorder (n = 2), hypochondriasis (n = 2), major depressive disorder (n = 1), and mania (n = 1). For all secondary diagnoses, the ADIS-IV-L clinical severity rating was 2 or more levels lower than the PDA rating. Participants accepted in the study with a secondary diagnosis had disorders that were not in immediate need of treatment as assessed by the psychiatrists.

A high percentage of patients (n = 31; 63.3%) were taking psychoactive medication. Medication needs of the patients were evaluated during the evaluation with the psychiatrist. Participants under pharmacological treatment for anxiety, at the time of the evaluation, were permitted to participate only after medication had been stable for 6 weeks prior to treatment. Participants were asked to maintain the same dosage throughout the treatment phase of the study to allow for evaluation of the effects of psychotherapy above the effects of these drugs (e.g., Brown & Barlow, 1995). Participants taking medication were not asked to discontinue pharmacotherapy before treatment since (a) many individuals would probably not participate because they would not want to stop taking their medication before treatment, and (b) discontinuing medication during treatment may lead to an increase in panic attacks which may affect responses given on baseline measures (Öst & Westling, 1995).

2.2 Treatment

Treatment was administered by experienced clinical psychologists. Co-therapists consisted of doctoral students in clinical psychology. They had experience in cognitive-behavior therapy, had been trained in administering the group treatment for PDA and were closely supervised by the second author of this study. All therapists followed a written manual which included the protocol for each session. There were a total of 6 groups that consisted of a maximum of 10 participants. Cognitive behavior group therapy was administered based on the Panic Control Treatment developed in SUNY Albany (Craske & Barlow, 1990). The treatment consisted of 14 weekly, 3-hour sessions and comprised five major components: (a) education and information concerning the nature, etiology and maintenance of panic; (b) cognitive restructuring (Beck, 1988) aimed at demystifying symptoms and fears and helping participants identify, monitor and change mistaken appraisals of threat that precipitate panic attacks and maintain avoidance behaviors; (c) training in diaphragmatic breathing as a way of reducing physical symptoms that often trigger panic attacks; (d) interoceptive exposure exercises designed to reduce fear of somatic sensations through repeated exposure to bodily sensations associated with panic; and (e) prolonged and repeated in vivo exposure to feared situations. Participants were also expected to practice techniques and read relevant material on PDA in between sessions.

2.3 Measures

2.3.1 Symptom measures

Participants completed a battery of self-reported questionnaires commonly used in PDA research. The following measures on symptom severity have demonstrated acceptable psychometric properties. A French version of these questionnaires was utilised in the current study.

Severity of cognitive panic symptoms was assessed by the Body Sensations Questionnaire (BSQ; Chambless et al., 1984) and Agoraphobia Cognitions Questionnaire (ACQ; Chambless et al., 1984). The BSQ is a 17-item questionnaire that measures level of fear concerning bodily sensations that have been experienced during a panic attack. The ACQ consists of 14 items measuring the frequency of catastrophic thoughts during a panic attack. Both measures are rated on a 5-point Likert-type scale. Coefficient alpha for the BSQ in this study was estimated at .88 and for the ACQ at .79. These two measures assess fear of fear as a consequence of panic experiences. The psychometric properties of the French-Canadian versions employed in this study are equivalent to those of the English version (Stephenson et al., 1998; Stephenson et al., 1999).

One of the three measures provided by the Mobility Inventory for Agoraphobia (MIA; Chambless et al., 1985) was used in this study: the severity of agoraphobic avoidance behavior when the person is alone. The MIA-Alone is a 26-item questionnaire rated on a 5-point Likert-type scale. This study calculated the coefficient alpha at .93. Psychometric properties of the French-Canadian version have been found to be similar to those of the English version (Stephenson et al., 1997).

Physical and cognitive symptoms experienced during the past week were assessed using the Beck Anxiety Inventory (BAI; Beck et al., 1988). This 21-item questionnaire, rated on a 4-point scale, examines the degree to which participants were affected by their symptoms over the past week. In this study, internal consistency was estimated at .93.

Depressive symptoms were measured using a French version of the Beck Depression Inventory-II (BDI-II; Beck et al., 1996). The BDI-II is composed of 21 items rating depressive symptoms for a two-week period, on a 4-point scale. In the current study, internal consistency for this measure was estimated at .91. In 1961 and 1978 the French-Canadian version of the BDI was validated (Gauthier et al., 1982; Bourque & Beaudette, 1982). There is no current validation study for the French-Canadian version of the BDI-II, however, we chose to use the latter in this study because there is greater consistency with the DSM-IV criteria for major depressive disorder.

2.3.2 Expectancy measures

All expectancy measures for this study were translated into French using forward and back translation techniques (Vallerand, 1989; see Table 2 for overall distribution of all expectancy measures). The following expectancy measures have not yet been validated for their psychometric properties.

2.3.2.1 Anxiety expectancy

A section of the Panic Attack Questionnaire (PAQ; Norton et al., 1986), containing 36 items, was used to assess anxiety expectancy. Participants rate on a scale of 0 (never) to 4 (very likely) how much they expect a future panic attack to occur in a particular situation regardless of whether or not they have previously experienced a panic attack in that situation. Internal consistency of the French version (Bélanger & Katerelos, 1998) of this questionnaire using the current sample was estimated at .91. This measure will be referred to as Panic Attack Questionnaire-Expectancy (PAQ-E).

2.3.2.2 Anxiety sensitivity

Anxiety Sensitivity Index (ASI; Reiss et al., 1986) is a 16-item questionnaire, rated on a 5-point Likert-type scale. It measures fear of anxiety and has been specifically associated with agoraphobia (see Taylor, 1993). The items assess the level of expected somatic, psychological or social harm that may occur as a result of anxiety symptoms. However, a history of panic attacks is not an essential component for developing negative beliefs about the harmful effects of anxiety. The internal consistency of the questionnaire has been estimated at .88 (Cox et al., 1996) and a two-week test-retest reliability has been computed at .75 (Reiss et al., 1986). Psychometric properties of the French-Canadian version have been found to be similar to those of the English version (Marchand et al., 1999). Internal consistency for the French translation of the ASI was calculated at .81 in this study.

2.3.2.3 Avoidance expectancy

An adaptation of the Mobility Inventory for Agoraphobia-Alone (MIA-A; Chambless et al., 1985) was used to assess prognostic expectations (with respect to avoidance behavior)(i.e., the probability of a therapeutic success). The Expectancy Mobility Inventory for Agoraphobia-Alone (EMIA-A) measures the degree of expected agoraphobic avoidance behavior following therapy (Katerelos et al., 1998). The same items as the MIA-A were administered along with the corresponding 5-point scale. However, the adapted version contains questions reformulated into expectancies (e.g., "After the treatment, I expect to…never avoid going to the movies"). With the current French sample and with the items reformulated into expectancies, internal consistency when alone was at 95.

2.4 Procedure

Participants recruited from advertisements in the local newspapers were screened using a brief telephone interview in order to determine suitability. Those who were considered appropriate for the study were invited to one of the clinics to take part in a structured interview. If the criteria for a primary diagnosis of PDA were satisfied according to the ADIS-IV-L, participants were evaluated by a psychiatrist from one of the two collaborating clinics to confirm the diagnosis. A battery of questionnaires was completed after the DSM-IV diagnosis of PDA had been confirmed. Those recruited directly from the clinics had already received a diagnosis of PDA by one of the psychiatrists. The ADIS-IV-L was subsequently administered in order to rule out an additional Axis I primary diagnosis and to confirm the initial DSM-IV diagnosis given by the psychiatrist. All participants provided informed consent prior to the structured interview with the ADIS-IV-L. Those who did not meet the criteria of the study were appropriately referred elsewhere.

Expectancies were assessed prior to therapy (T1) and after patients had completed 4 sessions (T2; initial treatment phase). Symptom severity was measured prior to therapy (T1), 4 sessions after therapy had begun (T2; initial treatment phase) and after the last session (T3). By session four, clients receive (a) education and information concerning the nature, etiology and maintenance of panic, as well as information on the impact PDA has on social functioning, daily activities, family and work; (b) symptom demystification, (c) training in diaphragmatic breathing, (d) basic coping strategies to deal with panic, and (e) information on the role of irrational thoughts in PDA.

3. Results

3.1 Sample characteristics

Of the 49 patients who began the treatment, 33 completed. An analysis of variance (ANOVA) detected no difference between dropouts and completers in symptomatology, expectancies, duration of PDA, gender or sociodemographic variables. In addition, analyses of variance did not reveal any significant differences between those who took medication and those who did not on gender, sociodemographic variables, pre-treatment expectancy measures nor on most symptom severity measures ($p > .05$). No significant differences were found between clients referred from either of the two clinics and those referred from the local newspapers on any sociodemographic or expectancy variable, and for most symptomatology variables ($p > .05$). However a univariate ANOVA revealed a significant main effect for group for the BDI-II measures $F(2, 45) = 4.1$, $P < .023$. Bonferroni post hoc comparisons demonstrated significantly higher BDI-II scores for the 8 participants selected from the Douglas Hospital Anxiety Clinic (M=24.1, SD=14.5) in contrast to those chosen from local newspapers (M=13.5, SD=9.2) ($p < .05$).

3.2 Dependent variables

The dependent variables (i.e., post-treatment measures; T3) approached a normal distribution. The means and standard deviations for the dependent variables were as follows: Body Sensations Questionnaire (BSQ) (M = 32.5, SD = 2), Agoraphobia Cognitions Questionnaire (ACQ) (M = 23.7, SD = 1.2), Beck Anxiety Inventory (BAI) (M = 11.4, SD = 1.9), Mobility Inventory for Agoraphobia-Alone (MIA-A) (M = 49.4, SD = 4.3) and the Beck Depression Inventory (BDI-II) (M = 8.2, SD = 1.3).

3.3 Predictors of pre-treatment (T1) symptom severity scores

Our first objective was to examine the impact of anxiety sensitivity (ASI), anxiety expectancy (PAQ-E) and avoidance expectancy (EMIA-A) on pre-treatment symptom severity. Stepwise regression analyses were conducted using data from the initial 49 participants in order to determine predictors of pre-treatment symptom severity. Correlations were calculated for the sample (see Table 1) and only measures that were significant at $p < .01$ were entered into the regression equations. The first regression analysis used the BSQ (T1) as the dependent variable. The findings revealed that the ASI (T1) significantly entered into the equation [$r2$ change = .44, $F(1, 46) = 35.9$, $P < .001$)]. The PAQ-E did not contribute to the prediction model.

The second regression analysis used the ACQ (T1) as the dependent variable. The ASI [$r2$ change = .09, $F(1, 45) = 8.1$, $P < .01$)] was once again the only significant predictor variable. The PAQ-E failed to significantly enter into the equation.

The third regression analysis examined to what degree the BAI (T1) was determined from expectancy scores. The findings revealed that PAQ-E (T1) [$r2$ change = .17, $F(1, 46) = 9.3$, $P < .01$)] significantly entered into the regression equation but the ASI failed to add to the prediction model.

A fourth regression analysis was performed to determine to what degree the MIA-A(T1) scores could be predicted from expectancy scores. The findings revealed that both the PAQ-E (T1) [$r2$ change = .24, $F(1, 47) = 14.8$, $P < .001$)] and the EMIA-A (T1) [$r2$ change = .08, $F(1, 46) = 5.2$, $P < .05$)] significantly entered into the equation.

The BDI-II (T1) was significantly correlated with one expectancy measure: the ASI ($r=.49$, $p < .001$).

None of the pre-treatment expectancy measures were significantly associated with duration of PDA and with number of panic attacks in the past month (p > .05).

Variables	Body Sensations Questionnaire	Agoraphobia Cognitions Questionnaire	Beck Anxiety Inventory	Mobility Inventory for Agoraphobia-Alone	Beck Depression Inventory
Anxiety Sensitivity Index	.66***	.66***	.37**	.11	.49***
Panic Attack Questionnaire-Expectancy	.37**	.43**	.37**	.49***	.18
Expectancy Mobility Inventory for Agoraphobia-Alone	.19	.32*	.21	.38**	.19

Note: Ns may vary from 47 to 49 due to missing data.
*$p < .05$, **$p < .01$, ***$p < .001$

Table 1. Correlations Between Pre-treatment Symptom Severity and Expectancy.

3.4 Pretreatment (T1) vs. initial treatment phase (T2): symptom severity and expectancy measures

In order to verify our second hypothesis indicating that initial treatment phase scores would be better predictors of outcome than pre-treatment scores, we first performed t-tests to determine whether there were any changes from pre- to initial treatment phase. There was considerable improvement from pre-treatment to session 4 (i.e., initial treatment phase) for all symptom severity and expectancy measures. One exception was noted for the Expectancy Mobility for Agoraphobia Inventory-Alone (EMIA-A). Changes in scores from pre-treatment to session 4, means, standard deviations, and ranges are presented in Table 2. All measures approximated a normal distribution.

	Pre-treatment Scores			Session 4 Scores				
Variables	*M*	*SD*	Range	*M*	*SD*	Range	*t*	*df*
Symptom Measures								
Body Sensations Questionnaire	50.4	14.5	17-85	42.6	15.1	19-75	2.86**	37
Agoraphobia Cognitions Questionnaire	35.7	9.4	17-60	30	9.7	17-58	4.05***	7
Beck Anxiety Inventory	28.1	14.8	0-55	16.4	10.6	1-41	5.11***	36
Mobility Inventory for Agoraphobia-Alone	85.7	24.2	46-130	67.6	28.2	31-129	7.23***	37
Beck Depression Inventory	16.4	10.1	2-44	12.7	10.4	0-36	-2.26*	37
Expectancy Measures								
Anxiety Sensitivity Index	34.1	10.8	11-58	25	11.6	2-48	4.68***	39
Panic Attack Questionnaire - Expectancy	72.8	24.7	8-120	52.3	23.8	0-117	5.22***	40
Mobility Inventory for Agoraphobia-Alone Expectancy	52.0	19.3	26-114	51.5	21.6	26-103	0.15	40

Note: Ns may vary from 37 to 41 due to missing data.
*$p < .05$, **$p < .01$, ***$p < .001$

Table 2. Changes in Independent Variables from Pre-treatment to Initial Treatment Phase.

3.5 Treatment outcome

Outcome data is provided for 33 patients. Significant improvements were detected from pre-treatment to post treatment scores on all symptom severity measures ($p < .001$). There was no significant relationship between duration of PDA and post-treatment measures ($p > .05$).

3.5.1 Predictors of pretreatment outcome

Consistent with our second objective, the effect of initial treatment phase scores (T2) in contrast to baseline scores (T1) on treatment outcome was examined. Multiple regression analyses were first performed for symptom severity measures and then for expectancy. Subsequent regression analyses were performed to verify our final objective aimed at determining the contribution of expectations over the effects of symptoms on treatment outcome. Only factors that were significantly correlated at a conservative alpha of .01 were entered into the regression equations (see Tables 3 and 4).

Variables	BSQ (T3)	ACQ (T3)	BAI (T3)	MIA-A (T3)	BDI-II (T3)
Pre-treatment (T1)					
Body Sensations Questionnaire	.34*	.28	.35*	-.05	.47**
Agoraphobia Cognitions Questionnaire	.30	.28	.33	.08	.36*
Beck Anxiety Inventory	.28	.25	.33	.21	.45**
Mobility Inventory for Agoraphobia-Alone	.07	.37*	.27	.72***	.14
Beck Depression Inventory	.61***	.49**	.40*	.31	.56***
Initial Treatment Phase (T2)					
Body Sensations Questionnaire	.63***	.43**	.24	.31	.16
Agoraphobia Cognitions Questionnaire	.47**	.47**	.21	.43*	.16
Beck Anxiety Inventory	.59***	.55**	.67***	.29	.50**
Mobility Inventory for Agoraphobia-Alone	.29	.28	.05	.77***	-.08
Beck Depression Inventory	.33	.30	.18	.08	.42*

Note: *Ns* may vary from 31 to 33 for post treatment data, 37 to 38 for mid-treatment data and 48 to 49 for pre-treatment data due to missing data and dropouts. BSQ = Body Sensations Questionnaire (T3); ACQ = Agoraphobia Cognitions Questionnaire; BAI= Beck Anxiety Inventory; MIA-A = Mobility Inventory for Agoraphobia-Alone; BDI = Beck Depression Inventory
*$p < .05$, **$p < .01$, ***$p < .001$

Table 3. Correlations between Dependent Variables and Independent Variables: Symptoms Measures

3.5.2 Multiple regression analyses with symptom severity measures

Hierarchical regression analyses were conducted to determine the extent to which variability in post-treatment (T3) symptomatology could be predicted from pre-treatment (T1) and initial treatment phase (T2) symptomatology measures. Initial treatment phase scores were entered into the first step followed by pre-treatment scores. The results in Table 5 demonstrate that overall, pre-treatment did not significantly add to the prediction of post-treatment severity, with the exception of the BDI-II. Since initial treatment phase scores significantly improved from baseline, this suggests that changes in symptomatology are better predictors of outcome than pre-treatment severity.

Variables	BSQ (T3)	ACQ (T3)	BAI (T3)	MIA-A (T3)	BDI-II (T3)	*M*	*SD*	Range
Pre-treatment (T1)								
Anxiety Sensitivity Index	.35	.18	.41*	.04	.47**	34.4	10.6	11-58
Panic Attack Questionnaire	.24	.27	.26	.35*	.10	73.1	23.5	8-120
Mobility Inventory for Agoraphobia-Alone Expectancy	.31	.23	.22	.41*	.19	52.9	18.5	26-114
Initial Treatment Phase (T2)								
Anxiety Sensitivity Index	.65***	.57***	.37*	.50**	.57***	24.7	11.6	2-48
Panic Attack Questionnaire	.76***	.59***	.52**	.55***	.43*	52.3	23.8	0-117
Mobility Inventory for Agoraphobia-Alone Expectancy	.52**	.55***	.30	.81***	.32	51.5	21.6	26-103

Note: *Ns* may vary from 31 to 33 for post-treatment, 37 to 38 for mid-treatment and 48 to 49 for pre-treatment data (i.e., *M, SD* and Range) due to missing data with treatment and dropouts between time. T3 = Post-treatment; BSQ = Body Sensations Questionnaire (T3); ACQ = Agoraphobia Cognitions Questionnaire; BAI= Beck Anxiety Inventory; MIA-A = Mobility Inventory for Agoraphobia-Alone; BDI = Beck Depression Inventory
*$p < .05$, **$p < .01$, ***$p < .001$

Table 4. Correlations between Dependent Variables and Independent Variables (i.e., Expectancy measures)

To determine which individual measures were the best predictors of post-treatment symptomatology, significant regression analyses were re-ran for the BSQ (T3), ACQ (T3), and the BDI (T3). Variables that did not significantly contribute to the initial model were removed from the equations.

Results for the BSQ post-treatment (T3), revealed that the BSQ (T2) [r2 change = .40, F(1, 28) = 18.3, P < .001)] and BAI (T2) [r2 change = .13, F(1, 27) = 7.6, P < .01)] were significant predictors in the model.

Results for the ACQ post-treatment (T3) revealed that the BAI (T2) [r2 change = .22, F(1, 28) = 7.7, P < .01)] and the ACQ (T2) [r2 change = .18, F(1, 27) = 8.1, P < .01)] were significant predictors of the ACQ (T3), accounting for 18% and10% of the variance respectively. A regression analysis was performed with factors that reached significance for the BDI-II post-treatment (T3). The BAI (T2) was entered into the first block and then the BDI-II (T1) was entered into the second. The findings revealed that pre-treatment depressive symptoms (BDI-II T1) [r2 change = .17, F(1, 27) = 7.63, P < .01)] contributed above and beyond the effects of initial treatment phase anxiety symptoms (BAI T2) [r2 change = .25, F(1, 28) = 9.38, P < .01)] in the prediction of post-treatment depressive symptoms (BDI-II T3). However, only pre-treatment depressive symptoms were significant predictors when the second model was retained. The BAI (T2) failed to reach significance. This suggests that severity in depression at baseline is a greater predictor of post-treatment depression when compared to any of the other measures taken after the fourth session (i.e., initial treatment phase).

The BAI post-treatment ratings (T3) were significantly correlated with one measure: the BAI scores at the initial treatment phase (i.e., session 4) (r = .67, p < .001).

Dependent Variables	Model	Predictor Variables	$R2$ change	F value for $R2$ change	dfs	Semi-partial $R2$
Body Sensations Questionnaire (T3)	1	BSQ (T2)	.53***	9.7	3, 26	.10*
		BAI (T2)				.13*
		ACQ (T2)				.00
	2	BDI-II (T1)	.06	4	1, 25	.06
Agoraphobia Cognitions Questionnaire (T3)	1	BAI (T2)	.40***	8.8	2, 27	.18**
		ACQ (T2)				.10*
	2	BDI-II (T1)	.03	1.4	1, 26	.03
Mobility Inventory for Agoraphobia-Alone (T3)	1	MIA-A (T2)	.59***	41.5	1, 29	.59***
	2	MIA-A (T1)	.02	1.7	1, 28	.02
Beck Depression Inventory (T3)	1	BAI (T2)	.25**	9.4	1, 28	.25**
	2	BDI-II (T1)	.21*	3.3	3, 25	.11*
		BSQ (T1)				.01
		BAI (T1)				.03

Note: *Ns* may vary from 30 to 31 due to missing data
BSQ = Body Sensations Questionnaire (T3); ACQ = Agoraphobia Cognitions Questionnaire; BAI= Beck Anxiety Inventory; MIA-A = Mobility Inventory for Agoraphobia-Alone; BDI = Beck Depression Inventory
*$p < .05$, **$p < .01$, ***$p < .001$

Table 5. Hierarchical Regression Analysis of Pre-treatment (T1) Symptomatology and Initial Treatment Phase (T2) Measures on Post-Treatment (T3) Symptomatology Measures

3.5.3 Multiple regression analyses with expectancy measures

In accordance with the second part of our second objective, hierarchical regression analyses were conducted to determine the extent to which variability in post-treatment symptomatology measures could be predicted from pre-treatment and initial treatment phase expectancy scores. Factors that were significantly correlated at the $p < .01$ level entered into the regression equations. Measures from the initial treatment phase (T2) were entered in the first block and baseline measures (T1) were entered in the second. Analyses were conducted for the BSQ (T3) and the BDI-II (T3) since they were the only measures that were significantly correlated ($p < .01$) with both pre-treatment and initial treatment phase expectancy measures (see Table 4). The results in Table 6 demonstrate that the initial phase session (T2; session 4) measures are significant predictors of the BSQ (T3) and the BDI-II (T3). Pre-treatment expectancy measures did not significantly add to the prediction model for these two dependent measures. To determine which initial treatment phase (T2) expectancy measures were the best predictors of post-treatment symptomatology, stepwise regression analyses were performed.

We first examined the degree to which BSQ (T3) scores could be predicted from initial treatment phase expectancy scores. The PAQ-E (T2), the ASI (T2), and the EMIA-A (T2)

were entered into the equation. The results showed that anxiety expectancy as measured by the PAQ-E (T2) accounts for significant variance in the BSQ (T3) [r2 change = .58, F(1, 30) = 41.4, P < .001)] , however, anxiety sensitivity (i.e., ASI T2) and avoidance expectancy (i.e., EMIA-A T2) failed to make a contribution to the model.

A stepwise regression analysis was performed to determine to what degree post-treatment agoraphobic cognitions (i.e., ACQ T3) scores could be predicted from the initial treatment phase (T2) scores. The PAQ-E (T2), the ASI (T2), and the EMIA-A (T2) were entered into the equation. The findings revealed that the PAQ-E (T2) [r2 change = .35, F(1, 30) = 16.2, P < .001)] and the EMIA-A (T2) [r2 change = .08, F(1, 29) = 4.3, P < .05)] each account for significant variance in the ACQ (T3) ratings (i.e., 13% and 8% respectively). The ASI (T2) did not enter significantly on the third step.

A stepwise regression analysis was conducted with EMIA-A (T2), PAQ-E (T2), and ASI (T2) as the independent measures and MIA-A post-treatment scores as the dependent measure. The findings showed that avoidance expectancy (i.e., EMIA-A T2) was the best predictor [r2 change = .66, F(1, 30) = 56.9, P < .001)]. The PAQ-E and the ASI failed to enter into the equation. When the EMIA-A (T2) was removed from the equation the ASI (T2) failed to enter into the equation and the PAQ-E (T2) explained a significant portion of the variance [r2 change = .31, F(1, 30) = 13.2, P < .001)].

The BAI post-treatment ratings were significantly correlated with one expectancy measure: the PAQ-E (T2) scores (r = .52, p < .01).

Dependent Variables	Model	Predictor Variables	*R2*	*R2* change	*F* value for *R2* change	*dfs*	Semi-partial *R2*
Body Sensations Questionnaire (T3)	1	PAQ-E (T2)	.60	.62***	15.2	3, 28	.43***
		ASI (T2)					.13
		EMIA-A(T2)					.07
	2	PAQ (T1)	.60	.01	.40	1, 27	.01
Beck Depression Inventory (T3)	1	ASI (T2)	.30	.31***	12.8	1, 29	.31***
	2	ASI (T1)	.40	.08	3.8	1, 28	.08

Note: *Ns* may vary from 31 to 32 due to missing data.
ASI = Anxiety Sensitivity Index; PAQ-E = Panic Attack Questionnaire-Expectancy; EMIA-A = Expectancy Mobility Inventory for Agoraphobia.
**p* < .05, ***p* < .01, ****p*< .001

Table 6. Hierarchical Regression Analyses of Pre-treatment (T1) and Initial TreatmentPhase (T2) Expectancy Measures on Post-treatment (T3) Symptom Severity Measures

3.5.4 Prediction of outcome measures

Consistent with our last objective, we examined the contribution of expectancies above and beyond the contribution of symptoms on the outcome of PDA following cognitive-behavior therapy. Hierarchical regression analyses were used to compare the utility of symptomatology versus expectancies in predicting symptomatology post-treatment scores. Initial treatment phase (i.e., T2 or session 4) symptom and expectancy variables that were identified in the previous sections as significant predictors of post-treatment (i.e., T3) symptom severity were entered into the equation. Symptom measures were entered in the first block followed by expectancy measures in the second. Findings revealed that the addition of expectancy measures significantly added to the prediction model for most dependent measures except for the BAI (T3) and the BDI-II (T3) scores (see Table 7).

To determine which individual measures were the best predictors of the symptom measures, stepwise regression analyses were performed.

The regression analysis for the BSQ (T3) revealed that anxiety expectancy after the fourth session (PAQ-E T2) was the best predictor of the BSQ [r2 change = .61, F(1, 28) = 44.1, P < .001)]. The BSQ (T2) and the BAI (T2) failed to enter into the equation.

Dependent Variables	Block	Predictor Variables	*R2* change	*F* value for *R2* change	*dfs*	Semi-partial *R2*
Body Sensations Questionnaire (T3)	1	BSQ (T2)	.53***	15.1	2, 27	.18**
		BAI (T2)				.13**
	2	PAQ-E (T2)	.14**	10.7	1, 26	.14**
Agoraphobia Cognitions Questionnaire (T3)	1	BAI (T2)	.40***	8.8	2, 27	.18**
		ACQ (T2)				.10*
	2	PAQ-E (T2)	.14*	3.6	2, 25	.02
		EMIA-A (T2)				.07
Mobility Inventory for Agoraphobia-Alone (T3)	1	MIA-A (T2)	.59***	41.5	1, 29	.59***
	2	EMIA-A (T2)	.12**	12	1, 28	.12**
Beck Anxiety Inventory (T3)	1	BAI (T2)	.47***	24.8	1, 28	.47***
	2	PAQ-E (T2)	.04	2	1, 27	.04
Beck Depression Inventory (T3)	1	BDI-II (T1)	.32***	14.2	1, 30	.32***
	2	ASI (T2)	.09	4.2	1, 29	.09H

Note: *Ns* may vary from 30 to 32 due to missing data.
BSQ = Body Sensations Questionnaire (T3); ACQ = Agoraphobia Cognitions Questionnaire; BAI= Beck Anxiety Inventory; MIA-A = Mobility Inventory for Agoraphobia-Alone; BDI = Beck Depression Inventory; ASI = Anxiety Sensitivity Index; PAQ-E = Panic Attack Questionnaire-Expectancy; EMIA-A = Expectancy Mobility Inventory for Agoraphobia.

*p < .05, **p < .01, ***p< .001; H *p* =.05

Table 7. Hierarchical Regression Analyses of Expectancy vs Symptomatology as Predictors of Post-Treatment Severity

We entered the BAI (T2), ACQ (T2), PAQ-E(T2) and the EMIA-A (T2) into a stepwise multiple regression analysis to determine the best predictor for the ACQ (T3). The PAQ-E

(T2) was the only significant predictor accounting for 37% of the variance [r2 change = .37, F(1, 28) = 16.4, P < .001)].

Finally, when the MIA-A (T2) and the EMIA-A (T2) are entered into a stepwise multiple regression with MIA-A (T3) as the dependent variable, the results show the EMIA-A (T2) enters significantly in the first step [r2 change = .65, F(1, 29) = 54.6, P < .001)], followed by the MIA-A (T2) [r2 change = .06, F(1, 28) = 5.7, P < .05)].

The above findings demonstrate that, for the most part, expectancies measured after four sessions (T2) are better predictors of PDA outcome, in contrast to initial treatment phase (T2) symptomatology.

4. Discussion

The objectives of this study were to examine (a) the relationship between expectancies (i.e., anxiety sensitivity and expectancy, and prognostic expectancy as measured by avoidance expectancy) and symptom severity (i.e., avoidance of specific situations, intensity of fear of somatic symptoms, frequency of agoraphobic cognitions, intensity of anxiety symptoms and levels of depressive symptoms) in panic disorder with agoraphobia (PDA) prior to treatment; (b) the impact of initial treatment phase scores in contrast to baseline scores on outcome; and (c) the contribution of expectancies above and beyond the contribution of symptoms on the outcome of PDA following a cognitive-behavior therapy.

Consistent with our first hypothesis, and similar to other studies (e.g., Cox et al., 1991; McNally, & Lorenz, 1987; Norton et al., 1999; Schmidt, et al., 1997) we found that baseline severity of PDA symptomatology was predicted by higher anxiety sensitivity, and greater expectations of anxiety and expectations of avoidance behavior. Our findings were independent of duration of PDA, suggesting that individuals with PDA may hold these strong beliefs about their symptoms regardless of how long they have had PDA. The experience of panic may further validate their beliefs surrounding the occurrence and consequences of anxiety symptoms and avoidance behaviors

As predicted in the first part of our second hypothesis, most of the initial treatment phase symptom scores were better predictors of PDA outcome. The only session 4 measure that did not significantly predict outcome was the BDI-II. Pre-treatment depressive symptoms were significant determinants of post-treatment scores on the BDI-II. This may suggest that regardless of the progress during group CBT for PDA, initial severity of depressive symptoms is the best predictor of mood following therapy. Clients suffering from PDA who also experience depressive symptoms may benefit from a therapy that includes a component aimed at addressing their depression.

Consistent with the second part of our second hypothesis, expectancies measured after session four were significant determinants of post-treatment PDA symptom severity. This suggests that clients who failed to make the cognitive shifts in expectancies after four sessions of therapy were more likely to have a poor outcome. Our results are also in line with the earlier theories posited by Perotti and Hopewell (1980) and Weiner (1982) (both cited in Garfield, 1986) that indicate after being exposed to several sessions of therapy, expectations may shift towards a positive direction if clients perceive improvement, or they may shift towards a negative direction if no benefits are noticed. However, we cannot conclude that expectancies shifted as a result of symptoms improving. It is likely that initial expectations and/or maladaptive beliefs were disconfirmed after being exposed to several components of therapy.

Our final objective examined the contribution of expectancies in contrast to symptomatology on the outcome of PDA. The findings revealed that the addition of expectancy measures significantly added to the prediction of most post-treatment symptom measures except for anxiety severity (i.e., BAI-T3) and depressive symptoms (i.e., BDI-II-T3). The best predictor of anxiety (i.e,. BAI-T3) at post-treatment was level of anxiety (BAI-T2) in the initial phase of treatment. This suggests that a reduction in anxiety symptoms following therapy is best predicted by the level of anxiety after four sessions of treatment rather than expectancies of experiencing a panic attack in a particular situation (i.e., PAQ-E). Perhaps examining prognostic expectancies specifically related to panic (i.e., the probability of therapeutic success with respect to experiencing various panic symptoms; e.g., "Following therapy, I expect my symptoms related to shortness of breath to diminish") rather than expectancies of experiencing panic attacks in a particular situation (i.e., PAQ-E) may have demonstrated greater predictability in post-treatment anxiety severity as measured by the BAI.

Post-treatment depressive symptoms were best predicted by baseline depressive symptoms. This implies that baseline severity and improvements from pre- to initial treatment phase in both PDA symptoms and expectancies are not predictive of post-treatment depressive symptoms. However, participants with lower levels of anxiety sensitivity after four sessions showed trends towards improvement in post-treatment depressive symptoms. This is consistent with other studies that demonstrate the relationship of anxiety sensitivity and depression (e.g., Schmidt et al., 1998; Taylor et al., 1996).

The remaining post-treatment symptom severity measures were best predicted by expectancy measures. A reduction in the fear of symptoms at the end of treatment (i.e., BSQ-T3) was best predicted by the level of expected anxiety (PAQ-E-T2) after clients had already been exposed to several components of therapy. A greater proportion of the variance in the post-treatment frequency of agoraphobic cognitions (i.e., ACQ-T3) was explained by avoidance expectancy (EMIA-A-T2), followed by anxiety severity (BAI-T2) after four sessions of therapy. This suggests that at the end of therapy, a decrease in the frequency of phobic cognitions during a panic attack appears to be determined by lower levels of expectancy to avoid a specific situation and by a decrease in anxiety-related symptoms after session four. Finally, post-treatment agoraphobic avoidance (MIA-T3) was best predicted by avoidance expectancies (EMIA-A-T2), followed by actual avoidance (MIA-A-T2).

The above findings appear to support the overprediction of fear model presented by Rachman (e.g., Rachman & Bichard, 1988; Rachman, 1994). The overprediction of fear implies that the predicted fear is greater than the actual experience of fear. Although we did not directly examine this phenomenon, there are some similarities in our findings. The clients in our study initially reported high levels of fear. However, after four sessions, their reported expectancy of experiencing panic attacks in several situations and their fear of anxiety-related sensations significantly diminished. These clients had not received any interoceptive or invivo exposure therapy at this point. It appears as though the majority of the participants in our study adjusted their expectations after they had received some corrective information with respect to their anxiety symptoms. Furthermore, greater accuracy in anxiety expectancies appeared to have had a better influence on most PDA outcome measures than the decrease in symptoms after four sessions. Another interesting finding was with respect to client's prognostic expectations (i.e., avoidance expectancy). There was no change from pre- to post-treatment. From the outset of therapy, most participants appeared to expect a fairly accurate outcome with respect to their avoidance behavior. When pre-treatment avoidance scores (M = 85.7) were compared with avoidance expectancy scores (M = 52), our findings revealed significantly less expected avoidance than actual avoidance ($p < .001$). They did not appear to underpredict what would happen at the end of therapy with respect to their avoidance since there was no significant difference between pre-treatment avoidance expectancy scores and post-treatment avoidance scores (M = 49.4; $p > .05$).

Overall, our results indicate that expectancies appear to be important predictors of PDA outcome following CBT. However, our findings did not detect anxiety sensitivity as an important determinant in PDA outcome. Anxiety sensitivity was detected as a good predictor of pre-treatment symptomatology. It may be suggested that anxiety sensitivity contributes to the development and relapse of PDA, but the effects of baseline and initial treatment phase anxiety sensitivity may not be evident until follow-up trials. Studies have demonstrated that ASI scores at the end of CBT for PDA predict relapse better than alternative measures (e.g., Brown & Barlow, 1995; Clarke et al., 1994). Future studies should also examine the impact of baseline and in-session anxiety sensitivity on relapse during follow-up.

The above findings demonstrate that addressing expectancies at the beginning of therapy may help clients gain a better understanding regarding some of the factors that contribute to their anxiety. Exposure therapy may function as a reality test for such individuals. Exposing oneself to the feared stimuli (i.e., bodily sensations and feared situations) will gradually disconfirm previous negative expectations related to the harmful consequences of anxiety sensations (e.g., Kirsch et al., 1983). Cognitive techniques (Beck, 1988) are also important in modifying expectations or beliefs regarding the harmful consequences of anxiety sensations. Similar to the conclusions made by Salkovskis, Clark and Gelder (1996), it appears to be more important to address "what is being avoided" rather than simply trying to habituate clients to their anxiety symptoms because if they continue to believe that their symptoms are dangerous, panic symptoms will persist regardless of whether they are controlled through breathing techniques or relaxation.

The measure of prognostic expectancy was adapted from the Mobility Inventory for Agoraphobia. Internal consistency of the measures was estimated but it is necessary to further validate it. Future studies should examine convergent validity of this measure in order to determine whether the questionnaires measured what it purported to measure.

5. Conclusion

Future research should assess expectancies prior to therapy and try to address some of these expectancies during the evaluation phase of treatment. For instance, providing clients with pre-treatment information on what should be expected in terms of the process and procedures of treatment and what the research has shown in terms of rate of improvement in PDA may result in an increase in treatment adherence and a decrease in levels of anxiety related to taking part in therapy (Deane et al., 1992; Webster, 1992). In light of the above findings, it appears important to examine how systematically modifying different types of expectations, as early as the beginning of the waiting period, by providing a pre-therapy modification expectancy video, can produce an impact on treatment outcome. Treatment improvement could also consist of addressing expectations early on in treatment, through a collaborative discussion-approach whereby clients' expectations and treatment objectives are identified in the initial session and a discussion process takes place between the therapist and the participants (Lazare et al., 1975). Combined, a pre-therapy video and a collaborative discussion-approach could be centred on modifying initial expectations, a common active ingredient in most therapies (Lambert et al., 1986; Muran et al., 1995). Finally, it is quite evident that expectations play a major role in clients suffering from PDA. Preparing clients for psychotherapy by a systematic modification of expectancies may be associated with improved outcome.

6. References

American Psychiatric Association (1994). *Diagnostic and Statistical Manual of Mental Disorders 4th ed.* Washington D.C.

Bachelor, A. & Salamé. (1992). Adaptation française du Counseling Evaluation Inventory. *Revue Canadienne des Sciences du Comportement, 24,* pp. 423-432.

Basoglu M., Marks I.M., Swinson R.P., Noshirvani H., O'Sullivan G., & Kuch K. (1994). Pre-treatment predictors of treatment outcome in panic disorder and agoraphobia treated with alprazolam and exposure. *Journal of Affective Disorders, 30(2),* pp. 123-132.

Barlow, D.H., Craske, M.G., Cerny, J.A., & Klosko, J.S. (1989). Behavioral treatment of panic disorder. *Behavior Therapy, 20,* pp. 261-282.

Beck, A.T. (1988). Cognitive approaches to panic disorder: Theory and therapy, In: *Panic: Psychological Perspectives,* S. Rackman & J.D. Maser, Lawrence Erlbaum, Hillsdale.

Beck A.T., Epstein, N., Brown, G., & Steer, R.A. (1988). An inventory for measuring clinical anxiety: Psychometric properties. *Journal of Consulting and Clinical Psychology,* 56, pp. 893-897.

Beck, A.T., Steer, R.A., & Brown, G.K. (1996). *Beck Depression Inventory Second Edition: Manual,* TX: Psychological Corporation, San Antonio.

Bélanger, C., & Katerelos, T.E. (1998). *Panic Attack Questionnaire-Expectancy.* Unpublished manuscript. Université de Québec à Montréal.

Black, D.W., Wesner, R., Bowers, W., & Gabel, J. (1993). A comparison of fluvoxamine, cognitive therapy, and placebo in the treatment of panic disorder. *Archives of General Psychiatry,* 50, pp. 44-50.

Bourque, P., & Beaudette, D. (1982). Étude psychométrique du questionnaire de dépression de Beck auprès d'un échantillon d'étudiants universitaires francophones. *Revue canadienne des sciences du comportement,* 14, pp. 211-218.

Brown, T.A., & Barlow, D.H. (1995). Long-term outcome in cognitive-behavioral treatment of panic disorder: Clinical predictors and alternative strategies for assessment. *Journal of Consulting and Clinical Psychology,* 63(5), pp. 754-765.

Chambless, D. L., Caputo, G. C., Bright, P., & Gallagher, R. (1984). Assessment of fear in agoraphobics: The Body Sensations Questionnaire and the Agoraphobic Cognitions Questionnaire. *Journal of Consulting and Clinical Psychology,* 52, pp. 1090-1097.

Chambless, D.L., Caputo, G.C., Jasin, S.E., Gracely, E.J., & Williams, C. (1985). The Mobility Inventory for Agoraphobia. *Behavior Research and Therapy,* 23, pp. 35-44.

Clark, D.M. (1986). A cognitive approach to panic. *Behavior Research and Therapy,* 24, pp. 461-470.

Clark, D.M., Salkovskis, P.M., Hackman, A., Middleton, H., Anastasiadis, P., & Gelder, M. (1994). A comparison of cognitive therapy, applied relaxation and imiparimine in the treatment of panic disorder. *British Journal of Psychiatry,* 164, pp. 759-769.

Cox, B.J., Endler, N.S., & Swinson, R.P. (1995). An examination of levels of agoraphobic severity in panic disorder. *Behavior Research and Therapy*, 33(1), pp. 57-62.

Cox, B.J., Endler, N.S., Norton, G.R., & Swinson, R.P. (1991). Anxiety sensitivity and nonclinical panic attacks. *Behavior Research and Therapy*, 29(4), pp. 367-369.

Cox, B.J., Parker, J.D.A. & Swinson, R.P. (1996). Anxiety sensitivity: Confirmatory evidence for a multidimensional construct. *Behavior Research and Therapy*, 34(7), pp. 591-598.

Cox, B.J., Swinson, R.P., Norton, G.R., & Kuch, K. (1991). Anticipatory anxiety and avoidance in panic disorder with agoraphobia. *Behavior Research and Therapy*, 29(4), pp. 363-365.

Craske, M.G., & Barlow, D.H.,(1990). *Therapist's guide for the mastery of anxiety and panic.* University of Albany, State University of New York: Center for Stress and Anxiety Disorders.

Craske, M.G., & Barlow, D. H. (1993). Panic Disorder and Agoraphobia. In D.H. Barlow (Ed.), *Clinical Handbook of Psychological Disorders* (2nd ed.) pp. 1-47, The Guilford Press, New York.

Craske, M.G., Brown, T.A., & Barlow, D. H. (1991). Behavioral treatment of panic: A two year follow-up. *Behavior Therapy*, 22, pp. 289-304.

Craske, M.G., Rapee, R.M., & Barlow, D.H. (1988). The significance of panic-expectancy for individual patterns of avoidance. *Behavior Therapy*, 19, pp. 577-592.

Deane, F.P., Spicer, J., & Leathem, J. (1992). Effects of videotaped preparatory information on expectations, anxiety, and psychotherapy outcome. *Journal of Consulting and Clinical Psychology*, 60(6), pp. 980-984.

de Beurs E, Lange A, van Dyck R, Koele P. (1995). Respiratory training prior to exposure in vivo in the treatment of panic disorder with agoraphobia: efficacy and predictors of outcome. *Austalian New Zealand Jouranl of Psychiatry*, 29(1), pp.104-113.

DiNardo, P.A., Brown, T.A., & Barlow, D.H. (1994). Anxiety Disorders Interview Schedule for DSM-IV: Lifetime version (ADIS-IV-L), Graywind Publications, Albany, NY.

Donnell, C.D., & McNally, R.J. (1990). Anxiety sensitivity and panic attacks in a nonclinical population. *Behavior Research and Therapy*, 29, pp. 83-85.

Ehlers, A. (1995). A 1-year prospective study of panic attacks: Clinical course and factors associated with maintenance. Journal of Abnormal *Psychology*, 104, pp. 164-172.

Fava, G., Zielezny, M., Savron, G., & Grandi, S. (1995). Long-term effects of behavioral treatment for panic disorder with agoraphobia. *British Journal of Psychiatry*, 166, pp. 87-92.

Frank, J.D. (1959). The dynamics of the psychotherapeutic relationship. *Psychiatry*, 22, pp. 17-39.

Garfield, S.L. (1986). Research on client variables in psychotherapy, In: *Handbook of psychotherapy and behavior change*, (3rd ed.), S.L. Garfield, & A.E. Bergin (Eds.), pp. 213-256, John Wiley & Sons, New York.

Gauthier, J., Morin, C., Thériault, F., & Lawson, J. S. (1982). Adaptation française d'une mesure d'auto-évaluation de l'intensité de la dépression. *Revue québécoise de psychologie*, 3, pp. 13-27.

Goldstein, A.P. (1962). Therapist-Patient Expectancies in Psychotherapy, Pergamon Press, New York.

Goldstein, A.P, & Shipman, W. (1961). Patient expectancies, symptom reduction, and aspects of the initial psychterapeutic interview. *Journal of Clinical Psychology*, 17, pp. 123-133.

Highlen, P.S., & Hill, C.E. (1984). Factors affecting client change in individual counseling: current status and theoretical speculations, In: *Handbook of Counseling Psychology*, S.D. Brown & R.W., Lent (Eds.), Wiley, New York.

Katerelos, T.E., Perreault, M., & Bélanger, C. (1998). The Expectancy Mobility Inventory for Agoraphobia-Alone. Unpublished manuscript, Université du Québec à Montréal.

Keijsers, G.P.J., Hoogduin, C.A.L., & Schaap, C.P. (1994). Prognostic factors in the behavioral treatment of panic disorder with and without agoraphobia. *Behavior Therapy*, 25, pp. 689-708.

Kirsch, I., Tennen, H., Wickless, C., Saccone, A.J., & Cody, S. (1983). The role of expectancy in fear reduction. *Behavior Therapy*, 14, pp. 520-533.

Klosko, J.S., Barlow, D.H., Tassinari, R.& Cerny, J.A.(1990). A comparison of alprazolam and behavior therapy in the treatment of panic disorder. *Journal of Consulting and Clinical Psychology*, 58, pp. 77-84.

Lambert, M.J., & Asay, T.P. (1984). Patient characteristics and their relationship to psychotherapy outcome , M. Hersen, L., Michelson, & A.S. Bellack (Eds), (pp. 313-359), Plenum Press, New York.

Lambert, M.J., Shapiro, D.A., & Bergin, A.E. (1986). The effectiveness of psychotherapy, In: *Handbook of psychotherapy and behavior change* (3rd ed.), S.L. Garfield, & A.E. Bergin (Eds.), (pp. 157-211), John Wiley & Sons, New York.

Lazare, A., Eisenthal, S., & Wasserman, L. (1975). The customer approach to patienthood: Attending to patient requests in a walk-in clinic. *Archives of General Psychiatry*, 32, pp. 553-558.

Maller, R.G., & Reiss, S. (1992). Anxiety sensitivity in 1984 and panic attacks in 1987. *Journal of Anxiety Disorders*, 6, pp. 241-247.

Marchand, L., Stephenson, R., Feeney, S., & Marchand, A. (1999). Validation factorielle de l'adaptation canadienne-française de l'Anxiety Sensitivity Scale. Poster session presented at the "congrès de l'Association Canadienne Française pour l'Avancement des Sciences (ACFAS)", Ottawa, Ontario, 10-14 mai.

Margraf, J., Barlow, D.H., Clark, D.M., & Telch, M.J. (1993). Psychological treatment of panic: Work in progress on outcome, active ingredients, and follow-up. *Behavior Research and Therapy*, 31(1), pp. 1-8.

McNally, R.J. (1992). Anxiety sensitivity distinguishes panic disorder from generalized anxiety disorder. *Journal of Nervous and Mental Disease*, 180, pp. 737-738.

McNally, R.J., & Lorenz, M. (1987). Anxiety sensitivity in agoraphobics. *Journal of Behavior Therapy and Experimental Psychiatry*, 18(1), pp. 3-11.

Muran, J.C., Gorman, B.S., Safran, J.D., Twining, L., Samstag, L.W., & Winston, A. (1995). Linking in-session change to overall outcome in short-term cognitive therapy. *Journal of Consulting and Clinical Psychology*, 63(4), pp. 651-657.

Norton, G.R., Dorward, J., & Cox, B.J. (1986). Factors associated with panic attacks in nonclinical subjects. *Behavior Therapy*, 17, pp. 239-252.

Norton, G.R., Pidlubny, S.R., & Norton, P.J. (1999). Prediction of panic attacks and related variables. *Behavior Therapy*, 30, pp. 319-330.

Öst, L.G., & Westling, B.E.(1995). Applied relaxation vs cognitive behavior therapy in the treatment of panic disorder. *Behavior Research and Therapy*, 33(2), pp. 145-158.

Perotti, L.P., & Hopewell, C.A. (1980). Expectancy effects in psychotherapy and systematic desensitization: A review. JSAS: Catalog of Selected Documents in psychology, 10 (Ms. No. 2052.).

Piper, W.E., & Wogan, M. (1970). Placebo effect in psychotherapy: an extension of earlier findings. *Journal of consulting and clinical psychology*, 34, pp. 447.

Pollack, M.H., Otto, M.W., Sachs, G.S., Leon, A., Shear, M.K., Deltito, J.A., Keller, M.B., & Rosenbaum, J.F. (1994). Anxiety psychopathology predictive of outcome in patients with panic disorder and depression treated with imipramine, alprazolam and placebo. *Journal of Affective Disorders*, 30, pp. 273-281.

Pollack, M.H., Otto, M.W., Tesar, G., Cohen, L.S., Meltzer-Brody, S., & Rosenbaum, J.F. (1993). Long-term outcome after acute treatment with clonazepam and alprazolam for panic disorder. *Journal of Clinical Psychopharmacology*, 13 pp. 257-263.

Rachman, S. (1994). The overprediction of fear: A review. *Behavior Research and Therapy*, 32(7), pp. 683-690.

Rachman, S., & Bichard, S. (1988). The overprediction of fear. *Clinical Psychology Review*, 8, pp. 303-312.

Reiss, S. (1991). Expectancy theory of fear, anxiety, and panic. *Clinical Psychology Review*, 11, pp. 141-153.

Reiss, S. & Havercamp, S. (1996). The sensitivity theory of motivation: Implications for psychopathology. *Behavior Research and Therapy*, 34(8), pp. 621-632.

Reiss, S., & McNally, R.J. (1985). The expectancy model of fear, In: *Theoretical issues in behavior therapy*, Reiss S. & Bootzin, R.R. (Eds.) (pp 107-121 Academic Press,). New York.

Reiss, S., Peterson, R.A., Gursky, D.M., & McNally, R.J. (1986). Anxiety sensitivity, anxiety frequency, and the prediction of fearfulness. *Behavior Research and Therapy*, 24, pp. 1-8.

Salkovskis, P.M., Clark, D.M., & Gelder, M.G. (1996). Cognition-behavior links in the persistence of panic. *Behavior Research and Therapy*, 34(5/6), pp. 453-485.

Schmidt, N.B., Lerew, D.R., & Jackson, R.J. (1997). Anxiety sensitivity in the pathogenesis of panic: Prospective evaluation of spontaneous panic attacks during acute stress. *Journal of Abnormal Psychology*, 106(3), pp. 355-364.

Schmidt, N.B., Lerew, D.R., & Joiner, T.E. Jr. (1998). Anxiety sensitivity and the pathogenesis of anxiety and depression: Evidence for symptom specificity. *Behavior Research and Therapy*, 36, pp. 165-177.

Shear, M.K., Pilkonis, P.A., Cloitre, M., & Leon, A.C. (1994). Cognitive behavioral treatment compared with nonprescriptive treatment of panic disorder. *Archives of General Psychiatry*, 51, pp. 395-401.

Southworth, S., & Kirsch, I. (1988). The role of expectancy in exposure-generated fear reduction in agoraphobia. *Behavior Research and Therapy*, 26(2), pp. 113-120.

Stephenson, R., Marchand, A., & Lavallée, M.-C. (1997). Validation de l'Inventaire de mobilité pour l'agoraphobie auprès de la population québécoise francophone. *Science et comportement*, 26, pp. 35-58.

Stephenson, R., Marchand, A., & Lavallée, M.-C. (1998). Validation du questionnaire des sensations physiques auprès de la population canadienne-française. *L'Encéphale*, 24, pp. 415-425.

Stephenson, R., Marchand, A., & Lavallée, M.-C. (1999). A Canadian French Adaptation of the Agoraphobic Cognitions Questionnaire: Cross-cultural validation and gender differences. *Scandinavian Journal of Behavior Therapy*, 28, pp. 58-69.

Taylor, S. (1993). The structure of fundamental fears. *Journal Behavior Therapy & Experimental Psychology*, 24(4), pp. 289-299.

Taylor, S., Koch, W.J., Woody, S.,& McLean, P.D. (1996). Anxiety sensitivity and depression: How are they related? *Journal of Abnormal Psychology*, 105(3), pp. 474-479.

Taylor, S., Koch, W.J., & McNally, R.J. (1992). How does anxiety sensitivity vary across the anxiety disorders? *Journal of Anxiety Disorders*, 7, pp. 249-259.

Taylor, S., Woody, S., Koch, W.J., McLean, P.D., & Anderson, K.W. (1996). Suffocation false alarms and efficacy of cognitive behavioral therapy for panic disorder. *Behavior Therapy*, 27, pp. 115-126.

Vallerand, R.J. (1989). Vers un méthodologie de validation trans-culturelle de questionnaires psychologiques: implications pour la recherche en langue Française. *Canadian Psychology*, 30, pp. 662-680.

Watt, MC., Stewart, S.H., & Cox, B.J. (1998). A retrospective study of the learning history origins of anxiety sensitivity. *Behavior Research and Therapy*, 36, pp. 505-525.

Webster, A. (1992). The effect of pre-assessment information on clients' satisfaction, expectation and attendance at a mental health day centre. *British Journal of Medical Psychology*, 65, pp. 89-93.

Weiner, B. (1982). An attributionally based theory of motivation and emotion: Focus, Range and Issues, In: *Expectations and actions: Expectancy-value models in psychology*, N.T. Feather (Ed.), (pp. 163-204), Lawrence Erlbaum Associates, Hillsdale, New Jersey.

Well, A., Clark, D.M., Salkovskis, P., Ludgate, J., Hackman, A., & Gelder, M. (1995). The role of in-situation safety behaviors in maintaining anxiety and negative beliefs. *Behavior Therapy*, 26, pp. 153-161.

Whittal, M.L., & Goetsch, V.L. (1997). The impact of panic expectancy and social demand on agoraphobic avoidance. *Behavior Research and Therapy*, 36(9), pp. 813-821.

Williams, S.L, & Falbo, J. (1996). Cognitive and performance-based treatments for panic attacks in people with varying degrees of agoraphobic disability. *Behavior Research and Therapy* 34(3), pp. 253-264.

16

Mulungu – Rainforest Anxiolytic

Patocka Jiri
Department of Radiology and Toxicology, Faculty of Health and Social Studies
University of South Bohemia Ceske Budejovice
Czech Republic

1. Introduction

There are over one hundred species of plants of the genus *Erythrina* in the tropics and many of them are native to the American continent (Neill 1988). *Erythrina* species are known to produce alkaloids, flavonoids and terpenes (Garcia-Mateos et al., 1998). As with other species of *Erythrina*, alkaloids appear to be one of the main constituents mulungu (Parsons and Palframan, 2010). Mulungu (*Erythrina mulungu*) is a branched tree native to Brazil, growing in rain-forestry of Amazonia. Since its flowers are the same red color as coral, the plant is sometimes also called "flor de coral" and in English literature "coral tree". The designation *Erythrina* also includes the species *Erythrina velutina*, endemic to the semi-arid regions of Northeastern Brazil, and *Erythrina mulungu*, a plant native to Southern Brazil.

In native herbal medicine, a leaf or bark decoction or tincture from mulungu has long been used in folk medicine due to their tranquilizing effects and as natural sedative. It is also anxiolytic and antibacterial (Garín-Aguilar et al., 2000). In both Brazil and Peru mulungu is used for epilepsy (Vasconcelos et al., 2007). Practitioners in the United States use mulungu to quiet hysteria from trauma or shock, as a mild sedative to calm the nervous system, to treat insomnia and promote healthy sleeping patterns. Anxiety disorders are among the most prevalent psychiatric diseases and mulungu offers novel therapy chance (Balbani et al., 2009; Patocka, 2009). Latest the present results suggest that *Erythrina* has anxiolytic-like effects on a specific subset of defensive behaviors, particularly one that has been related in clinical terms to generalized anxiety. These observations support the popular use of extracts of the plant as tranquilizing agents.

2. Ethnobotany

Erythrina is a genus of flowering plants in the pea family, *Fabaceae*. It contains about 130 species, which are distributed in tropical and subtropical regions worldwide. They are trees, growing up to 30 m in height. The generic name is derived from the Greek word ερυθρός (*erythros*), meaning "red", referring to the flower color of certain species. These trees are religious for some ethnic minority and are used as floral emblems in many countries. For example Cockspur Coral Tree (*E. crista-galli*) is the national flower of Argentina and Uruguay. The Coastal Coral Tree (*E. caffra*) is the official city tree of Los Angeles, California. The state trees of Mérida and Trujillo in Venezuela are "bucaré ceibo" (*E. poeppigiana*) and Purple Coral Tree ("bucaré anauco", *E. fusca*), respectively. *E. variegata* is used as floral emblem in Yonabaru, Okinawa. Some coral trees are used widely as street and park trees, especially in tropical countries. These trees are very suitable as "frame tree" for vanilla vines to grow up on or are used as "shade trees" in coffee or cocoa plantations (Westley and Powell, 1993). The plants of the genus *Erythrina* were used in Pre-Columbian America in traditional medicine (Towle, 2007) to calm agitation and for insomnia and other disorders of the nervous system.

3. Ethnopharmacology

Pharmacological assays performed with the alkaloids of *Erythrina americana* have shown anticonvulsant, hypnotic and analgesic effects (Garín-Aguilar et al., 2000; Koné et al., 2004). The species *Erythrina glauca* and *Erythrina lysistemon* have been reported to possess antiviral, antibacterial, and estrogenic activity (Ito, 1999; Tanee et al., 2007). Furthermore, analgesic and anti-inflammatory effects were observed for an aqueous extract of the stem bark of *Erythrina senegalensis* (Saidu et al., 2000).

Erythrina mulungu, tree high up to 10 m, is at home in South America. In Brasilia it is known as *colorines, chilicote* or *tzompanquahuitl* (Agra et al. 2007). In herbal medicine, a leaf or bark decoction or tincture from mulungu is considered to calm agitation and other disorders of the nervous system, including insomnia (Rodrigues and Carlini, 2003; Vasconcelos et al., 2007). Mulungu also decreased blood pressure and normalize heart arythmia (Begossi et al., 2004). There have also been some reports on the therapeutic use of the plant's inflorescence by herbal practitioners (Onusic et al. 2003). In Pre-Columbian civilizations decoction from the bark of this tree was used for suppression of fight fear and wartime hardship (Duke, 2008). At present, mulungu is used in the area of South America, mainly in Brasilia and Peru, as sedative and also in epilepsy (Teixeira-Silva et al., 2008).

People's healers and some practitioners in The United States use mulungu to quiet hysteria from trauma or shock, as a mild, hypnotic sedative to calm the nervous system, to treat insomnia and promote healthy sleeping patterns, to regulate heart palpitations, and to treat hepatitis and liver disorders. Nevertheless, despite its wide popular utilization, the supposed therapeutic properties of *Erythrina mulungu* only recently began to be evaluated in preclinical studies.

4. Chemistry of *Erythrina* constituents

The chemicals constituents of mulungu have been studied extensively after modern medical science find health potential of this biomedicine. In this biological material have been found large amounts of novel flavonoids, triterpenes, and alkaloids (Da-Cunha et al., 1996; Majinda et al., 2005; Cui et al., 2009). The genus *Erythrina* is very rich in secondary metabolites particularly of the flavonoids class. A literature survey showed the presence of flavanones, flavonols, chalcones, cinnamoylphenols, stilbenoids, isoflavones, isoflavans, isoflavanones, pterocarpans, isoflav-3-enes, 3-phenoxychromones, coumastans, 3-phenyl-coumarins, lignans, cinnamate esters, simple phenolics, triterpenes, sesquiterpenes, long-chain carboxylic acids, and long-chain alcohols (Majinda et al., 2005). Flavonoids represent a group of very active chemicals with various properties and are almost always present in *Erythrina* species.

The most considerable group of biologicaly active compounds of mulungu are alkaloids (Ozawa et al. 2009). The alkaloids have been found in 78 of 107 species in the genus

Erythrina; mulungu is documented with 20 isoquinoline alkaloids (Tanaka et al., 2008; Parsons and Palframan, 2010). The alkaloids accumulated not only at the end of maturation in the seeds but also in young tissues. On a dried basis, a high content of alkaloids was observed in flowers and dry seeds in comparison to low levels in dry pods. The highest concentrations were found in the mature seeds (García-Mateos et al., 1996). Many of these have demonstrated anti-inflammatory, cardioactive, narcotic, and sedative activities (Parsons and Palframan, 2010).

The pivotal structure of erythrinan alkaloids is tetraheterocyclic nitrogen compound with tetrahydroisoquinoline moiety called erythrinane (**I**) (Amer et al., 1991). Compounds of these structure were known for a long time (Koniuszy et al., 1949), but until medical science research of mulungu ignified concern over these alkaloids. Heft of erythrinan alkaloids are derivatives of **I** substituted at nucleus A and D by hydroxyl or alkoxy groups. The most considerable erythrinan alkaloids are erysotrine (**II**), erythravine (**III**), erysodine (**IV**), and erysopine (**V**) (Fig. 1) (Flausino et al., 2007a,b). For ever new erythrinan alkaloids are recovered (Tanaka et al., 2008; Cui et al., 2009, Parsons and Palframan, 2010).

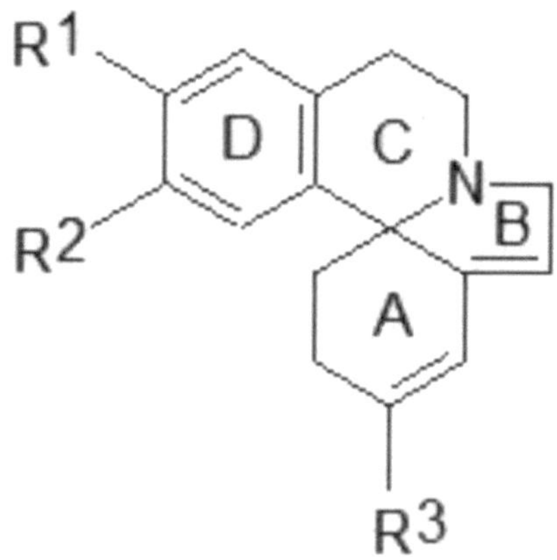

Alkaloid	R¹	R²	R³
I	H	H	H
II	OCH_3	OCH_3	OCH_3
III	OCH_3	OCH_3	OH
IV	OH	OCH_3	OCH_3
V	OH	OH	OCH_3

Fig. 1. Chemical structures of erythrinan alkaloids. Erythrinan alkaloids are derived from tetraheterocyclic nitrogen compound with tetrahydroisoquinoline moiety called erythrinane (**I**). Heft of erythrinan alkaloids are derivatives of **I** substituted at nucleus A and D by hydroxyl or alkoxy groups. The most considerable erythrinan alkaloids are erysotrine (**II**), erythravine (**III**), erysodine (**IV**), and erysopine (**V**).

5. Toxicology

Mulungu is relatively safe remedy. Acute oral toxicity (LD_{50}) of aqueous extract of stem bark of *E. variegata* was 425 mg/kg in mice (Pitchaiah et al., 2010). Lollato et al. (2010) estimated for extracts of *E. speciosa* LD_{50} value for mice as being higher than 2000 mg/kg.
The toxicity of chloroform stem bark extract of *Erythrina senegalensis* DC, a medicinal plant with anti-inflammatory activity, was studied in vivo and in vitro by Udem and co-workers (2010). The LD_{50} intraperitoneal of the extract was 526 mg/kg after an acute toxicity test (24 h). A brine shrimp lethality test with the extract gave LC_{50} of 60.86 ppm. The chronic studies revealed alterations in the levels of biochemical markers of hepatic and cardiac damage. The alterations were, however, not significant except in the group fed the highest inclusion of the extract (1.0 g extract/kg feed) where significant ($p < 0.05$) increases in the activities of alanine aminotransferase, aspartate aminotransferase, and alkaline phosphatase were observed. Hematological assessments of mice in this group showed significant ($p < 0.05$) decreases in the red blood cell count and the packed cell volume. Increases in the relative weights of the liver and heart were also significant ($p < 0.05$). Lipid peroxidation product levels assayed as malondialdehyde was significantly ($p < 0.05$) elevated in the groups fed 0.5 and 1.0 g/kg of feed at day 84. Significant histopathological changes like myocardial hemorrhages and degeneration of hepatocytes were observed in the heart and liver respectively.
Mulungu is less toxic than most of synthetic tranquilizers, e.g. LD_{50} value for diazepam in mice at peroral administration is 49 mg/kg (Hogskilde et al., 1987). To evaluate the acute toxicity of the aqueous extract of *Erythrina velutina* leaves, which is frequently used in folk medicine as a tranquilizer, adult Wistar rats were treated *per os* with the limit dose of 5 g/kg of the extract and then observed for 14 consecutive days. No animals died and no signs of toxicity were detected either during the behavioral observations or at the autopsies, what indicates a reasonable lack of toxicity for the extract (Craveiro et al., 2010).

6. Biological activity

The traditional use of mulungu for anxiety and stress has been validated by researchers in a few studies, where it was shown to alter anxiety-related responses (Flausino et al. 2007a,b). An animal model (correlating to human generalized anxiety disorder, as well as panic disorder) was undertaken on a water-alcohol extract of mulungu (Vasconcelos et al. 2004; Ribeiro et al. 2006; Flausino et al. 2007a). Vasconcelos and co-workers (2004) studied the effects of hydroalcoholic extracts of both *Erythrina velutina* and *Erythrina mulungu* on the behavior of female mice submitted to the open-field test and to the elevated plus-maze after oral or intraperitoneal administration. The highest doses (800 mg/kg, oral, and 400 mg/kg, intraperitoneal) of the hydroalcoholic extracts decreased locomotor activity both in the open-field and in the elevated plus-maze test. The authors concluded that these results supported, at least in part, the popular use of the two species of *Erythrina* as tranquilizers in Brazilian folk medicine. Another study (Dantas et al., 2004) performed with intraperitoneal administration of an aqueous *Erythrina velutina* extract showed that the extract prolonged the duration of sleep induced by sodium pentobarbital at higher doses and blocked the acquisition of foot shock memory at lower doses. These results led the authors to propose that *Erythrina velutina* might interfere with the mnemonic process and might have a sedative action (Dantas et al., 4004).

The researchers reported that the mulungu extract had an effect similar to the commonly-prescribed anti-anxiety drug diazepam (Onusic et al. 2003; Ribeiro et al. 2006; Teixeira-Silva et al. 2008). Raupp and co-workers (2008) administered orally the hydroalcoholic extract of the stem bark of *Erythrina velutina* in mice submitted to the following tests: elevated plus-maze, forced swim, spontaneous locomotor activity, and habituation to active chamber. Chlordiazepoxide and imipramine were used as standard drugs. In the elevated plus-maze test, chronic, but not acute, *Erythrina velutina* (100 mg/kg) administration increased the percentage of open arm entries, an effect also seen in both acute and chronic treatments with chlordiazepoxide (7.5 mg/kg). In the forced swim test, only imipramine (25 mg/kg) decreased immobility time. Impairment of habituation was seen only with acute imipramine administration and with the lowest doses of *Erythrina velutina* extract tested in acute (10 mg/kg) and chronic (50 mg/kg) administrations. These results suggest that chronic administration of the hydroalcoholic extract of the stem bark of *Erythrina velutina* exerts an anxiolytic-like effect on mice, and it could serve as a new approach for the treatment anxiety, although it may have an amnesic effect at low doses.

It was suggested in many studies that the alkaloids in *Erythrina* may alter GABAergic neurotransmission (Ribeiro et al, 2006; Teixeira-Silva et al. 2008; Khanum and Razack, 2010). GABA acts as a neurotransmitter in the brain and abnormalities with its function is implicated in diseases including epilepsy, anxiety, and depression. Nevertheless, mechanism of anxiolytic effect of erythrina alkaloids is evidently different from diazepines. These alkaloids induced contractions seem to involve $GABA_A$ receptor activation, acetylcholine release, muscarinic receptor activation, augmentation of Ca^{2+} entry through L-type calcium channels, and calcium release from the intracellular stores. These findings provide further support for *Erythrina velutina* traditional uses (Carvalho et al. 2009).

Hydroalcoholic extracts from the stem bark of *rythrina velutina* and *Eerythrina mulungu* have anticonvulsant effects only in the strychnine-induced seizure model, suggesting their possible action in glycine system and a potentiation of pentobarbital sleeping time, suggesting depressant action in the CNS (Vasconcelos et al. 2007). Data of Dantas and co-workers (2004) showed that the crude extract of *E. velutina* at lower doses interferes with mnemonic process for different tasks, while at higher doses, the sedative and neuromuscular blocking actions are the main effects. Anticonvulsant profile of erythrina alkaloids was recently studied by Faggion et al. (2011). They isolated the alkaloids (+)-erythravine and (+)-11-α-hydroxy-erythravine from the flowers of *Erythrina mulungu* and evaluated the action of these compounds against chemically induced seizures in rats (Faggion et al. 2011). These results showed that the administration of different doses of (+)-erythravine inhibited seizures evoked by bicuculline, pentylenetetrazole, and kainic acid at maximum of 80, 100, and 100%, respectively, whereas different doses of (+)-11-α-hydroxy-erythravine inhibited seizures at a maximum of 100% when induced by bicuculline, NMDA, and kainic acid, and, to a lesser extent, pentylenetetrazole (60%). All animals were protected against death when treated with different doses of (+)-11-α-hydroxy-erythravine in the tests using the four chemical convulsants. Identical results were obtained when using (+)-erythravine in the tests of bicuculline, NMDA, and pentylenetetrazole, and, to a lesser extent, kainic acid.

Further research has validated the traditional use of mulungu as an antimicrobial agent for throat and urinary infections. Mulungu has demonstrated antibacterial activity against *Escherichia coli, Staphylococcus aureus,* and antimycobacterial activity against *Mycobacterium fortuitum* and *M. smegmatis* (Virtuoso et al., 2005; Ferreira de Lima et al., 2006). Some isoflavonoids, mainly erycristagallin (3,9-dihydroxy-2,10-di(gamma,gamma-dimethylallyl)-6a,11a-dehydropterocarpan), isolated from *Erythrina variegata* have antibacterial activita against cariogenic oral bacteria (Sato et al., 2003). The findings indicate that erycristagallin has a potential as potent phytochemical agent for prevention of dental caries by inhibiting the growth of cariogenic bacteria and by interfering with incorporation of glucose responsible for production of organic acids.

Two new compounds with antibacterial effect, erybacin A and erybacin B, were isolated from the roots of *Erythrina herbacea*. Their structures were established on the basis of spectroscopic analyses. Erybacin A is a rare, naturally occurring 1-hydroxy-1,3-diphenylpropan-2-one derivative. The isolated compounds were evaluated for their antibacterial activity against 13 strains of methicillin-resistant *Staphylococcus aureus* (MRSA). The new compound erybacin B showed a potent bactericidal activity against MRSA (Tanaka et al., 2010b).

Hydroalcoholic extracts from the stem bark and leaves of *Erythrina velutina* and *Erythrina mulungu* have also antinociceptive effects which was not reversed by naloxone, i.e. these are independent of the opioid system (Vasconcelos et al., 2003; Marchioro et al., 2005).

Alkaloid erysodine is a competitive antagonist at neuronal nicotinic acetylcholine receptors (Mansbach et al., 2000). The potent and competitive nature of erysodine's antagonism together with its ability to enter the brain after systemic administration suggest that erysodine may be a useful tool in characterizing neuronal nicotinic acetylcholine receptors (Decker et al., 1995). Recent findings show that erysodine and also dihydro-beta-erythroidine are potent and selective competitive inhibitors of alpha4beta2 nicotinic acetylcholine receptors (Iturriaga-Vásquez et al., 2010).

Erythrinan alkaloids cristanine A and cristanine B were isolated from the bark of *Erythrina crista-galli*. In Brazil, the bark of the title tree is used for the treatment of rheumatism and hepatitis as well as for sedation and hypnogenesis. However, the title alkaloids cristanine A and B are inactive concerning the inhibitory activity on lipopolysaccharide-induced nitric oxide production (Ozawa et al., 2010). Probably erythrinan alkaloids are also responsible for the antiinflammatory and analgesic effects of the ethanolic extract of Erythrina indica (Rajeev eta l. 2010). *Erythrina indica* leaves are traditionally used in Kerala to treat inflammation, ulcers, earache etc.

7. Current practical use of *Erythrina*

Mulungu, drug from the tree *Erythrina mulungu,* is not very widely known or used in advanced countries. Mostly appearing as an ingredient in only a few herbal formulas for anxiety or depression. *Erythrina* plants produce alkaloids, flavonoids and terpenes and are commonly used in folk medicine due to their tranquilizing effects. Currently, the most widely prescribed medications for anxiety disorders are benzodiazepines. However, the clinical uses of benzodiazepines are limited by their side effects such as psychomotor impairment, potentiation of other central depressant drugs and dependence liability. Therefore, the development of new medications processing anxiolytic effect without the complications of benzodiazepines would be of great importance in the treatment of anxiety related disorders.

The use of herbal medicines by physicians in Europe, Asia, and America, exploring their traditional remedies to find a suitable cure of these 'mind affecting diseases' and herbal medicines are often considered to be gentle and safe alternative to synthetic drugs. Nevertheless, till this time no relevant clinical study exist.

Recently many studies of other *Erythrina* species from different parts of world appeared. These studies show that bioactive products of these trees may be useful in modern medicine also in other statements. From the bark of *Erythrina addisoniae* new flavonoids of stilbenoide type were isolated. These compounds are strong imhibitors of viral neuraminidases. Quite new compound, which is a formylated stilbenoid derivative, exhibited strong inhibition of both influenza H1N1 and H9N2 neuraminidases with IC_{50} values of 8.80 ± 0.34 µg/mL and 7.19 ± 0.40 µg/mL, respectively (Nguyen et al., 2010).

From the bark of *Erythrina abyssinica* has been isolated new coumestans and benzofurans with stimulatory effects on AMP-activated protein kinase (AMPK) (Nguyen et al., 2010) which has been proposed as a therapeutic target for the treatment of metabolic syndrome including obesity and type-2 diabetes. These results suggest that benzofurans and coumestans may be new lead compounds for regulating the AMPK enzyme. Prenylated flavanones from the same of source inhibited protein tyrosine phosphatase PTP1B activity in an *in vitro* assay with IC_{50} values ranging from 15.2 ± 1.2 to 19.6 ± 2.3 µM, whereas very known potent inhibitor of PTP1B known as RK-682 (Hamaguchi et al., 1995) used as a positive control displayed an IC_{50} value of 4.7 ± 0.5 µM (Long et al., 2010).

Two new dimethylpyrano-isoflavones, named erymildbaedin A and B, were isolated from the stem bark of *Eyrthrina mildbraedi* - Cameroonian medicinal plant. Some of them strongly inhibited the growth of human breast, prostate, and endometrial adenocarcinoma cell lines (Tchokouaha et al. 2010).

Another flavonoids with the antibacterial activity were isolated from *Erythrina caffra*, deciduous subtropical tree indigenous to South Africa. All the compounds were active against both Gram-negative and Gram-positive bacteria. The minimum inhibitory concentration values obtained (MIC) ranged from 3.9 µg/mL to 125 µg/mL (Chukwujekwu et al., 2010). A new bis-isoflavonoid, biseryvarin A, was isolated from the roots of Erythrina variegata. Biseryvarin A is the first dimeric isoflavonoid possessing isoprenoid groups from the genus Erythrina. Biseryvarin A showed low activity MRSA. The methanol extract of the bark of *Erythrina variegata* showed significant anti-malarial activity toward *Plasmodium falciparum in vitro* using the lactate dehydrogenase assay. The ethyl acetate fraction showed the most activity, exhibiting equipotency against both strains of parasite with IC_{50} of 23.8 µg/mL against 3D7 and 9.3 µg/mL against K1. Furthermore, by using the anti-malarial activity to follow separation, the ethyl acetate fraction was separated by combination of column chromatography to yield an active compound. The chemical structure of active compound was determined on the basis of spectroscopic evidences and comparison with those previously reported and identified as an isoflavonoid, warangalone. The warangalone showed anti-malarial activity against both strains of parasite used with IC_{50} of 4.8 µg/mL against 3D7 and 3.7 µg/mL against K1 (Herlina et al., 2009). Next flavonoids were isolated from *Erythrina vogelii*, a Cameroonian medicinal plant (Ali et al. 2010), in *Erythrina senegalensis* were found hepatoprotective flavonoids (Njayou et al., 2010) with low toxicity (Atsamo et al., 2010). Flavonoids of pterocarpane-type with antibacterial, antiplasmodial and cytotoxic activities, were isolated from the stems of *Erythrina fusca* (Innok et al., 2010).

8. References

Agra MF, Baracho GS, Nurit K, Basilio IJLD, Coelho VPM. Medicinal and poisonous diversity of the flora of "Cariri Paraibano", Brazil J Ethnopharmacol 2007; 111: 383-395.

Ali MI, Ahmed Z, Waffo AF, Ali MS. Flavonoids from Erythrina vogelii (Fabaceae) of Cameroon. Nat Prod Commun. 2010; 5(6): 889-892.

Amer ME, Sharmma M, Freyer AJ. The tetracyclic arythrina alkaloids. J Nat Prod 1991; 54(2): 329-363.

Atsamo AD, Nguelefack TB, Datté JY, Kamanyi A. Acute and subchronic oral toxicity assessment of the aqueous extract from the stem bark of *Erythrina senegalensis* DC (Fabaceae) in rodents. J Ethopharmacol, Article in Press.

Balbani AP, Silva DH, Montovani JC. Patents of drugs extracted from Brazilian medicinal plants. Expert Opin Ther Pat 2009; 19(4): 461-473.

Begossi A, Hanazaki N, Tamashiro JY. Medicinal plants in the atlantic forest (Brazil): knowledge, use, and conservation. Human Ecology 2004; 30: 281-299.

Carvalho AC, Almeida DS, Melo MG, Cavalcanti SC, Marçal RM. Evidence of the mechanism of action of *Erythrina velutina* Willd (Fabaceae) leaves aqueous extract. J Ethnopharmacol 2009; 122: 374-378.

Chukwujekwu JC, Van Heerden FR, Van Staden J. Antibaczerial activity of flavonoids from the stem bark of *Erythrina caffra* thunb. Phytother Res 2010; 25(1): 46-48.

Craveiro ACS et al. Toxicidade aguda do extrato aquoso de folhas de Erythrina *velutina* em animais experimentais. Rev. Bras. Farmacogn. 2008; 18: 739-743.

Cui L, Thuong PT, Fomum ZT, Oh WK. A new erythrinan alkaloid from the seed of *Erythrina addisoniae*. Arch Pharm Res 2009; 11(10): 233-2241.

Da-Cunha EV, Dias C, Barbosa-Filho JM, Gray AI. Eryvellutinone, an isoflavone from the stem bark of *Erythrina vellutina*. Phytochemistry 1996; 43(6): 1371-1373.

Dantas MC, De Oliveira FS, Bandeira SM, Batista JS, Silva CD Jr, Alves PB, Antoniolli AR, Marchioro M. Central nervous system effects of the crude extract of *Erythrina velutina* on rodents. J Ethnopharmacol. 2004; 94(1): 129-133.

Decker MW, Anderson DJ, Brioni JD, Donnelly-Roberts DL, Kang CH, O'Neill AB, Piattoni-Kaplan M, Swanson S, Sullivan JP. Erysodine, a competitive antagonist at neuronal nicotinic acetylcholine receptors. Eur J Pharmacol 1995; 280(1): 79-89.

Duke JA. Dukes Handbuch of Medicinal Plants of Latin America. CRC Press, 2008, 832 s. ISBN 1420043161

Faggion SA, Cunha AO, Fachim HA, Gavin AS, Dos Santos WF, Pereira AM, Beleboni RO. Anticonvulsant profile of the alkaloids (+)-erythravine and (+)-11-α-hydroxy-erythravine isolated from the flowers of *Erythrina mulungu* Mart ex Benth (Leguminosae-Papilionaceae). Epilepsy Behav 2011 Feb 1. [Epub ahead of print]

Ferreira de Lima MR, de Souza Luna J, dos Santos AF, Caño de Andrade MC, Goulart SantAna AE, Genet JP, Marquez B, Neuville L, Moreau N. Anti-bacterial activity of some Beazilian medicinal plants. J Ethnopharmacol 2006; 105(1-2): 137-147.

Flausino OA, de Avila Santos L, Verli H, Pereira AM, Bolzani VS, Nunes-de-Souza RL. Anxiolytic effects of erythrinian alkaloids from *Erythrina mulungu*. J Nat Prod 2007b; 70: 48-53.

Flausino OA, Pereira AM, da Silva Bolzani V, Nunes-de-Souza RL Effects of erythrinian alkaloids isolated from *Erythrina mulungu* (Papilionaceae) in mice submitted to animal models of anxiety. Biol Pharm Bull 2007a; 30: 375-378.

García-Mateos R, Lucas B., Zendejas M, Soto-Hernández M, Martínez M, Sotelo A. Variation of total nitrogen, non-protein nitrogen content, types of alkaloids at different stages of development in *Erythrina americana* seeds. J Agric Food Chem 1996; 44(10): 2987-2991.

Garcia-Mateos R, Soto-Hernández M, Kelly D. Alkaloids form six *Erythrina* species endemic to Mexico. Biochem System Ecol 1998; 26: 545-551.

Garín-Aguilar MA, Luna JER, Soto-Hernández M, Valencia del Toro G, Vásquez MM. Effect of crude extracts of *Erythrina americana* Mill. on aggressive behavior in rats. J. Ethnopharmacol 2000; 69: 189-196.

Hamaguchi T, Sudo T, Osada H. RK-682, a potent inhibitor of tyrosine phosphatase, arrested the mammalian cell cycle progression at G1 phase. FEBS Lett 1995; 372(1): 54-58.

Herlina T, Supratman U, Soedjanaatmadja MS, Subarnas A, Sutardjo S, Abdullah NR, Hayashi H. Anti-malarial compound from the stem bark of Erythrina variegata. Indo J Chem 2009; 9(2): only on-line
http://pdm-mipa.ugm.ac.id/ojs/index.php/ijc/article/viewArticle/526

Hogskilde S, Nielsen JW, Carl P., Angelo H, Bredgaard Sorensen M. The anticonvulsive activity and toxicity of diazepam in three different formulatuions. An experimental study in mice. Acta Anaesth Scand 1987; 31(4): 289-291.

Innok P, Rukachaisirikul T, Phongpaichit S, Suksamrarn A. Fuscacarpans A - C, new pterocarpans from the stems of *Erythrina fusca*. Fitoterapia 2010; 81(6): 518-523.

Ito K. Studies on the alkaloids of *Erythrina* plants. [Article in Japanese] Yakugaku Zasshi. 1999; 119(5): 340-356.

Iturriaga-Vásquez P, Carbone A, García-Beltrán O, Livingstone PD, Biggin PC, Cassels BK, Wonnacott S, Zapata-Torres G, Bermudez I. Molecular determinants for competitive inhibition of alpha4beta2 nicotinic acetylcholine receptors. Mol Pharmacol 2010; 78(3): 366-375.

Khanum F, Razack S. Anxiety - Herbal treatment: A review. Res Rev Biomed Biotech 2010; 1(2): 83-89.

Koné WM, Atindehou KK, Terreaux C, Hostettmann K, Traoré D, Dosso M. Traditional medicine in north Côte-d'Ivoire: screening of 50 medicinal plants for antibacterial activity. J Ethnopharmacol 2004; 93(1): 43-49.

Koniuszy F, Wiley PF, Folkers K. *Erythrina* alkaloids; studies on the constitution of erysodine erysovine and erysopine. J Am Chem Soc 1949; 71:875-878.

Lollato G, Scarminio IS, Moreira EG. Behavioral effects of aqueous and dichloromethane extracts of *Erythrina speciosa* Andrews, Fabaceae, leaves in mice. Rev Bras Farmacognosia 2010; 20(6): 939-944.

Long C, Sun LH, Tantoh ND, Tanyi MJ, Ho KY, Van LT, Hung NP, Keun OW. New prenylated flavanones from Erythrina abyssinica with protein tyrosine phosphatase 1B (PTP1B) inhibitory activity. Planta Medica 2010; 76(7): 713-718.

Majinda RRT, Wanjala CCW, Juma BF. Bioactive non-akaloidal cinstituents from the genus *Erythrina*. Stud Natural Prod Chem 2005; 32(12): 821-853.

Mansbach RS, Chambers LK, Rovetti CC. Effects of the competitive nicotinic antagonist erysodine on behavior occasioned or maintained by nicotine: comparison with mecamylamine. Psychopharmacology (Berl) 2000; 148(3): 234-242.

Marchioro M, Blank Mde F, Mourão RH, Antoniolli AR. Anti-nociceptive activity of the aqueous extract of *Erythrina velutina* leaves. Fitoterapia 2005; 76(7-8): 637-642.

Neill DA. Experimental studies on species relationships in *Erythrina* (Leguminosae: Papilionoideae). Ann Missouri Botanical Garden, 1988; 75: 886-969.

Nguyen PH, Na M, Dao TT, Ndinteh DT, Mbafor JT, Park J, Cheong H, Oh WK. New stilbenoid with inhibitory activity on viral neuraminidases from Erythrina addisoniae. Bioorg Med Chem Lett 2010; 20(22): 6430-6434.

Nguyen PH, Nguyen TNA, Dao TT, Kang HW, Ndinteh DT, Mbafor JT, Oh WK. AMP-Activated protein kinase (AMPK) activation by benzofurans and coumestans isolated from Erythrina abyssinica. J Nat Prod. 2010; 73(4): 598-602.

Njayou F, Moundipa P, Donfack J, Chuisseu D, Tchana A, Ngadjui B, Tchouanguep F. Hepato-protective, antioxidant activities and acute toxicity of a stem bark extract of Erythrina senegalensis DC. I J Biol Chem Sci 2010; 4(3): only on-line http://www.ajol.info/index.php/ijbcs/article/view/60503

Onusic GM, Nogueira RL, Rereira AMS, Flausino OA, Jr., de Barros Viana M. Effects of chronic treatment with a water-alcohol extrat from *Erythrina mulungu* on anxiety-related response in rats. Biol Pharm Bull 2003; 26(11): 1538-1542.

Ozawa M, Etoh T, Hayashi M, Komiyama K, Kishida A, Ohsaki A. TRAIL-enhancing activity of Erythrinan alkaloids from *Erythrina velutina.* Bioorg Med Chem Lett 2009;19:234-236.

Ozawa M, Kawamata S, Etoh T, Hayashi M, Komiyama K, Kishida A, Kuroda C, Ohsaki A. Structure of new erythrinan alkaloids and nitric oxide production inhibitors from Erythrina crista-galli. Chem Pharm Bull 2010; 58: 1119-1122.

Parsons AF, Palframan MJ. *Erythrina* and related alkaloids. Alkaloids Chem. Biol. 68, 39-81, 2010.

Patocka J. Mulungu - Anxiolytics from an Amazonian rainforest. [Article in Czech]. Psychiatrie 2009; 13: 89-91.

Pitchaiah G, Viswanatha GL, Srinath R, Nandakumar K, Dayabaran D, Florance EJ. Anxiolytic and anticonvulsant activity of aqueous extract of stem bark of *Erythrina variegata* in rodents. Int J Parm Tech Res 2010; 2(1): 40-48.

Rajeev VE, Latha PG, Anuja GI, Suja SR, Sini S, Shine VJ, Shyamal S, Krishnakumar NM, Shikha P, Liji J, Rajasekharan S. Antiinflammatory and analgesic properties of Erythrina indica Lamb. Med Plants 2010; 2(3):

Raupp IM, Sereniki A, Virtuoso S, Ghislandi C, Cavalcanti e Silva EL, Trebien HA, Miguel OG, Andreatini R. Anxiolytic-like effect of chronic treatmemnt with Erythrina velutina extract in the elevated plus-maze test. J Ethopharmacol 2008; 118(2): 295-299.

Ribeiro MD, Onusic GM, Poltronieri SC, Viana MB. Effect of *Erythrina velutina* and *Erythrina mulungu* in rats submitted to animal models of anxiety and depression. Braz J Med Biol Res 2006; 39: 263-270.

Rodrigues E, Carlini E: Possíveis efeitos de plantas utilizadas por duas culturas brasileiras (quilombolas e índios) sobre o sistema nervoso central. Arq Bras Fitomed Cient 2003; 1: 147-154.

Saidu K, Onah J, Orisadipe A, Olusola A, Wambebe C, Gamaniel K. Antiplasmodial, analgesic, and anti-inflammatory activities of the aqueous extract of the stem bark of *Erythrina senegalensis*. J Ethnopharmacol 2000; 71(1-2): 275-280.

Sato M, Tanaka H, Fujiwara S, Hirata M, Yamaguchi R, Etoh H, Tokuda C. Antibacterial property of isoflavonoids isolated from *Erythrina variegata* against cariogenic oral bacteria. Phytomedicine 2003; 10(5): 427-433.

Tanaka H, Hattori H, Tanaka T, Sakai E, Tanaka N, Kulkarni A, Etoh H. A new *Erythrina* alkaloid from *Erythrina herbacea*. Nat Med (Tokyo) 2008; 62: 228-231.

Tanaka H, Sudo M, Hirata M, Etoh H, Sato M, Yamaguchi R, Sakai E, Chen IS, Fukai

T. A new biisoflavonoid from the roots of Erythrina variegata. Nat Prod Commun. 2010; 5(11): 1781-1784.

Tanaka H, Sudo M, Kawamura T, Sato M, Yamaguchi R, Fukai T, Sakai E, Tanaka N. Antibacterial constituents from the roots of Erythrina herbacea against methicillin-resistant Staphylococcus aureus. Planta Med. 2010b; 76(9): 916-919.

Tanee FS, Njamen D, Magne NCB, Wanji J, Zierau O, Fomum ZT, Vollmer G. Estrogenic effects of the ethyl-acetate extract of the stem bark of *Erythrina lysistemon* Hutch (Fabaceae). Phytomedicine 2007; 14(2-3): 222-226.

Teixeira-Silva F, Santos FN, Sarasqueta DFO, Alves MFS, Neto VA, Moreira de Paula C, Santos Estevan C, Antoniolli AR, Marchioro M. Benzodiazepine-like effects of the alcohol extract from *Erythrina velutina* leaves: Memory, anxiety, and epilepsy. Pharm Biol 2008; 46: 321-328.

Towle MA. The Ethnobotany of Pre-Columbian Peru. Transaction Publisher, Rutgers, The State University, 2007. 180 pages. ISBN: 978-0-202-30930-9.

Vasconcelos SM, Lima NM, Sales GT, Cunha GM, Aguiar LM, Silveira ER, Rodrigues

AC, Macedo DS, Fonteles MM, Sousa FC, Viana GS. Anticonvulsant activity of hydroalcoholic extracts from *Erythrina velutina* and *Erythrina mulungu*. J Ethnopharmacol 2007; 110(2): 271-274.

Vasconcelos SM, Macedo DS, de Melo CT, Paiva Monteiro A, Rodrigues AC, Silveira

ER, Cunha GM, Sousa FC, Viana GS. Central activity of hydroalcoholic extracts from *Erythrina velutina* and *Erythrina mulungu* in mice. J Pharm Pharmacol 2004; 56(3): 389-393.

Vasconcelos SM, Rebouças Oliveira G, Mohana de Carvalho M, Rodrigues AC, Rocha

Silveira E, Maria França Fonteles M, Florenço Sousa FC, Barros Viana GS. Antinociceptive activities of the hydroalcoholic extracts from *Erythrina velutina* and *Erythrina mulungu* in mice. Biol Pharm Bull 2003; 26(7): 946-949.

Udem SC, Obidoa O, Asuzu IU. Acute and chronic toxicity studies of Erythrina senegalensis DC stem bark extract in mice. Comp Clin Pathol 2010; 19(3): 275-282.

Virtuoso S, Davet A, Dias JFG, Cunico MM, Miguel MD, Oliveira AB, Miguel OG. Preliminar\y study of the antibacterial activity of *Erythrina velutina* Willd. Fabacae (Leguminosae) bark. [Article in Portuguese] Rev Bras Farmacogn 2005; 15(2): 137-142.

Westley SS, Powell MH. Erythrina in the New and Old Worlds. NFTR Special Issue, Bangkok, 1993, 370 pages. ISBN: 974-8434-55-9.